Handbook of
DIGESTIVE
DISEASES

Anil Minocha, MD, FACP, FACG

Professor of Medicine
Director of Digestive Diseases
University of Mississippi Medical Center
Jackson, Mississippi

D1558753

SLACK
INCORPORATED

An innovative information, education, and management company
6900 Grove Road • Thorofare, NJ 08086

Published by: SLACK Incorporated
                     6900 Grove Road
                     Thorofare, NJ 08086 USA
                     Telephone: 856-848-1000
                     Fax: 856-853-5991
                     www.slackbooks.com

Printed in the United States of America.

Minocha, Anil.
  The handbook of digestive diseases / Anil Minocha.
      p. ; cm.
  Includes bibliographical references.
  ISBN 1-55642-665-8 (pbk.)
  1. Digestive organs--Diseases--Handbooks, manuals, etc.
  [DNLM: 1. Digestive System Diseases--Handbooks. WI 39 M666h 2004] I. Title.
RC802.M5673 2004
616.3--dc22

                          2004004328

Last digit is print number: 10 9 8 7 6 5 4 3 2 1

DEDICATION

With pride and love, I dedicate this book to my daughter Geeta, the light of my life; to my loving parents, Kamla and Ram S. Minocha, for their constant encouragement and dedication that shaped my life; and to my entire Minocha family for their patience, love, and understanding without which the book could not have been written.

CONTENTS

Section Eight: Large Intestine

Section Nine: Diagnostic and Therapeutic Modalities

Section Ten: Miscellaneous Topics

ACKNOWLEDGMENTS

This book has been an enormous "solo" project that would not have been possible without the teachings, assistance, and cooperation of many friends, senior colleagues, teachers, and thought-leaders with whom I have interacted throughout my career and who have selflessly shared their knowledge and wisdom that carries me through this day.

I am deeply indebted to the numerous expert friends and colleagues who have reviewed the contents of the book and provided me with important feedback and helpful suggestions. In particular, I would like to express my deep sense of gratitude to Thomas Abell, MD; Bhupinder Anand, MD; Farshid Araghizadeh, MD; Maher Azzouz, MD; Adil Bharucha, MD; Roger Blake, MD; Alan Buchman, MD; Randall Burt, MD; Lawrence Brandt, MD; Michael Camilleri, MD; Jennifer Christie, MD; Poonputt Chotiprasidhi, MD; Ray Clouse, MD; Sheila Crowe, MD; Richard deShazo, MD; Douglas Drossman, MD; Chris Friedrich, MD, PhD; Susan Galandiuk, MD; Robert Halpert, MD; Harold Henderson, MD; Jorge Herrera, MD; Peter Kahrilas, MD; Bret Lashner, MD; Kalyana Lavu, MD; Scott Malinowski, PharmD; Stephen McClave, MD; Roy Orlando, MD; C. S. Pitchumoni, MD; Satish Rao, MD; Douglas Rex, MD; Arvey Rogers, MD; Sitesh Roy, MD; Lawrence Schiller, MD; Reza Shaker, MD; Gagan Sood, MD; and last but not the least, Christina Surawicz, MD. The high quality of the text is primarily due to their help and guidance; the errors are all mine.

I am greatly indebted to my publisher, John Bond, and the acquisitions editor, Carrie Kotlar, for providing me with this unique opportunity to contribute to my passion of medical education and high quality patient care. Finally, it was the project editor, Robert Smentek, and his team who successfully converted a bland manuscript into a book that readers can easily read and assimilate. I am grateful to him for doing his best to make me—and my book—look good.

ACKNOWLEDGEMENTS

ABOUT THE AUTHOR

Anil Minocha, MD currently serves as Professor of Medicine and Director, Division of Digestive Diseases at the University of Mississippi Medical Center in Jackson, Mississippi. In addition to an active involvement in patient care and research, he also serves as the Program Director for the Gastroenterology Fellowship Program.

Dr. Minocha is board-certified in gastroenterology, internal medicine, and geriatrics. In addition to gastroenterology, he is fellowship-trained in clinical pharmacology and medical toxicology. He is also a Fellow of the American College of Physicians and American College of Gastroenterology.

Dr. Minocha is the former gastroenterology editor for *Veterans Health Systems Journal* and a medical editor of the *Gastroenterology Textbook of eMedicine*. He also serves as a manuscript reviewer for a variety of peer-reviewed medical journals. In addition to writing several books for physicians and the lay public, he has authored or coauthored over 70 publications in peer-reviewed scientific literature.

The author invites any comments or criticisms of the book that you might have.

PREFACE

The education of the doctor which goes on after he has his degree is, after all, the most important part of his education.

John Shaw Billings

Medicine is an art, not a science, and our vast fund of knowledge is increasing exponentially. Time is of the essence when a patient is sitting in an office waiting for decisions about the plan of management of his or her digestive complaints, and there may not be enough time to shuffle through the pages of a voluminous text book. This book fulfills the need for a quick, concise, complete, and up-to-date source of practical and unclouded clinical information, allowing a physician to develop a plan of action in an expeditious manner in any setting.

A unique and distinctive characteristic of this book is that while many other books may list management options, this book actually includes decision-making processes, as well as the generic and brand names of the commonly used products for a particular disorder along with the recommended doses. This feature eliminates the need for the physician to read several different books or the PDR for different pieces of information. The bottom line is that this book is a quick, one-stop shop for quickly needed information.

At the end of each chapter, I have also provided pearls that highlight important teaching points and/or common errors to avoid with respect to that disorder. In addition, each chapter is followed by bibliographies for those interested in a more exhaustive reading of the subject.

To achieve the goal of providing a condensed version of the state of knowledge for a broad audience, I have presented what I think is the mainstream consensus, while touching on the controversies surrounding various issues. While this book is an abbreviated version of a standard text book, it is by no means a substitute for a reference textbook or the wisdom of the thought-leaders. Robert Hutchinson once said, "It is unnecessary—perhaps dangerous—in medicine to be too clever." This advice still holds true.

As for myself, this book has been a lot of hard work, but it has been a lot more fun!

COMMON GASTROINTESTINAL COMPLAINTS

Chapter

1 *Dysphagia*

Approximately 30 to 40 pairs of muscles, and at least six pairs of nerves, are involved in facilitating the movement of food from the mouth to the stomach. Adding to the complexity is the fact that swallowing has to be coordinated with respiration in order to prevent aspiration. A functional or an anatomic defect at any level can lead to dysphagia.

EPIDEMIOLOGY

The overall prevalence of dysphagia in the general population is about 7%. The prevalence of dysphagia among subjects greater than 50 years of age varies from 16 to 30% and may be as high as 60% in acute hospital wards and nursing homes.

TYPES OF DYSPHAGIA

Swallowing function is comprised of three phases:
1. Oral
2. Pharyngeal
3. Esophageal

Dysphagia may be classified into two types: *Oropharyngeal dysphagia,* in which the problem lies in the oropharynx; and *Esophageal dysphagia,* in which the problem lies in the esophagus.

Oropharyngeal Dysphagia

PATHOGENESIS

Oropharyngeal dysfunction may be classified into four categories:

1. Inability or excessive delay in initiating swallowing.
2. Aspiration of food.
3. Nasopharyngeal regurgitation.
4. Presence of food residue after swallowing.

Dysphagia can be caused by numerous factors including:

1. Iatrogenic (chemotherapy and neuroleptics, head and neck surgery).
2. Infections (diphtheria, botulism, Lyme disease, syphilis, and viral or fungal mucositis).
3. Metabolic causes (amyloidosis, Cushing's syndrome, thyrotoxicosis, Wilson's disease).
4. Myopathic problems (connective tissue disorders, myasthenia gravis, myotonic dystrophy, sarcoidosis).
5. Paraneoplastic syndromes.
6. Neurological disorders (brain stem tumors, head trauma, stroke, cerebral palsy, Huntington's disease, multiple sclerosis, polio and postpolio syndrome, tardive dyskinesia, Parkinson's disease and dementia).
7. Structural causes (cricopharyngeal achalasia, Zenker's diverticulum, cervical webs, head and neck tumors).
8. Hyper- and hypothyroidism.
9. Oral ulcerations due to Crohn's and Behcet's disease.
10. Poor dentition and ill-fitting dentures.

Amongst the elderly subjects, the causes are typically neuromuscular in origin in approximately 80% of the cases.

Clinical Manifestations

Patients can usually point out the site of the problem (eg, oropharynx). They may complain of food accumulating in the mouth, inability to initiate swallowing, or describe aspiration. Patients may also have difficulty with chewing. They may drool and suffer from aspiration, cough, and have choking spells during meals.

Patients complaining of dysphagia for both solids and liquids and their ability to expectorate rather than vomit out the food suggests oropharyngeal rather than esophageal dysphagia.

Oropharyngeal dysphagia should be distinguished from not only esophageal dysphagia, but also from globus sensation and hyposalivation or xerostomia. These distinctions can usually be made on the basis of history.

Globus sensation or globus hystericus is a sensation of a lump or fullness in the throat which does not affect or impede the swallowing processes. Swallowing, in fact, may improve the symptoms.

Oropharyngeal dysphagia due to hyposalivation occurs due to loss of lubrication from saliva.

Physical examination involves performing a general physical examination in addition to an attempt to identify any neuromuscular or systemic disorders that may be causing the dysphagia as well as its complications. Assistance by a speech language pathologist is valuable.

DIAGNOSIS

The underlying cause is usually apparent in most cases on the basis of clinical assessment. A videofluoroscopic evaluation of oropharyngeal function is of paramount importance. A nasal endoscopy is performed in some centers which helps identify not only the structural lesions of the oropharynx, but also assesses the swallowing function and the oropharyngeal reflexes. Presence or absence of aspiration can also be determined by this technique. A direct or indirect laryngoscopy should be performed in patients suspected of having structural oropharyngeal lesions. Manometry and mano-fluorography is used in select centers, but their clinical contribution is limited.

TREATMENT

Treatment depends upon the cause and the goal of feeding if the cause can not be effectively treated. Three types of dysfunction can be categorized:

1. Severe dysfunction with the risk for severe aspiration requiring nonoral feeding and even tracheotomy.
2. Structural dysfunction amenable to cricopharyngeal myotomy.
3. Dysfunction amenable to dietary modification and swallowing therapy.

Treatment of Structural Problems

Endoscopic dilatation is carried out for cricopharyngeal strictures. Surgery or chemoradiation therapy may be useful in oropharyngeal tumors.

The significance of cricopharyngeal bar identified on radiography is controversial, although cricopharyngeal myotomy may relieve dysphagia in select cases. Cervical osteophytes are common in elderly subjects; surgery should only be undertaken in patients with severe dysphagia in whom all other causes have been excluded and conservative management has failed.

Small lateral pharyngeal diverticula can be seen in patients with or without dysphagia; improvement in dysphagia may occur after surgical ligation or removal of these diverticula. Diverticulectomy is undertaken for Zenker's diverticulum along with cricopharyngeal myotomy to prevent recurrence. Endoscopic myotomy has also been used.

Dilatation or myotomy for cervical esophageal webs yields mixed results.

Treatment of Patients at Risk for Aspiration

In patients with high risk of aspiration pneumonia, gastrostomy feedings may be required; however, its benefit remains to be established since the risk of aspiration of oropharyngeal secretions is not reduced by gastrostomy. In severe cases, surgical procedures to reduce or eliminate aspiration may be needed. Jejunal feeding may or may not improve airway safety.

Management of Patients with Cardiovascular Accident

Most stroke-related dysphagia improves in 10 to 15 days. Although it may be better to avoid gastrostomy during this period, considerations of risks, costs, and benefits of transfer of the patient from the hospital to a nursing home may overshadow the clinical considerations and lead to early gastrostomy placement in select cases.

Swallowing Therapy

This includes dietary modification and adjustments in the swallowing posture or swallowing technique. The goal is to strengthen the weak oropharyngeal muscles in order to improve the speed and coordination of the swallowing processes with minimal aspiration. While dietary modifications have the strongest scientific basis for its effectiveness, swallowing therapy is frequently used because of biological plausibility, low cost, and no risk.

Esophageal Dysphagia

PATHOGENESIS

Esophageal dysphagia may be caused by a variety of disorders, for example, strictures or narrowing due to gastroesophageal reflux disease (GERD), esophageal rings, tumors, lye ingestion, pill esophagitis, radiation and infectious esophagitis; mediastinal diseases (enlarged heart, aortic aneurysm, lung tumors, mediastinal masses, lymphoma); infections (tuberculosis and histoplasmosis); and motility disorders (achalasia, scleroderma, etc).

CLINICAL FEATURES

Patients usually complain of dysphagia primarily to solid foods, whereas those with neuromuscular disorders have dysphagia to both solids and liquids. Patients are only 70% accurate in localizing the site of the problem. In the remainder, they point to the neck. The location pointed out by the patient suggests that the lesion is either at or above that site and it is only rarely below that site.

Schatzki's Ring

Patients usually have intermittent and nonprogressive dysphagia. This often occurs during a meal in a restaurant, and as such, the term Steak-house syndrome has been used. Patients may go without symptoms for months or even years between the episodes.

Esophageal Stricture

Benign strictures cause gradually progressive dysphagia with a history of heartburn obtained in 75% of the cases. In contrast, malignant strictures may cause rapidly progressive dysphagia, and is associated with weight loss. Ingestion of medications like doxycycline, potassium, nonsteroidal anti-inflammatory drugs (NSAIDs), quinidine, or alendronate suggest the possibility of stricture due to pill-esophagitis.

Patients who are immune-compromised are more likely to get infectious esophagitis due to *Candida, Cytomegalovirus (CMV)*, or *Herpes simplex* virus, although odynophagia is more likely under these circumstances than dysphagia alone. Infectious esophagitis does not typically cause a severe stricture.

Neuromuscular Dysfunction

Collagen vascular disorders like scleroderma and systemic lupus erythematosus (SLE) cause neuromuscular dysfunction resulting in dysphagia to both solids and liquids. Achalasia presents with long-standing dysphagia; weight loss may be present in some cases.

Physical Findings

Physical examination is unremarkable in many cases. It is important to assess the nutritional status as well as to look for any systemic disorder or signs of malignancy.

INVESTIGATIONS

Barium Swallow vs Endoscopy

Barium swallow with a barium pill is more sensitive than endoscopy for detection of esophageal narrowing, especially if the lumen is greater than the diameter of the endoscope. It also provides information on causes of extrinsic compression.

Some experts consider endoscopy to be a more cost effective first step and proceed directly to esophagogastroduodenoscopy (EGD) rather than performing a barium study. Endoscopic evaluation is recommended for patients with esophageal dysphagia not only to establish and confirm the diagnosis of an obstruction, inflammation, infection, or malignancy, but also for therapeutic purposes (ie, biopsies and esophageal dilatation can be undertaken if necessary).

Role of Esophageal Manometry

Esophageal manometry is useful in cases of suspected esophageal motility disorders like achalasia, diffuse esophageal spasm (DES) and collagen vascular diseases. Manometry should be used selectively since its effect upon altering the outcome in neuromuscular disorders except achalasia is controversial.

Findings in achalasia include esophageal aperistalsis and failure of the lower esophageal sphincter to relax in response to swallow. Secondary achalasia as a manifestation of cancer of the lung or gastric cardia needs to be ruled out before treating achalasia as idiopathic.

Radionuclide Studies

Esophageal transit scintigraphy is primarily used for research purposes.

TREATMENT

Treatment depends upon the cause.

Benign Stricture

Strictures are treated with aggressive acid suppression as well as esophageal dilation. Simple strictures greater than 12.0 mm in size can be dilated using mercury bougies, polyvinyl bougies, or balloons. Complex strictures which are narrow or tortuous should be dilated using dilators over the guide wire or through-the-scope (TTS) balloon dilators. Aggressive acid suppression should continue for patients in whom dysphagia resolves and no further dilation is needed.

If dysphagia persist or returns, repeat endoscopy should be undertaken to confirm the presence of any mucosal lesions as well as for a repeat dilatation. Patients may continue to require dilatation intermittently on as needed basis.

In patients in whom dysphagia persists despite repeated dilation or returns quickly, consider a local injection of corticosteroids. Intralesional injection of corticosteroid involves injection of triamcinolone (Kenalog 40.0 mg/mL) 0.25 mL in each of four quadrants. Other experts dilute the drug and give 0.5 mL (1:1 dilution with sterile saline) or 1 mL (1:3 dilution) into each quadrant at the narrowest region of the stricture.

Self-bougienage and surgery are undertaken as a last resort.

Schatzki's Ring

Patients should be treated by using a single large dilator for disruption of the ring along with aggressive acid suppression. Although there is no good scientific data, I do not recommend a graded dilation starting with smaller diameter and advancing to larger diameter. Repeated dilatation on an as needed basis may be required.

If dysphagia persists or returns quickly, manometry should be considered to look for a treatable motility disorder. Repeat endoscopy should be undertaken to confirm healing of esophagitis and to look for persistence of the ring. If the ring is persistent, further abrupt dilatation, pneumatic dilation, endoscopic therapy, or surgery should be considered.

Achalasia

Treatment depends upon patient preference, skill of the endoscopist and the surgeon, as well as the patient's condition (ie, whether the patient is good or poor operative risk). Both pneumatic dilatation and surgical myotomy are effective and can be undertaken in patients who are good operative risks. Patients who fail pneumatic dilation once are candidates for repeat dilation using a larger diameter balloon for a total of up to three pneumatic dilatations. Persistent failure of pneumatic dilation should prompt surgical myotomy.

Patients who are poor operative risks may be considered for medical therapy using nitrates or calcium channel blockers and periodic dilation with a large diameter dilator.

If dysphagia persists or is quick to return, injection of botulinum toxin into the lower esophageal sphincter should be undertaken. The effect of botulinum toxin usually lasts for about 6 months and then treatment can be repeated. If dysphagia persists despite botulinum toxin, consider gastrostomy, pneumatic dilation, or surgical myotomy.

Patients with a severely dilated esophagus due to longstanding achalasia may not benefit from above measures and frequently require esophagectomy.

PEARLS

- ○ Although not applicable to all cases, patients with oropharyngeal dysphagia usually have more difficulty swallowing liquids than solids. Patients with esophageal dysphagia present with the same degree of difficulty for solids and liquids or with solid foods more than liquids.
- ○ Feeding through gastrostomy does not reduce the incidence of aspiration pneumonia in patients with oropharyngeal dysphagia.
- ○ Barium swallow with a barium pill is superior to endoscopy for detecting esophageal stricture; however, endoscopy without performing a barium study may be more cost-effective.

BIBLIOGRAPHY

Lind CD. Dysphagia: evaluation and treatment. *Gastroenterol Clin North Am.* 2003;32(2):553-75.

Chapter 2

Noncardiac Chest Pain

Noncardiac chest pain (NCCP) is defined as an angina-like substernal chest pain unrelated to the heart. Since microvascular angina is one of the etiologies contributing to NCCP, angina-like chest pain may be a more appropriate term.

EPIDEMIOLOGY

As many as 35% of coronary angiograms performed in the United States are entirely normal. Based on the magnitude of coronary angiograms performed annually, the incidence of new cases of NCCP is about 500,000 per year. However, this may be an underestimation because it includes only the cases where cardiac catheterization has been performed, whereas many patients undergo less invasive workup. This disorder accounts for as much as $2 billion cost annually to the health care system.

PATHOPHYSIOLOGY

The esophagus is believed to be involved in as many as 60% of the cases. The mechanisms involved are not well understood and may include the presence of noxious stimulus in the esophagus, a lowering of sensory pain threshold, or an abnormality of the nervous system. GERD plays a predominant role. Esophageal motility disorders are found only in a minority of cases and there is a poor relationship between symptoms and the occurrence of an episode of esophageal dysmotility. Visceral hypersensitivity may be involved. These patients have lower pain threshold to balloon distention compared to controls.

Although termed NCCP, cardiac causes may still cause "noncardiac" chest pain. There is a high prevalence of microvascular angina or syndrome X. Other potential cardiac etiologies include pericarditis and mitral valve prolapse.

Psychiatric disorders include panic disorder, anxiety, and somatization. Musculoskeletal disorders like fibromyalgia and costochondritis occur in about 10% of cases.

No single etiology may be able to explain the chest pain for most people since there is a high frequency of psychiatric, esophageal, and cardiac abnormalities overlapping in many of the same patients.

CLINICAL FEATURES

Patients complain of a substernal, squeezing chest pain, which may be associated with nausea and vomiting. This pain may possibly radiate to the jaw, neck, back, or arms. It is frequently difficult to distinguish a cardiac from a noncardiac source. An esophageal etiology is suggested by pain without radiation, lasting for several hours and days, and has a positive response to antacids and acid-suppressive therapy. Association with dysphagia, regurgitation, and heartburn also points to GERD.

DIAGNOSIS

History and physical examination cannot reliably distinguish between cardiac and noncardiac source of pain. Cardiac etiology must always be excluded first since both cardiac and esophageal etiology may coexist in the same patient, and a cardiac cause can be fatal. Cardiac evaluation appropriate for age and risk factors should be undertaken including a noninvasive or invasive test, although coronary angiography is standard.

Once a cardiac etiology has been excluded, attention should focus on the esophagus with the predominant target being GERD. Esophageal tests available include 24-hour pH monitoring, upper endoscopy, esophageal manometry, and provocative testing. A 24-hour pH monitoring combined with symptom analysis provides the best diagnostic yield. The role of impedance plethysmography is evolving.

The usefulness of esophageal manometry is controversial because of the lack of temporal relationship between episodes of dysmotility and the pain. Provocative tests like Bernstein's test and edrophonium test are usually not done these days. These provocative tests have low sensitivity but high specificity of 70 to 90%. Balloon distention test attempts to identify patients with visceral hyperalgesia.

A proton pump inhibitor (PPI) test using a twice a day dose of a PPI has a highly positive predictive value if the patient's symptoms abate in 14 days. In the absence of an esophageal diagnosis, a psychiatric evaluation may be required.

DIFFERENTIAL DIAGNOSIS

In addition to the common potential causes of NCCP, one should not forget other conditions like biliary colic and peptic ulcer disease. Chest pain may also occur as the result of chronic obstructive pulmonary disease (COPD) and asthma.

MANAGEMENT

Management includes identification of the cause, exclusion of a cardiac etiology, and reassurance about an excellent prognosis.

GERD responds well to treatment with acid suppressive therapy. Beta-blockers, nitrates, and calcium channel blockers have been tried for esophageal motility disorders, as well as for microvascular angina with limited success. Studies using smooth muscle relaxants have shown conflicting results.

Musculoskeletal conditions respond to the use of appropriate analgesics and NSAIDs. Tricyclic antidepressants, as well as selective serotonin reuptake inhibitors (SSRIs), are effective for panic disorder.

Low doses of tricyclic antidepressants like imipramine (Tofranil 20.0 to 50.0 mg/day) or amitriptyline (Elavil 25.0 to 50.0 mg/day) are effective in reducing the severity and frequency of chest pain episodes irrespective of the underlying cause of pain.

Cognitive behavioral therapy has been shown to be of benefit. Thoracic longitudinal myotomy has been used in rare cases of severe refractory chest pain due to nutcracker esophagus.

SUGGESTED STRATEGY

A rational approach to management includes exclusion of cardiac etiology as the first step. Once a cardiac etiology has been excluded, attempts should be made to classify the pain into esophageal, musculoskeletal, and/or psychological causes. If an esophageal etiology is suspected, an empiric trial of a twice-a-day PPI should be undertaken. In responders, the treatment may be continued as maintenance.

In nonresponders, an EGD and/or 24-hour pH monitoring with symptom analysis should be done. If the 24-hour pH monitoring and EGD are normal, an empiric trial with tricyclic antidepressants is appropriate. Esophageal manometry and provocative testing should be undertaken in selected cases if tricyclic antidepressants fail. Calcium channel blockers may be tried if a severe motility disorder other than achalasia is identified.

In patients whose clinical features suggest musculoskeletal etiology, look for trigger points and the reproducibility of the chest pain.

Anti-inflammatory and local therapies are helpful in such cases. If a psychological dysfunction is suspected, panic disorder and depression should be ruled out. A short course of benzodiazepines may be appropriate but long-term management may require assistance from a mental health professional.

PROGNOSIS

Long-term mortality of patients in whom coronary angiogram has been normal is less than 1% at 10 years. However, the morbidity is high because of frequent visits to the physicians, as well as the emergency rooms; frequent coronary angiograms; limitation of activity and inability to work; and continued use of health care resources despite negative cardiac evaluation.

PEARLS

○ Cardiac etiology must always be excluded to a reasonable degree of certainty since both gastroesophageal reflux disease and coronary artery disease may coexist in the same patient.

○ Gastroesophageal reflux disease, and not esophageal spasm, is the predominant esophageal cause of noncardiac chest pain.

○ Gastroesophageal reflux disease is the most common treatable cause of noncardiac chest pain.

BIBLIOGRAPHY

Minocha A. Non-cardiac chest pain: where does it start? *PostGraduate Medicine.* 1996;100:107-114.

Chapter

3 *Nausea and Vomiting*

Nausea is a sensation of impending vomiting whereas vomiting itself is a well-coordinated motor act that results in expulsion of upper gastrointestinal (GI) contents in retrograde fashion. Vomiting is usually, but not always, preceded by nausea.

Rumination occurs when the gastric contents come up to the oropharynx followed by chewing again and are then reswallowed. It is effortless and occurs in the absence of the coordinated neuromuscular activity seen in vomiting; in humans, it is often labeled as pseudorumination.

Cyclic vomiting syndrome is characterized by repeated and persistent episodes of nausea and vomiting lasting for hours or days. Patients are symptom-free between the episodes. There is often a personal or family history of migraine.

PATHOGENESIS

Nausea is usually associated with the disruptions of normal electromechanical function along with an increase of endogenous epinephrine and norepinephrine as well as other changes of the autonomic nervous system (ANS).

Vomiting is a protective reflex that is normally regulated by a combination of neural, hormonal, and GI factors. Multiple well-coordinated events occur during the act of vomiting, including relaxation of the stomach and the lower esophageal sphincter, retrograde contraction in the distal stomach and proximal small bowel, contraction of abdominal muscles, along with contraction of cricopharyngeus followed by its relaxation just before vomiting.

ETIOLOGY

Nausea and vomiting can be conceptualized as due to central, extrinsic (to the gut) or intrinsic/enteric causes. The differential diagnosis is complex and diverse and includes infectious or eosinophilic gastroenteritis, postoperative vomiting, alcoholism, congestive heart failure, cyclic vomiting syndrome, pregnancy, mechanical obstruction (gastric outlet obstruction, intestinal obstruction), infections, dysmotility (GERD, gastroparesis, intestinal pseudo-obstruction), endocrine and metabolic disorders (diabetes mellitus, hypo- and hyperthyroidism, hypo- and hyperparathyroidism, Addison's disease, and renal failure), medications (chemotherapy, NSAIDs, digoxin, antidepressants and psychotropic agents), radiation therapy, intraabdominal inflammatory conditions (peptic ulcer, cholecystitis, pancreatitis, hepatitis, Crohn's disease), central nervous system (CNS) disorders (brain tumor, abscess, meningitis or infarction, motion sickness, labyrinthitis, Meniere's disease), and psychogenic disorders (anxiety neurosis, depression, anorexia-bulimia syndrome).

CLINICAL FEATURES

History often provides clues to the underlying cause. Acute onset of symptoms occurs due to infections, medications, or acute exacerbation of a chronic medical condition like diabetes mellitus. A number of patients with diabetic gastropathy (which can include both delayed and rapid emptying) present with cyclical symptoms, much like the migraine-related cyclic vomiting syndrome.

Chronic nausea and vomiting is seen in patients with gastroparesis, intestinal pseudo-obstruction and related GI neuromuscular disorders; most have dyspeptic symptoms regularly.

Abdominal pain is seen in infectious and inflammatory conditions like peptic ulcer disease, cholecystitis, or pancreatitis.

Vomiting soon after eating points to gastroparesis, gastric outlet obstruction, or pseudorumination. Vomitus containing undigested food from several hours or days before suggests outlet obstruction or a primary esophageal disorder such as achalasia. Feculent vomitus suggests intestinal obstruction or gastrocolic fistula.

Complaint of abdominal distention suggests intestinal obstruction. Upper GI bleed may occur because of the underlying cause of vomiting (eg, peptic ulcer, pancreatitis) or a result of forceful vomiting causing a Mallory-Weiss tear.

INVESTIGATIONS

These are tailored according to the clinical presentation and the pathology suspected. Anatomic disorders such as peptic ulceration or partial small bowel obstruction (SBO) must always be considered, realizing that the presentation of SBO or intusseception may not be straightforward.

Studies include CBC, comprehensive metabolic profile, serum amylase, and lipase, as well as abdominal x-ray series. Right upper quadrant ultrasound and HIDA scan are helpful in hepatobiliary and pancreatic disorders. Miscellaneous tests done in select cases include pregnancy test, thyroid function tests, serologic markers for collagen vascular disorders, dedicated small bowel barium study, and an abdominal CT scan. GI motor function and physiology can be assessed by gastric emptying time and electrogastrography, along with small intestinal manometry.

TREATMENT

General Management

Management includes nutritional and symptomatic therapy in addition to the treatment of underlying cause. A low-residue, low-fat, and predominantly liquid diet is helpful. The underlying disorder should be aggressively corrected (eg, correction of hyperglycemia in diabetes mellitus). In addition to other possible indications of underlying disorders, patients with evidence of dehydration should be hospitalized.

Prokinetics

Prokinetic agents (metoclopramide 10.0 to 20.0 mg qid, domperidone 10.0 to 30.0 mg qid, and cisapride 10.0 to 20.0 mg qid) are useful as antiemetics especially in cases of gastroparesis. Erythromycin is effective as a prokinetic, but suffers from tachyphylaxis; other macrolide analogues are being investigated. Tegaserod also has significant effects on the upper GI tract, although it is currently approved in the United States for constipation-predominant irritable bowel syndrome (IBS) in females. See Chapter 33 for details on treatment of gastroparesis.

Symptomatic Control

Nonspecific control of symptoms is achieved by using antiemetics. Combination of drugs with different mechanisms of action is beneficial in severe cases. Serotonin antagonists like ondansetron (Zofran) 4 to 10.0 mg IV or 8.0 mg PO tid, dolasetron 12.5 mg IV, or granisetron (Kytril) 10.0 mcg/kg IV qd or 1.0 mg PO bid are effective; the latter are primarily used for chemo-/radiation-induced or postoperative vomiting.

Phenothiazines (promethazine 25.0 mg PO/IV q 4 to 6 hours or 8.0 to 15.0 mg/h IV infusion; prochlorperazine 5.0 to 10.0 mg PO qid or 5.0-10.0 mg IV q 6 hours) alone or in combination with other agents are useful in a variety of disorders. The dose should be titrated to the side effect of sedation.

Muscrinic agents are used primarily in motion sickness. Options include scopolamine (Transderm Scop) 1 patch 4 hours prior to event and meclizine (Antivert 25.0 to 50.0 mg starting before trip) and repeated every day as needed.

Other options of antiemetics include trimethobenzamide (Tigan 300.0 mg PO tid or 200.0 mg IM tid), dronabinol (Marinol), and droperidol (Inapsine); the use of the latter is limited by its side effects.

Acid-Suppression

This is frequently undertaken especially in severe cases. H_2RAs or PPIs may be used depending upon the severity of symptoms.

Miscellaneous Treatments

Tricyclic antidepressants and sumatriptan are reported to be helpful in cyclic vomiting syndrome, as they can be in migraine. Clonidine may be helpful in some patients with gastroparesis.

Powdered ginger-root (250.0 mg qid), pyridoxine (10.0 to 50.0 mg PO q 6 hours), doxylamine (Unisom 25.0 mg PO bid), acupuncture, and acupressure are beneficial in nausea and vomiting associated with pregnancy. Refractory cases of hyperemesis gravidarum may benefit from a short-course of corticosteroids and parenteral nutrition.

Patients with chronic symptoms who are unable to tolerate oral feeds may need enteral feedings via a jejunostomy tube with or without a venting gastrostomy. Some patients may be candidates for implantable gastric electrical stimulation (GES) device. Surgical resections and drainage procedures are not helpful. Psychiatric evaluation may be needed in select patients.

COMPLICATIONS

Fluid and electrolyte disturbances, malnutrition, purpura, loss of dental enamel, dental caries, esophagitis, Mallory-Weiss tear, and even Boerhaave's syndrome may be seen. Many patients with chronic nausea and vomiting may suffer from complications of long-term intravenous access including thrombosis and infection.

PEARLS

- ○ Nausea and vomiting are symptoms and aggressive efforts should be made to define and treat the underlying disorder.
- ○ Many patients have an underlying GI neuromuscular disease.
- ○ Gastric electrical stimulation device is useful in severe gastroparesis.

BIBLIOGRAPHY

Quigley EM, Hasler WL, Parkman HP. AGA technical review on nausea and vomiting. *Gastroenterology.* 2001;120(1):263-86.

Rashed H, Abell TL, Familoni BO, Cardoso S. Autonomic function in cyclic vomiting syndrome and classic migraine. *Dig Dis Sci.* 1999;44:74s-78s.

Koch KL, Frissora CL. Nausea and vomiting during pregnancy. *Gastroenterol Clin North Am.* 2003;32(1):201-34.

Chapter

Belching

Dictionaries describe belching or eructation as "the voiding of gas or a small quantity of acidic fluid from the stomach through the mouth." Aerophagia means swallowing of air. It primarily occurs while eating, drinking, chewing gum, and smoking, and increases exponentially during anxiety. Belching in anxious persons is an extension of "normal" aerophagia and belching. While breathing in, the patients suck air into the esophagus in addition to the trachea.

PATHOGENESIS

Normally the air in stomach is passed downstream into the intestines. Belching occurs when the stomach air, instead of going down, goes up into the esophagus and is expelled through the mouth. As in GERD, this process requires that the lower esophageal sphincter (LES) relax to allow the regurgitation of air upward into the esophagus and then out through the mouth making a sound.

Belching after a meal, especially a big meal, may be normal. It occurs as a result of air being swallowed while eating. In addition, a lot of swallowed air accumulates in the stomach in between meals. The food once it reaches the stomach, displaces the air already present there. Postparandial belching is facilitated by LES relaxation from foods like onions, mint, tomatoes, and alcohol.

Cultural acceptance of belching varies. While considered to be uncouth in the western society, a belch after a hearty meal is considered to be a compliment for the chef in some Eastern cultures.

Chronic belching is generally not due any organic disorder. Rather, it is a learned process, albeit subconsciously. In most cases, air is swallowed into the esophagus as described above, but is promptly expelled out as a belch even before it has had a chance to reach the stomach. This develops into a habit in anxious persons.

Magenblase syndrome is a poorly defined disorder that involves increased fullness and bloating due to a collection of gas in the stomach after a meal as described above. The symptoms resolve after the patient belches.

CLINICAL FEATURES

Many patients believe that the belching is an indicator of disease of the digestive system. Frequently, they ascribe relief of their digestive symptoms actually caused by other disorders to belching.

Measures to decrease aerophagia frequently prescribed in chronic belching (but which may be of limited benefit) include eating slowly; not chewing gum; and avoiding carbonated beverages, mint, onions, chocolates, and alcohol. Stress reduction and relaxation is the key.

PEARLS

○ Belching is a normal phenomenon and is an extension of "normal" aerophagia and belching.

BIBLIOGRAPHY

Rao SS. Belching, bloating, and flatulence. How to help patients who have troublesome abdominal gas. *Postgrad Med.* 1997;101(4):263-9, 275-8.

Chapter

5 *Hiccups*

These commonly occur after a large meal or alcohol ingestion, and are frequently subjected to numerous home-remedies.

PATHOGENESIS

Hiccups occur as a result of intermittent and involuntary spasmodic contraction of inspiratory muscles associated with abrupt airway closure at the glottis, which produces the audible sound.

ETIOLOGIC FACTORS

Prolonged hiccups may be caused by foreign bodies in the ear canal, cervical tumors, neurologic disorders, diabetes, uremia, alcoholism, and inflammatory or neoplastic lesions in the chest like tuberculosis, pleurisy, and cancer. Medications like corticosteroids and benzodiazepines have been implicated, but convincing evidence is lacking.

GI causes include GERD, and gastric outlet obstruction. GERD is frequently the result—and not the cause—of hiccups.

CLINICAL FEATURES

Most hiccups are short-lived and resolve spontaneously. Chronic hiccups are defined as those persisting for greater than 48 hours. Prolonged and persistent hiccups can persist for days, and even months to years, creating problems of chronic fatigue, sleep disturbances, depression, weight loss, and even suicide.

INVESTIGATIONS

These should be tailored to the overall presentation. These may include CBC, comprehensive metabolic profile, upper-endoscopy, laryngoscopy, x-rays, and/or CT of the chest and abdomen. An MRI of the brain may be undertaken as last resort. No cause is found in majority of the cases. Fluoroscopy should be performed to evaluate diaphragmatic movements.

TREATMENT

Treatment should be directed at the cause. However, no cause can be identified in many cases.

Home Remedies

These include breath holding, drinking water, rebreathing into a bag, and Valsalva maneuver.

Medical Treatment

Pharyngeal stimulation with a nasogastric tube may be of benefit. Firm pharyngeal stimulation in a fasting state has been advocated. Medications used include baclofen (5.0 to 20.0 mg tid), metoclopramide, chlorpromazine, haloperidol, amitriptyline, carbamazepine, dilantin, and nifedipine.

Surgery

Phrenic nerve ablation may be needed in select cases. Phrenic nerve stimulation by surgically placed electrodes is in its infancy.

PEARLS

○ Most hiccups are short-lived and resolve spontaneously or in response to simple home remedies.
○ Majority of chronic hiccups are idiopathic in origin.

BIBLIOGRAPHY

Friedman NL. Hiccups: a treatment review. *Pharmacotherapy.* 1996;16(6):986-95.

Thompson DF, Landry JP. Drug-induced hiccups. *Ann Pharmacother.* 1997;31(3):367-9.

Chapter

6 *Dyspepsia*

Dyspepsia is defined as an upper abdominal discomfort that may be associated with nausea, vomiting, fullness, bloating, or early satiety. Although some experts include heartburn as one of the associations, the presence of heartburn alone is not considered to be dyspepsia.

EPIDEMIOLOGY

Prevalence estimates vary depending upon the population studied and the definition used. Annual prevalence is estimated to be 25%. The number increases to 40% if patients with frequent heartburn are also included.

ETIOLOGY

As many as 15% to 25% of the patients with dyspepsia have peptic ulcer disease, while GERD is the cause in 5% to 15%. Biliary tract disease, pancreatitis, medications, gastroparesis, infections, and malignancies are rare causes. As many as 50% to 80% of the patients are characterized as functional dyspepsia (see Chapter 31).

CLINICAL FEATURES

Three patterns of symptoms are described:
1. Ulcer-like dyspepsia characterized by burning or epigastric pain relieved with antacids or acid blockers.
2. Dysmotility like dyspepsia has predominance of nausea, vomiting, bloating, and early satiety.
2. Unspecified or mixed.

There is a marked overlap between the three groups, and about half of the patients can be classified into more than one subgroup.

Symptoms alone have poor predictive value for the diagnosis found during endoscopy.

Physical examination is usually unremarkable. Epigastric tenderness may be seen in some cases. Presence of occult blood in stool raises concerns for a slowly bleeding peptic ulcer disease or malignancy.

Diagnosis

CBC, comprehensive metabolic profile (including liver function tests), and thyroid function tests are usually normal. In young patients, multiple strategies for investigating dyspepsia in the absence of alarm symptoms (ie, weight loss and bleeding) have been suggested and remain embroiled in controversy. Various options include:

1. Empiric trial of antisecretory drug therapy.
2. Initial endoscopy.
3. Noninvasive serological testing for *H. pylori* (Hp) followed by treatment if positive.
4. Empiric eradication of Hp.
5. Testing for Hp in patients undergoing endoscopy, ultimately eradicating it if infection is present.

Endoscopy is the standard for the diagnosis of mucosal disease including ulcers, reflux esophagitis, and cancer, but it is expensive, invasive, and not cost-effective in young patients without alarm symptoms. Empiric treatment with acid suppression provides rapid symptomatic relief in large number of patients; however, a high rate of symptom recurrence and the possibility of inappropriate long-term medication use make this option less desirable.

Empiric eradication of Hp results in financial savings, but is not favored by most experts. Testing for Hp and performing endoscopy in patients with a positive test is not cost-effective.

Testing for Hp and eradicating it, if positive, is the initial step recommended by many professional societies for patients younger than 45 years of age without any alarm symptoms. This strategy increases the chances of antibiotic resistance.

Barium studies are cheaper than endoscopy, but less accurate for the diagnosis of peptic ulcer disease, and are not routinely recommended. Gallbladder ultrasound in patients with dyspeptic symptoms but without typical biliary pain should be avoided, since the presence of gallstones in such patients can lead to unnecessary surgery. Although gastroparesis is found in 30 to 80% of the patients, prokinetic drugs provide inconsistent relief of symptoms.

DIFFERENTIAL DIAGNOSIS

Patients with a duodenal ulcer typically have pain 2 to 5 hours after meals or on an empty stomach. They also tend to wake up around midnight with pain. However, the classic symptoms tend to occur in less than 50% of the patients. About 20% of the patients report weight gain.

GERD manifests with heartburn and regurgitation; symptoms are often relieved with antacids.

Patients with gastric malignancy usually have alarm features like weight loss, bleeding, anemia, and/or dysphagia, in addition to abdominal pain. Gastroparesis may be seen in patients with a history of diabetes mellitus, hypo- or hyperthyroidism, and hyperparathyroidism. Medications associated with dyspepsia include iron, NSAIDs, bisphosphonates, and antibiotics. Although scientific data is lacking, food intolerances are frequently implicated by the patients.

Biliary pain is acute, severe, epigastric, and/or right upper quadrant pain lasting for at least 1 hour and may radiate to back or scapula; it is associated with nausea, vomiting, sweating, and restlessness. The patient is typically pain-free between the episodes.

Cholelithiasis by itself does not cause dyspeptic symptoms in the absence of biliary colic or other complications. Although there is a huge overlap of functional dyspepsia and IBS, patients with IBS have disturbed bowel habit in addition to the abdominal pain.

RECOMMENDED APPROACH

If history suggests GERD, biliary pain, IBS, aerophagia, or medication-induced symptoms, then the patient should be managed appropriately by targeting the diagnosis.

The various strategies for management of uninvestigated dyspepsia continue to be mired in controversy and should be tailored to the individual patient and the likelihood of Hp infection. Patients less than 45 years of age presenting with dyspeptic symptoms, but without predominant GERD symptoms, ingestion of NSAIDs, or any other alarm symptoms (weight loss, bleeding, recurrent vomiting, anemia, or dysphagia) should be tested for Hp using a noninvasive test. Hp eradication should be carried out in patients who test positive for it. Patients who do not respond to Hp eradication therapy should undergo endoscopy.

Patients who initially test negative for Hp should undergo an empiric trial of acid suppression, preferably a proton pump inhibitor. If symptoms persist despite acid suppressive therapy or if symptoms occur rapidly after cessation of treatment, endoscopy should be performed.

Because the incidence of peptic ulcer disease due to Hp is declining, some experts recommend acid suppression as the initial step, followed by testing for Hp in patients who fail to resolve with acid suppressive therapy.

PEARLS

○ Majority of patients with typical symptoms of peptic ulcer disease are found to have functional dyspepsia.

○ Investigation of dyspepsia should be based upon the patient's age and clinical features including presence or absence of alarm symptoms.

BIBLIOGRAPHY

Delaney BC, Moayyedi P, Forman D. Initial management strategies for dyspepsia. *Cochrane Database Syst Rev*. 2003;(2):CD001961.

Chapter

 Acute Abdominal Pain ▬▬▬

The abdomen is a Pandora's box. Abdominal pain may be visceral, somatoparietal, or referred. History and physical examination lack sensitivity and specificity in localizing the source of the pain. A rational approach to management requires an understanding of the mechanisms, as well as the causes and associations of the pain, typical patterns, and typical clinical presentations. The majority of patients do not present with a typical picture, especially elderly subjects and the immune-comprised host.

CAUSES OF PAIN BY LOCATION

• *Right upper quadrant pain*: hepatitis, cholecystitis, biliary colic, cholangitis, pancreatitis, pneumonia, subdiaphragmatic abscesses.

• *Right lower quadrant pain*: appendicitis, pelvic inflammatory disease, ectopic pregnancy, inguinal hernia.

• *Epigastric pain*: peptic ulcer disease, GERD, gastritis, pancreatitis, myocardial infarction, pericarditis, ruptured aortic aneurysm.

- *Periumbilical pain*: ruptured aortic aneurysm, early appendicitis, gastroenteritis, SBO.
- *Left upper quadrant pain*: pancreatitis, gastric ulcer, acute gastritis, splenic infarction, abscess.
- *Left lower quadrant*: diverticulitis, pelvic inflammatory disease, ectopic pregnancy, inguinal hernia, inflammatory bowel disease (IBD), IBS.
- *Diffuse abdominal pain*: gastroenteritis, mesenteric ischemia, metabolic causes (diabetic ketoacidosis and porphyria), malaria, bowel obstruction, peritonitis, IBS.

PRINCIPLES OF LOCALIZATION OF PAIN

1. Most digestive pain is focused in the midline, except in the gallbladder and ascending and descending colon.
2. Pain is perceived in the spinal segment consistent with the location at which the nerves enter the spinal cord. Since nerves from the small intestine enter the spinal cord between T8 and L1, its pain is felt in the periumbilical region.
3. Pain may be perceived in the cutaneous dermatome sharing the same spinal cord level as the visceral input. Thus pain of cholecystitis may be felt in the scapular region. Once peritoneal inflammation occurs, the pain then localizes to the right upper quadrant.
4. Abdominal pain may arise from extra-abdominal sites (eg, *Herpes zoster*, myocardial infarction, pneumonia, esophagitis, uremia, porphyria, acute adrenal insufficiency, sickle cell anemia, hypersensitivity reaction to insect bites, lead poisoning, muscular contusion, or heat stroke).
5. The specificity for associations of pain with its location is the highest for epigastric pain seen with gastroduodenal diseases, right subcostal and right upper quadrant pain seen in hepatobiliary diseases, and mid-lower abdominal pain due to gynecological causes.

HISTORY

History is of paramount importance and provides important clues.

Pain Characteristics

Dull, aching, and poorly localized visceral pain usually arises from distention or spasm of a hollow organ (eg, early intestinal obstruction or choledocholithiasis). Pain that is sharp and localized occurs due to peritoneal irritation, as seen in acute appendicitis.

Pain of pancreatitis is steady with a gradual worsening, whereas a rupture of viscous with acute peritonitis is sudden in onset and quickly reaches its maximal intensity.

Burning or gnawing pain occurs in GERD or peptic ulcer disease, whereas colicky pain is seen in gastroenteritis and intestinal obstruction.

Pain Severity

The severity of the pain provides few clues since it depends upon subjective report from the patient, as well as host factors like age and immune-status. In general, pain of mesenteric ischemia, biliary colic, and renal colic is severe, whereas patients with gastroenteritis tend to present with a less severe pain.

Pain Radiation

Pain due to pancreatitis radiates to the back, while renal colic pain radiates to the groin.

Associated Factors

Patients with chronic mesenteric ischemia tend to develop pain within 1 hour of eating. In contrast, patients with duodenal ulcer get relief upon eating and the pain recurs within a few hours once the stomach is empty. Diffuse cramps associated with diarrhea may point to gastroenteritis. Pain associated with abdominal distension may suggest intestinal obstruction.

PHYSICAL EXAMINATION

General Examination

Vital signs provide vital information. This includes measurement of orthostatic changes if possible. Hypotension and shock may be seen in patients with intestinal obstruction, peritonitis, and bowel infarction because of third-spacing and intravascular volume depletion. Presence of jaundice points to hepatobiliary disease.

Inspection

Inspection includes observing the patient's position, as well as his or her general level of comfort. Patients with pancreatitis are usually seen sitting up and leaning forward to relieve their pain. Patients with peritonitis lie still on their back since motion causes pain. Patients with renal colic are restless and in agony.

Abdominal distention and audible bowel sounds may be appreciated. High pitch bowel sounds may be heard in early intestinal obstruction.

Auscultation

Bowel sounds are absent in advanced peritonitis and intestinal pseudo-obstruction. Early bowel obstruction may manifest with the high pitched bowel sounds. Presence of bowel sounds does not exclude intestinal pseudo-obstruction.

Percussion

Gentle percussion is less painful and is the preferred method for testing rebound tenderness, rather than deep palpation and withdrawal. Percussion also helps to identify ascites, liver span, and abdominal mass.

Palpation

Distract the patient while performing palpation, especially if a psychogenic component is suspected. Guarding and rigidity are seen in patients with peritoneal inflammation, but it may be localized in case of localized peritonitis due to diverticular abscess or appendicitis.

A rectal and pelvic examination is part of complete physical examination of patients with acute abdominal pain. A rectal exam identifying fecal impaction may provide the diagnosis of obstruction in elderly subjects. Tenderness on rectal exam may be elicited in retrocecal appendicitis as well as pelvic inflammatory disease. Stools should be check for occult blood.

INVESTIGATIONS

The depth and breadth of work-up depends upon the clues from the history and physical examination, and whether patient is stable. Lack of findings on history and physical examination in elderly and immune-compromised subjects should be interpreted with caution.

A CBC and differential may point towards an infectious or inflammatory process. A comprehensive metabolic profile can help exclude metabolic causes. Liver function tests, serum amylase, lipase, abdominal x-rays, chest x-ray, EKG, and urinalysis are usually obtained initially. A urine pregnancy test should be done in women of child-bearing age.

Abdominal x-ray series including chest x-ray, supine, and upright abdominal x-ray may provide clues to evidence of obstruction or perforation. A CT scan is helpful when the differential diagnosis includes a variety of infectious, inflammatory, and ischemic etiologies.

Ultrasound is helpful when a gallbladder disease or a gynecological disease is suspected. Ultrasound also aids in the evaluation of suspected appendicitis, although a CT scan is the test of choice. An MRI does not play any role in the investigation of acute abdominal pain with the exception of MRCP, which helps evaluate the bile ducts and pancreatic ducts.

COMMON ACUTE ABDOMINAL PAIN SYNDROMES

1. *Biliary colic*: Uncomplicated cholelithiasis is usually asymptomatic. Biliary colic usually occurs due to impaction of stone in the cystic duct frequently preceded by a fatty meal. The pain is not colicky but steady. It is usually deep and aching, but can be sharp and severe. There is transient elevation of liver enzymes. AST/ALT may go as high as 1800 IU/L. Pancreatic enzymes may be elevated. The pain lasts for a few hours and then resolves completely. Persistence of pain beyond 6 hours should raise a suspicion for cholecystitis. Persistence of the abnormal liver tests raises the possibility of a persistent stone in the common bile duct or alternate etiologies.

2. *Acute cholecystitis*: Pain is localized in the right upper quadrant or epigastrium and may be referred to the scapula. There is associated nausea, vomiting, and fever. Physical exam shows tenderness in right upper quadrant. Murphy's sign may be positive. HIDA scan shows a lack of filling of gallbladder.

3. *Acute cholangitis*: It results from impaction and obstruction of the bile duct and is characterized by fever, jaundice, and abdominal pain. Labs show elevated serum bilirubin and alkaline phosphatase. Ultrasound may show a dilated common bile duct.

4. *Acute pancreatitis*: The most common causes are alcoholism and gallstones. A bout of acute pancreatitis usually arises 1 to 3 days after drinking. Patients complain of pain in the upper abdomen, which may be in the right upper quadrant, epigastrium, or left abdomen with radiation to the back. Pain is rapid in onset and reaches maximum intensity within an hour. Acute pancreatitis may be painless in about 5% of the cases. Pancreatic enzymes are elevated. Serum amylase rises 2 to 12 hours after onset of symptoms and declines over the next 3 to 5 days. In contrast, serum lipase persists much longer. Greater than 3-fold increase in serum ALT suggest a biliary etiology. CT scan is superior to ultrasound for evaluation of pancreas (see Chapter 60).

5. *Splenic abscess and infarct*: Pain occurs in the left upper quadrant and is associated with fever and tenderness. It should be considered in patients with risk for embolism (eg, atrial fibrillation).

6. *Acute appendicitis*: Initially the pain is periumbilical, which eventually localizes to the right lower-quadrant with evidence of localized peritoneal signs. Occasionally patients may complain of generalized abdominal pain. Patients with a retrocecal appendix may only complain of dull achy pain without any localized tenderness. A good history and physical examination is usually sufficient for diagnosis in most cases. A urinalysis should be obtained to exclude urinary tract infection. Pelvic cultures may be helpful in sexually-active menstruating women. A pregnancy test should be done in women of child-bearing age to exclude ectopic pregnancy. Of note, 30% of patients with acute appendicitis do not show any leukocytosis; however, most of them do show left shift. Imaging studies are only required if the diagnosis is in doubt. A CT scan is the test of choice (see Chapter 72).

7. *Diverticular disease*: Uncomplicated diverticulosis is asymptomatic. Painful diverticular disease may present with abdominal cramps, bloating, and a feeling of incomplete or difficult evacuation and irregular defecation. Physical exam is unremarkable. Diverticulitis on the other hand occurs as a result of microscopic or macroscopic perforation of the diverticulum, which quickly seals off. Most patients present with a left lower-quadrant pain. In Asian countries, right-sided diverticulitis is more common. Patients may present to the physician several days after the onset which helps to distinguish it from any other abdominal complaints. Localized tenderness is seen. CBC shows leukocytosis. Endoscopic evaluation and barium enema are relatively contraindicated especially in acute severe diverticulitis and the treatment is usually based on clinical grounds. The studies are only undertaken if the diagnosis is in doubt. However, once an episode of acute diverticulitis is resolved, patient should undergo a colonoscopic evaluation in about 4 to 8 weeks to exclude any other disorder mimicking diverticulitis including a malignancy (see Chapter 78).

8. *Nephrolithiasis*: There is a wide spectrum of pain which may be minimal to severe, eventually requiring hospitalization and parenteral pain control. Pain waxes and wanes in paroxysms lasting from 10 to 60 minutes. Pain may be in the flank or may radiate to the testicle or tip of the penis or labia. The location of

the pain can change as the stone migrates. A CT scan is the test of choice. Ultrasound may be undertaken in patients who wish to avoid radiation especially pregnant women or women of child bearing age.

9. *Pelvic inflammatory disease*: It is characterized by lower abdominal pain especially during menstruation or sexual intercourse. It occurs more commonly between the ages of 15 and 25 years. Those at risk include African Americans, those with multiple sex partners, and those with a male sex partner who has a sexually transmitted disease. Pain is usually bilateral. Additional features may include uterine bleeding, new onset of vaginal discharge, proctitis, fever, and chills. Ectopic pregnancy, ruptured ovarian cyst, torsion of the fallopian tubes, and endometriosis should be excluded.

10. *Chronic mesenteric ischemia*: There is postparandial pain associated with weight loss and sometimes nausea, vomiting, and diarrhea. It may be seen in patients with atherosclerosis or may be a manifestation of systemic vasculitis. Angiography is the test of choice (see Chapter 100).

11. *Acute mesenteric ischemia*: Abdominal pain is acute, severe, diffuse, and out of proportion to the physical findings. There may be frank hematochezia or only heme-positive stools. Angiography provides diagnosis as well as therapeutic options (see Chapter 99).

12. *Acute intestinal obstruction*: It causes acute, severe, and diffuse abdominal pain. Etiologies include adhesions, incarcerated hernia, intussusception, or volvulus. Adhesions account for 80 to 95% of the cases. Fecal impaction may sometimes present as obstruction especially in case of elderly or those with neurological or developmental disorders. Patients complain of abdominal pain, nausea, vomiting, abdominal distention, and lack of passage of flatus. Abdominal x-ray series shows dilated bowel with multiple air-fluid levels (see Chapter 77).

MANAGEMENT

General Measures

Stable patients seen in ambulatory settings usually do not require any aggressive investigations. Patients with acute abdomen, on the other hand, should go to the emergency room and be admitted. They should take nothing by mouth. Intravenous fluids and electrolytes are administered while the investigations are pending. A surgical consult should be obtained.

Pain Control

Narcotics for pain control should be avoided early in the case because they cloud the assessment and decision-making process. Patients with biliary colic or acute cholecystitis get benefit from parenteral NSAIDs like ketorolac (15.0 to 30.0 mg IV or IM q 6 hours).

Specific Management

Treatment beyond intravenous fluids and pain control depends upon the etiology of the pain. Patients with evidence of diffuse peritonitis required emergent surgical consultation.

PEARLS

- ○ Typical clinical and laboratory features of acute abdominal pain may be absent in about 30% of the cases, especially in elderly and immune-compromised subjects.
- ○ Rectal and pelvic exam should be performed in all cases of acute abdomen.
- ○ A pregnancy test should be performed in all women of child-bearing age.

BIBLIOGRAPHY

Sharp HT. The acute abdomen during pregnancy. *Clin Obstet Gynecol.* 2002;45(2):405-13.

Gore RM, Miller FH, Pereles FS, Yaghmai V, Berlin JW. Helical CT in the evaluation of the acute abdomen. *Am J Roentgenol.* 2000;174(4):901-13.

Chapter

8 *Upper Gastrointestinal Bleeding*

Upper GI bleeding is a major cause of morbidity and mortality, as well as utilization of health care resources. It accounts for over 100 hospitalizations per 100 000 population and is more common in males. The elderly are especially at high-risk.

ETIOLOGY

Peptic ulcer disease accounts for 55% of the cases. Risk factors for bleeding in peptic ulcer disease include Hp infection, NSAIDs, severe stress of sickness in ICU patients (stress gastropathy), and gastric hyperacidity.

Varices are the cause in 14% of upper GI hemorrhage and variceal bleeding carries a mortality rate of 30% for each episode. Arteriovenous malformations are the diagnosis in 6%, whereas Mallory-Weiss tears, erosions, and tumors each are the cause in about 5% cases.

Uncommon causes of upper GI bleed include Dieulafoy's lesion, gastric antral vascular ectasia (GAVE), portal hypertensive gastropathy, hemobilia, hemosuccus pancreaticus, and upper GI tumors.

CLINICAL FEATURES

Patients usually present with hematemesis or coffee ground-like emesis and/or melena. Instillation of 50 to 100 mL of blood into the stomach results in melena; on the other hand, patients losing 100 mL of blood per day may have normal appearing stools.

DIAGNOSIS

Gastric lavage of frank blood or coffee ground-like material is diagnostic. However, lavage may be negative if the bleeding has stopped or the source of bleeding is beyond the pylorus and the pylorus is closed.

The presence of bilious material on gastric lavage suggests that there is no active upper GI bleeding. Hematochezia may be seen in 5 to 10% of the patients with severe upper GI hemorrhage. Such cases are usually accompanied by hemodynamic compromise. Endoscopy is undertaken for diagnostic as well as therapeutic purposes.

INITIAL MANAGEMENT

Rapid assessment of hemodynamic status and resuscitation are more important than the precise diagnosis of the cause of bleed. Large bore intravenous access should be accomplished quickly. Stat labs should be drawn for at least a CBC, basic metabolic panel, and coagulation profile. Patients with shock, orthostatic hypotension, drop of hematocrit greater than 6%, transfusion requirement of greater than two units, or continued active bleeding should be admitted to the ICU for close monitoring. Aggressive resuscitation with stabilization as much as possible is essential to minimize complications.

Transfusions

Elderly patients or those with severe comorbidity like coronary artery disease should have blood transfusions to maintain a hematocrit above 30%. Young and otherwise healthy subjects may be transfused to the extent of 20% or above.

Patients with continued bleeding in the presence of coagulopathy (INR greater than 1.5) or low platelet count less than 50 000/mm^2 should be given fresh frozen plasma and platelets respectively.

Role of Gastric Lavage

The impact of nasogastric lavage on the outcome remains to be established. Gastric lavage using a large-bore orogastric tube removes blood and blood clots and facilitates endoscopy as well as reduces the risk for aspiration. Use of prokinetic prior to endoscopy may accomplish the same objective.

Airway Protection

Endotracheal intubation should be considered in patients with continuing active bleed and altered mental status.

Initial Medical Management

Octreotide is effective in controlling active variceal bleeding due to varices and reducing risk for rebleeding after endoscopic control of the hemorrhage. Its role in nonvariceal upper GI hemorrhage is controversial and I recommend its use as an adjunctive treatment before endoscopy or if endoscopy is unsuccessful or unavailable. I also recommend intravenous PPI infusion to be started as soon as possible prior to endoscopy.

SPECIFIC DIAGNOSIS

EGD allows a precise diagnosis as well as opportunity for therapeutics. A single dose of metoclopramide 20.0 mg IV or erythromycin 250.0 mg IV may be given 20 to 120 minutes prior to endoscopy to hasten gastric emptying of the blood and clots, thereby improving visibility and the quality of endoscopic visualization.

Angiography or RBC bleeding scan may occasionally be helpful. Endoscopic ultrasound may help distinguish between gastric varices and large gastric folds. Upper GI barium studies are contraindicated in the presence of acute GI bleed.

TREATMENT OF BLEEDING ULCERS

Risk Stratification

Endoscopy allows for risk stratification of the patients. For example, patients with active arterial bleeding are likely to rebleed in 90% of the cases on medical management alone, nonbleeding visible vessel in 50%, and adherent clot in about 25% of cases. On the other hand, an ulcer with a clean base rebleeds in less than 5% of the cases. Persistent oozing from an ulcer without a visible vessel has a rebleeding rate of 10 to 20%.

Endoscopic Strategy Based on Risk Stratification

Endoscopic therapy improves outcome in patients with active bleeding as well as nonbleeding visible vessels. Ulcers with a clean base or flat pigmented spot should not be treated endoscopically. The management of adherent clot is controversial. Clots that can not be removed by aggressive irrigation carry a 25% risk for rebleeding. While some experts manage these patients medically, others attempt to remove the clot by ensnaring and then treating it based on the underlying ulcer pathology.

Endoscopic Treatments

Endoscopic treatments for bleeding peptic ulcers include electrocoagulation, injection therapy, hemostatic clips, a fibrin sealant or glue, or cauterization. Usually a combination of injection therapy with epinephrine 1/10 000 locally followed by thermal coagulation is performed. Endoscopic clips control bleeding in the manner similar to surgical ligation. The role for fibrin sealant needs to be defined.

Iatrogenic Complications

Treatment related complications include aspiration, hypoventilation, hypotension, perforation or worsening of bleeding. Use of greater than 30 mL of epinephrine 1/10 000 and/or greater than 5 pulses of thermal coagulation increases the risk for perforation.

Failure of Endoscopic Therapy

Risk factors for failure of endoscopic therapy include presentation with active hemorrhage, shock, gastric ulcers along the lesser curvature, and posterior duodenal bulb ulcers. NSAID use, coagulopathy, previous peptic ulcer disease, or severe coronary artery disease do not correlate with the outcome of endoscopic therapy.

Nonmedical, Nonendoscopic Treatments

Angiography and/or surgery should be considered in patients with failure of endoscopic therapy. In patients in whom ulcer bleeding was controlled but has recurred, a repeat endoscopy should be performed and patients referred to surgery if bleeding persist or recurs after two therapeutic endoscopies. Patients should also be considered for surgery if they continue to be hemodynamically unstable despite administration of greater than 2 to 3 units of blood transfusion, recurrent hemorrhage despite two attempts at therapeutic endoscopies, shock associated with recurrent hemorrhage, and continued slow bleeding requiring greater than 3 units of blood transfusion per day.

Relative indications for surgery include elderly patients, severe comorbidity, chronic gastric ulcer as the cause of bleeding, and refusal of a blood transfusion. In the absence of randomized controlled trials, the type of emergency surgery for bleeding ulcer is based on the surgeon's preference and expertise. The basic surgery involves oversewing of the ulcer. In addition to oversewing, some surgeons perform a truncal vagotomy with pyloroplasty, whereas others advocate a vagotomy plus antrectomy.

Risk for Rebleeding

Risk of rebleeding after discharge from the hospital is 1% per month. Acid suppressive therapy helps in reducing the risk. In patients with Hp infection, eradication of Hp reduces recurrence. Patients with bleeding due to NSAIDs benefit from NSAID prophylaxis in case the NSAID needs to be continued.

TREATMENT OF VARICEAL BLEEDING

Medical treatment options for control of acute variceal bleed include intravenous vasopressin plus nitroglycerin, intravenous octreotide, and balloon tamponade. Endoscopic therapies include sclerotherapy (5% ethanolamine, 5% sodium morrhuate, or 1 to 3% sodium tetradecyl sulfate), variceal band ligation, or combination of the two. Sclerotherapy carries higher risk of complications than variceal banding. Variceal band ligation is preferred over sclerotherapy for preventing recurrence as well as for reducing mortality. Thermal coagulation may worsen the bleeding in patients with varices.

Management of bleeding gastric varices is difficult. Nonbleeding gastric varices should be treated only as part of investigative protocols. Bleeding due to gastric varices may be controlled by intravariceal injections of sclerosants. Patients with uncontrolled variceal bleed or frequent recurrences are candidates for transjugular intrahepatic porto-systemic shunts (TIPS). Complications of TIPS include encephalopathy, shunt occlusion, and shunt migration.

Surgery for Variceal Bleeding

Surgery is rarely employed for acute variceal bleed due to high mortality. Options include portosystemic shunts, esophageal transaction and devascularization. The only hope for cure is liver transplantation. Although, portosystemic shunts reduce the risk of bleeding, they increase the risk for the encephalopathy just like TIPS. Esophageal transection and devascularization has been used for acute bleeding in the literature but is rarely used. Splenectomy should be performed in patients with isolated gastric varices due to splenic vein thrombosis.

Primary Prophylaxis of Varices

Primary prophylaxis for esophageal varices should be undertaken using propranolol or nadolol. Goal is reduction in heart rate by 25%. In patients with large esophageal varices, endoscopic band ligation may be beneficial.

Prevention of Recurrent Variceal Rebleed

Control or elimination of the underlying risk factors is important for reducing recurrent bleeding. Over two-thirds of the patients will rebleed unless the varices are obliterated. The risks for rebleeding from varices can be reduced by eradication of varices by sclerotherapy or preferably banding. The use of nonselective beta-blockers like propranolol may further decrease the risk for rebleeding and improve survival. Bleeding from esophageal varices is usually a marker for advanced liver disease and majority of the patients die within 1 year because of bleeding or hepatic decompensation.

TREATMENT OF MALLORY-WEISS TEAR

This usually occurs in the distal esophagus at the level of gastroesophageal junction. The most common cause is retching or vomiting, although these symptoms may not present in about 50% of the cases.

Endoscopy is the diagnostic method of choice. Most tears heal within 24 to 48 hours and may not be visible if endoscopy is performed thereafter. Differential diagnosis includes esophageal ulceration due to acid reflux, infectious esophagitis, or pill-induced esophagitis. Endoscopic treatment is undertaken for active bleeding at the time of endoscopy and includes injection therapy with epinephrine 1:10,000 as well as a thermal coagulation. The esophagus may be very thin at the site of tear, and as such, sclerosants and repeated coagulation should be avoided. Angiographic arterial embolization or surgery may be rarely needed in cases in which bleeding cannot be controlled. Medical treatment with H_2RAs, PPIs, or sucralfate is frequently used but is of unproven benefit. Rebleeding from Mallory-Weiss tear is rare in the absence of portal hypertensive gastropathy.

PEARLS

○ EGD can characterize an ulcer and predict the risk for rebleeding.

○ Octreotide has been shown to be of benefit for variceal as well as nonvariceal upper GI bleeding.

BIBLIOGRAPHY

Eisen GM. An annotated algorithmic approach to upper gastrointestinal bleeding. *Gastrointest Endosc.* 2001;53(7):853-8.

Chapter

9 *Lower Gastrointestinal Bleeding* ▬▬▬▬▬

Lower GI bleeding refers to blood loss from a GI source distal to the ligament of Treitz frequently resulting in hemodynamic instability, anemia, and/or transfusion requirements.

EPIDEMIOLOGY

About 14% of Americans report some kind of rectal bleeding; however most do not seek medical attention. Rate of hospitalization for lower GI bleeding is 21 per 100 000 persons per year in the United States. Males are at higher risk than females.

CLINICAL FEATURES

Patients usually present with passage of bright red or maroon colored blood and/or clots per rectum. Melena, although usually a sign of upper GI bleeding, can occur from a colonic source—especially the right colon. Similarly, hematochezia may occur as a result of severe upper GI bleeding in about 10% of the cases.

ETIOLOGY

Internal hemorrhoids are the most common cause of lower GI bleeding in individuals below the age of 50. In the remaining individuals, the etiology includes diverticulosis (20 to 50%), colon polyps or cancer (15 to 25%), colitis or various kinds of ulcers (10 to 25%), and angiodysplasia or vascular ectasia (5 to 37%). Anorectal disorders like hemorrhoids, fissures, and solitary rectal ulcer syndrome each account for about 5 to 10% of the cases. In individuals above the age of 65, angiodysplasia may be the most common cause.

DIFFERENTIAL DIAGNOSIS

Diverticulosis causes massive, painless bleed usually arising from the right colon. Diverticular bleeding and acute diverticulitis usually do not occur concurrently. Patients at risk for diverticular bleeding include those with a low fiber diet, those who take NSAIDs, elderly subjects, and those suffering from constipation. Fecal occult blood positive stools should not be attributed to diverticulosis.

In contrast to the arterial bleeding in diverticulosis, the bleeding in angiodysplasia tends to be less severe. Over 80% of the patients with untreated angiodysplasia tend to rebleed. There is no relationship between angiodysplasia and aortic stenosis.

Colitis is usually idiopathic chronic inflammatory bowel disease (ulcerative colitis or Crohn's disease) in young individuals, whereas ischemic colitis is more likely in elderly subjects. Infectious colitis may occur due to *E. coli O157:H7, Campylobacter, Salmonella, Yersinia,* or *Entameba histolytica*.

Colon cancer accounts for about 10% of the cases for hematochezia in patients above the age of 50 years, but is uncommon below that age.

Hemorrhoids do not cause problems in most individuals, but may present with GI bleeding that is rarely massive enough to require blood transfusions. Bleeding due to hemorrhoids is painless, whereas fissures are painful. Blood is usually on the side of the stool or only on the toilet paper. Bleeding due to radiation proctitis may occur as an early or late complication of radiation therapy to the pelvic region.

Iatrogenic bleeding following a biopsy or polypectomy is rare and is usually self-limited. It may be delayed by 7 to 28 days.

DIAGNOSIS AND MANAGEMENT

Young patients who are hemodynamically stable and not actively bleeding may be investigated as outpatients. Patients who are hemodynamically unstable and have significant comorbid conditions, persistent bleeding requiring multiple transfusions, or evidence of acute abdomen should be hospitalized.

Immediate Management

The management starts with resuscitative measures including intravenous fluids and blood products as needed. Patients with INR greater than 1.5 or a platelet count less than 50 000/mm³ should receive fresh frozen plasma and platelets respectively. Maintain the hematocrit at 30% for high-risk individuals especially elderly subjects, whereas 20 to 25% may be acceptable in young, healthy individuals. Plain abdominal x-rays should be undertaken if any perforation or obstruction is suspected.

Etiology of acute hematochezia may be an upper GI source in up to 10% of the cases. As such, insertion of nasogastric tube and lavage to exclude an upper GI source is recommended. Upper endoscopy should be the initial test if there is fresh blood or coffee ground-like aspirate, and should be considered for patients in whom bilious fluid is not obtained. Upper endoscopy may especially be attractive in patients with massive hematochezia who are otherwise hemodynamically compromised if the nasogastric aspirate has not yielded bilious material.

In all other cases, colonoscopy is the initial test of choice. Once a source has been identified during colonoscopy, it should be treated accordingly. Some experts perform colonoscopy without any purgation while most prefer a rapid colonic cleansing with 1 gallon of polyethylene glycol (PEG) solution given via nasogastric tube over 2 hours. Metoclopramide 10.0 mg IV or erythromycin 250.0 mg IV given at the start of colonic cleansing may increase the effectiveness of lavage.

If colonoscopy is not possible due to the severity of bleeding, arteriography and a surgical consultation should be undertaken.

RBC Bleeding Scan vs Angiography

Patients suspected of slow intermittent bleed may benefit from a tagged RBC bleeding scan. The accuracy rates varies from 25 to 90%. RBC scan should be obtained only after colonoscopy has been undertaken. However, it may be undertaken prior to angiography. Angiography is only positive if there is active bleeding of greater than 0.5 to 1.0 mL per minute. The advantages of angiography include that it does not require colonic cleansing and its localization is accurate. In addition, therapeutic interventions can be undertaken in the form of vasopressin infusion or embolization.

Investigation of Obscure Source

Small bowel evaluation may be needed in patients that have had negative results in upper and lower endoscopy. These include a small bowel enteroscopy and enteroclysis. Enteroclysis is superior to small bowel series for evaluation of bleeding. A radionuclide scan for Meckel's diverticulum may be undertaken in young patients with acute lower GI bleeding.

Specific Treatment

Treatment depends upon the cause. Cauterization of bleeding from a diverticulum or arteriovenus malformation (AVM) is effective. Patients with radiation proctitis respond well to laser or argon plasma coagulator (APC) therapy. Solitary rectal ulcer syndrome should be treated as a case of constipation with the goal of effective and regular defecation. In some cases, no precise cause or source may be found; such patients may benefit from subtotal colectomy.

PEARLS

O   Melena may occur from lower GI source, especially right colon.

O   Severe hematochezia may be due to upper GI source in up to 10% of the cases.

BIBLIOGRAPHY

Eisen GM. An annotated algorithmic approach to acute lower gastrointestinal bleeding. *Gastrointest Endosc.* 2001;53(7):859-63.

Chapter 10 Occult and Obscure Gastrointestinal Bleeding

Occult GI bleeding is defined as heme-positive stools and/or the presence of unexplained iron deficiency anemia. Obscure GI bleeding on the other hand is defined as a overt or occult bleeding which persists despite negative endoscopic evaluation (usually colonoscopy and EGD).

EPIDEMIOLOGY

While data on obscure-occult bleeding are sparse, only about 0.5 to 1.5% of overt acute GI bleeding remain obscure after evaluation.

ETIOLOGY

The most common cause of iron deficiency anemia is blood loss. The most likely cause is GI bleeding, although menstrual blood loss should be a strong consideration in premenopausal women. While the focus of fecal occult blood testing is colorectal cancer, the source of blood may be anywhere in the GI or respiratory tracts.

Small Intestinal Causes

The source of blood loss may be the small intestine in patients who have a normal upper endoscopy and colonoscopy. Causes include angiodysplasia, tumors, medication-induced ulcers, and hemobilia. Celiac disease may cause heme-occult positive stools in as many as 50% of the cases. Five to 12% of the patients with iron deficiency anemia may have small intestinal biopsy findings consistent with celiac disease.

Anemia in Menstruating Females

In addition to fecal occult blood positive stools, investigations should be carried out in premenopausal women in following cases:

1. The anemia is disproportional to the menstrual blood loss.
2. Presence of abdominal symptoms.
3. Family history of GI malignancies, especially in patients over age 40.

DIAGNOSIS

History should focus on the use of anticoagulants and other medications that may injure GI mucosa like NSAIDs, potassium, alendronate, etc. Look for signs of cutaneous manifestations of disorders like Peutz-Jeghers syndrome (pigmented spots on lips), celiac sprue (dermatitis herpetiformis), neurofibromatosis (neurofibromas and Café au lait spots), Gardner's syndrome (sebaceous cysts and osteomas), and Cronkite-Canada syndrome (abnormalities of hair and nails).

Care should be taken as not to ascribe fecal occult blood positive stools to diverticulosis or esophageal varices—both of which usually cause massive GI bleeding.

DIAGNOSTIC STRATEGY

The work-up of the patients who take NSAIDs or anticoagulants or who abuse alcohol is the same as those without history of such ingestion.

Colonoscopy vs EGD

In case of occult blood loss (ie, FOBT-positive stools), a dilemma frequently faced by a physician is whether to evaluate the colon or upper GI tract first. This is complicated by the fact that a finding seen on one procedure may not necessarily represent the true cause for bleeding and there may be a concomitant source of bleeding in another part of the GI tract. Except in young patients without family history of colon cancer and without symptoms referable to the upper GI tract, most gastroenterologists prefer to start with a colonoscopy.

Colonoscopy

Colonoscopy is required in all patients with iron deficiency anemia and/or FOBT-positive stools. Premenopausal women with fecal occult blood negative stools who are asymptomatic and without family history of GI malignancy may not need colonoscopy.

EGD

Controversy exists with respect to the timing of upper endoscopy and under what conditions it should be performed. The role of evaluation of upper GI tract should not be underestimated, since the source of GI blood loss is more likely to be found on upper endoscopy than colonoscopy.

In general, I recommend upper endoscopy at the same time as colonoscopy. If a definite bleeding source that accounts for all the findings is found during colonoscopy, the upper endoscopy need not be carried out. This includes colonic malignancy. On the other hand, if there is a source like internal hemorrhoids or a nonbleeding polyp, an upper endoscopy should be undertaken. Upper GI series and barium enema have low sensitivity and do not offer the therapeutic option.

Evaluation of Small Intestine

In the presence of negative upper endoscopy and colonoscopy, the GI loss is presumed to be from small intestine. However, because of the difficulty in identifying small intestinal lesions with currently available tests, evaluation of small intestine is not always necessary unless the bleeding is significant enough to require transfusions.

Small bowel series or preferably enteroclysis should be the initial test of choice for evaluation of small intestine. The role of wireless capsule endoscopy, although promising needs to be established. A small bowel enteroscopy should be considered in patients in whom the above work-up continues to be negative. Patients with persistent requirement for blood transfusions may benefit from intraoperative enteroscopy during exploratory surgery in order to exclude AVMs, ulcers, small bowel neoplasms, etc, as a source of GI bleeding.

Scintigraphy

Radio-isotope bleeding scans may be helpful in localizing the source of bleeding, although the data is not clear. For a positive result, it requires bleeding at the rate of at least of 0.1 mL/minute. Results of delayed scans obtained at 12 to 24 hours after injection should be interpreted with caution since there may be pooling of blood from different sites in the GI tract. Radionuclide Meckel's scan is occasionally used as part of work-up but it only indicates the presence of gastric mucosa in the Meckel's diverticulum, and not whether it is the source of bleeding.

Angiography

The exact role of angiography in obscure bleeding has not been established. The test requires an active bleeding of at least 0.5 to 1.0 mL/minute for the test to be positive. Anticoagulants and vasodilators have been used to precipitate bleeding and improve the yield of angiography; however, the utility of this technique remains to be established. Avoidance of meperidine or its reversal during endoscopy may unmask an angiodysplasia that may not have been visible because of vasoconstriction.

TREATMENT

Medical and Endoscopic Management

Treatment is directed at the cause. Endoscopic therapy using thermal contact probes, injection therapy, and argon plasma coagulation are useful for angiodysplasia and GAVE. Angiotherapy using vasopressin infusion, as well as embolization for overt small intestinal bleeding sources, is beneficial in select cases—but not without potential for serious or life threatening complications. Octreotide (50.0 to 100.0 mcg SC; two to three times a day) helps reduce blood loss from intestinal angiodysplasia.

Patients may require iron supplementation and periodic transfusions. Hormonal therapy with estrogen has been used for angiodysplasia but has not been found to be of benefit in randomized controlled trials.

Role of Surgery

Surgery is required for most bleeding tumors. Exploratory laparotomy and bowel resection may be needed in patients with continued bleeding and high transfusion requirements. The success rate is the highest if the segmental bowel resection has been undertaken following localization by angiography. Blind total colectomy without preoperative localization in the presence of massive lower intestinal bleeding is associated with a mortality of 10 to 30%.

PROGNOSIS

Prognosis is excellent in early stages. The long-term outcome depends on the etiology for the bleeding such as cancer. Intraoperative endoscopy directed therapy results in reduction of GI blood loss in 40 to 70% of the patients.

PEARLS

○ GI blood loss is the most common cause of iron deficiency anemia.
○ The work-up of the patients who are taking NSAIDs or anticoagulants or who abuse alcohol is the same as those without history of such ingestion.

BIBLIOGRAPHY

Zuckerman GR, Prakash C, Askin MP, Lewis BS. AGA technical review on the evaluation and management of occult and obscure gastrointestinal bleeding. *Gastroenterol.* 2000;118:201-221.

Chapter
11   *Acute Diarrhea*

DEFINITION

Although diarrhea is technically defined as greater than 200.0 g/day of stool weight, this definition is of little clinical value. Clinically, it may be defined as three or more loose or watery stools per day or a decrease in consistency and increase in frequency of bowel movement for an individual patient. Most patients with diarrhea have three to seven bowel movements per day, although the number may reach 20 or more in cases of severe infectious diarrhea and certain tumors. Diarrhea persisting for greater than 2 weeks is termed as persistent diarrhea, whereas when it extends beyond 1 month, it is termed as chronic diarrhea. Most acute diarrhea lasts less than 4 days.

EPIDEMIOLOGY

Diarrhea is the second most common cause of death worldwide, and the most common cause of death amongst children. Food-borne diseases account for 76 million illnesses, 325 000 hospitalizations, and 5000 deaths each year in the United States. This is however an under-estimation since acute diarrhea may occur due to nonfood borne ill-nesses also. Similarly, gastroenteritis is cited as the reason for over 450 000 hospital admissions each year in the United States.

Diarrhea accounts for 1.5 million outpatient visits, and more than $1 billion in direct medical costs in addition to the indirect costs.

ETIOLOGY

Small Bowel vs Large Bowel Diarrhea

Small bowel infectious diarrhea usually presents with large vol-ume, watery stools with abdominal cramps, and weight loss. WBCs are absent in the stool. The large bowel diarrhea on the other hand presents with frequent small volume stools that may be associated with fever plus blood or WBCs in the stool.

DIAGNOSTIC CLUES

Immune-Competent Patients

Small bowel diarrhea is usually noninflammatory and may be caused by bacteria (*Salmonella, E. coli, Clostridium perfringens, Staphylococcus aureus, Bacillus cereus,* and *Vibrio cholerae*), viruses (*Rotavirus* and *Norwalk agent*), or protozoa (*Cryptosporidium, Microsporidium, Isospora, Cyclospora,* and *Giardia*). Colonic diarrhea, which is frequently inflammatory, may be caused by bacteria (*Campylobacter, Shigella, Clostridium difficile, Yersinia, Vibrio para-haemolyticus, Enteroinvasive E. coli*), viruses (*CMV, Adenovirus, Herpes simplex*), and protozoa (*Entamoeba histolytica*).

Salmonella, Cryptosporidia, Microsporidia, Campylobacter, and *CMV* may involve both small and large bowel. Offending pathogen can be isolated from stool culture in 5 to 40% of the cases.

Salmonella is the most common cause of food-borne illness in the United States and is associated with ingestion of poultry, eggs, and milk products. Shigella-causing dysentery is the second most common and is commonly seen in daycare centers. *Campylobacter* may cause watery or hemorrhagic diarrhea, depending on whether the small or large bowel is involved.

E. coli 0157:H7 is a common cause of acute hemorrhagic colitis and is associated with ingestion of undercooked ground beef, as well as unpasteurized apple cider. It may also lead to hemolytic-uremic syndrome (HUS) and thrombotic thrombocytopenic purpura (TTP).

Vibrio cholerae causes small bowel diarrhea, whereas *Vibrio parahaemolyticus* leads to colonic diarrhea, and is related to consumption of shellfish. Cyclospora may cause diarrhea that may last greater than 3 weeks and is associated with fatigue, as well as myalgias along with diarrhea.

Rotavirus is a common cause of acute diarrhea in infants, whereas Norwalk agent causes diarrhea in older children and adults.

Immune-Compromised Patients

Patients with history of lymphoma, bone marrow transplantation, and HIV are at greater risk for development of diarrhea. As many as 60% of AIDS patients in the West and 95% in the developing countries have diarrhea. Infections in immune-compromised patients include *Cryptosporidium, Isospora belli, Cyclospora, Microspordia, Salmonella, Campylobacter, Shigella, Mycobacterium avium complex, CMV, Herpes,* and *Adenovirus*.

Cryptosporidium diarrhea in HIV-infected patients with well-preserved CD4 cell counts is self-limited, just as it is in non-HIV patients.

Noninfectious Diarrhea

While most acute diarrhea is infectious, noninfectious causes include drugs (misoprostol), drug and food sweeteners (sorbitol), food allergies, IBD, endocrine diseases (thyrotoxicosis, diabetes mellitus), and tumors (VIPoma, carcinoid syndrome).

Nosocomial Diarrhea

Nosocomial diarrhea develops after the patient has been admitted to the hospital for greater than 3 days. It may be due to tube feeding, medications, or infections. Diarrhea may occur up to 3 weeks after cessation of the offending medication.

CLINICAL FEATURES

Most cases of acute diarrhea are self-limited. Less than 25% of patients seek medical attention. Medical evaluation is indicated in the presence of dehydration, bleeding, fever, greater than six loose stools per 24 hours, more than 2 days of illness, and severe abdominal pain in patients above the age of 50, as well as in elderly and immune-compromised patients.

DIAGNOSIS

Detailed history and comprehensive physical exam is of paramount importance. Stools should be checked for occult blood and fecal leukocytes. Serum chemistries may reflect dehydration as well as fluid and electrolyte imbalance.

Role of Endoscopy

Endoscopy is rarely needed and should be performed to distinguish IBD from infectious diarrhea, for diagnosis of *C. difficile* infection in whom stool tests are not available or are negative despite high index of suspicion, and in immune-compromised patients. Endoscopy may also be performed in patients in whom ischemic colitis is suspected but the diagnosis has not been established on clinical or radiological grounds.

Stool Cultures

The value of stool cultures is controversial. They are of no value in patients with nosocomial diarrhea, but may be helpful in immune-compromised patients as well those with severe comorbidities or concurrent inflammatory bowel disease. Negative stool cultures may be required for some occupations like food handlers prior to being permitted to return to work. Most labs only look for *Salmonella, Campylobacter*, and *Shigella*. Thus *Aeromonas, Yersinia*, and *Enterohemorrhagic E. coli* (ETEC) are likely to be overlooked unless specifically requested.

Stools for Ova and Parasites

Testing stools for ova and parasites is not cost-effective in most cases. It may be helpful in patients with persistent diarrhea, diarrhea of foreign travel, diarrhea in daycare workers, homosexual or HIV-infected patients, or bloody diarrhea in the absence of fecal leukocytes. In contrast to bacterial pathogens, parasitic excretion is intermittent, and as such three specimens on three consecutive days should be sent for examination.

DIFFERENTIAL DIAGNOSIS

Presence of fever indicates invasive diarrhea with *Salmonella, Shigella, Campylobacter, C. difficile, Enteric viruses*, or *E. histolytica*. Diarrhea due to *Staphylococcus aureus* or *Bacillus cereus* occurs within 6 hours of ingestion because of preformed toxin. Diarrhea in *Clostridium perfringens* occurs 8 to 14 hours following ingestion. *E. coli* and viruses usually cause diarrhea after about 15 hours of ingestion. Recent antibiotic use suggests antibiotic-associated diarrhea with or without *C. difficile* infection.

TREATMENT

General Measures

Hydration and maintaining electrolyte balance form the cornerstone of treatment. Antibiotics are not required in most cases.

The oral hydration solution recommended by the World Health Organization is adequate in most cases. It contains per 1 L of water, 3.5 g sodium chloride, 2.5 g sodium bicarbonate, 1.5 g potassium chloride, and 20.0 g of glucose or 40.0 g of sucrose. However, it is underutilized in the West. An equivalent home recipe is 0.5 teaspoon of salt, 0.5 teaspoon of baking soda, and 4.0 tablespoons of sugar in 1 L of water. Rice water may also be used.

Use of Antibiotics

Empiric antibiotic therapy is indicated in patients with fever, bloody diarrhea, greater than eight stools per day, dehydration, symptoms lasting greater than 1 week, immune-compromised patients, presence of fecal leukocytes, prior to consideration for hospitalization. Options for empiric therapy include oral quinolone like norfloxacin 400.0 mg PO bid, ofloxacin 400.0 mg bid or ciprofloxacin 500.0 mg PO bid. Antibiotics are unlikely to be effective in ETEC including *E. coli O157:H7, Salmonella,* or *Yersinia* without sepsis and mild to moderate traveler's diarrhea.

Metronidazole 250.0 to 500.0 mg PO qid should be given to patients with presumed *C. difficile* infection. The duration of therapy is tailored according to the pathogen isolated.

Antimotility Agents

Drugs such as loperamide or diphenoxylate may be used in patients in whom there is no fever and the stools are not bloody. Initially, give loperamide 4.0 mg followed by 2.0 mg after each unformed stool (not to exceed 16.0 mg/day for 2 days) or give diphenoxylate 4.0 mg bid to qid for up to 2 days. These agents should not be administered to patients with *E. coli 0157:H57* or *C. difficile colitis.* Pepto-Bismol 30 mL or 2 tablets q 4 to 6 hours PRN may help.

Miscellaneous Agents

Probiotics are helpful in *C. difficile* diarrhea, traveler's diarrhea, and acute diarrhea in children. Nutrition during acute diarrhea may include boiled potatoes, rice, wheat with salt, crackers, bananas, yogurt, and soup. Products containing lactose should be avoided even in patients with no history of lactose intolerance.

PEARLS

- ○ Antibiotics are not required in most cases of acute diarrhea.
- ○ Most cases of acute diarrhea are self-limited.
- ○ Stool cultures are not of value in patients with nosocomial diarrhea.

BIBLIOGRAPHY

Manatsathit S. Guideline for the management of acute diarrhea in adults. *J Gastroenterol Hepatol.* 2002;7(Suppl):S54-71.

Guerrant RS, Van Gilder T, Steiner TS. Practice guidelines for the management of infectious diarrhea. *Clinical Infectious Diseases.* 2001;32(3):331-51.

Chapter
12 *Traveler's Diarrhea*

As many as 40 to 60% of subjects traveling to developing countries may develop traveler's diarrhea. The course is very benign and self-limited. Travel to Asia, Africa, South and Central America, and Mexico is associated with the highest risk for traveler's diarrhea, whereas northern Europe, Australia, New Zealand, Canada, Singapore, and the United States are the lowest risks.

PATHOGENESIS

Risk factors include:
1. Immune-compromised patients
2. Hypochlorhydria due to acid suppressive medications
3. Patients with gastroduodenal surgery

Most cases occur due to ingestion of contaminated food or water. The most common pathogen is enterotoxigenic *E. coli*. Other bacteria implicated are *Campylobacter*, *Salmonella*, and *Shigella*. Scientific data for occurrence of diarrhea due to spices and changes in the climate or time zones is lacking. Parasitic infections including *Giardia* and *Cyclospora* may rarely be involved.

CLINICAL FEATURES

Symptoms include nausea, vomiting, diarrhea, abdominal cramps, malaise, loss of appetite, and low-grade fever. Blood or pus in stool is rare. Most illnesses resolve within 1 to 5 days.

PREVENTION

Making informed choices about food, ingested fluids, and water purification during travel can prevent traveler's diarrhea. Routine prophylactic use of antibiotics is controversial.

Ice in drinks is not safe unless made from boiled or filtered water. Alcohol cannot sterilize water. Carbonated beverages are safer than noncarbonated ones. If bottled water is not available, boil water for 5 to 15 minutes or add 2 drops of 5% sodium hypochlorite to a quart of water or 5 drops of tincture of iodine to a quart of water. Compact water filters can also be used.

Avoid fruit salads, lettuce, and chicken salads. Fruits peeled just before eating are safe. Bottled drinks should be consumed from the bottle with a straw rather than from a glass. Table buffets are risky.

PROPHYLAXIS

Use of prophylactic medications although effective is not routinely recommended because of concerns of cost as well as side effects. Exceptions include patients with prior gastric surgery, severe IBD, severe cardiovascular or renal disease or severe-immune compromised state such as HIV or organ transplant. Options include ciprofloxacin 500.0 mg qd or bid, norfloxacin 400.0 mg/day, or Pepto-Bismol 30 mL or 2 tablets qid. There are concerns for salicylate toxicity with use of high doses of Pepto-Bismol. Probiotic *Lactobacillus GG* has also been shown to be effective.

TREATMENT

Treatment of traveler's diarrhea involves fluid replacement to maintain adequate hydration status, antibiotics, and antidiarrheal agents. Oral hydration is effective in most cases. Packets of oral hydration solution mixed with clean water should be used or a similar solution may be prepared by using 0.5 teaspoon of salt, 0.5 teaspoon of baking soda, and 4 tablespoonfuls of sugar to 1 L of water.

Antibiotics are indicated in patients with moderate to severe diarrhea or those associated with fever, blood or mucus in stools.

Ciprofloxacin 500.0 mg twice a day for 1 to 2 days is effective. Bismuth subsalicylate (Pepto-Bismol) 4 tablets every 30 minutes until diarrhea resolves (with a maximum of 8 doses) can be effective but there are concerns for salicylate toxicity. Antidiarrheal agents like loperamide and diphenoxylate (Lomotil) are also effective but should be avoided in patients with invasive diarrhea unless under medical supervision. An empiric course of antiprotozoal therapy (metronidazole 500.0 mg PO tid) may be tried in patients not responsive to antibacterial and antimotility agents.

PEARLS

- ○ Routine antibiotic prophylaxis for traveler's diarrhea is not recommended.
- ○ Parasitic infections are a rare cause of traveler's diarrhea.

BIBLIOGRAPHY

Ansdell VE, Ericsson CD. Prevention and empiric treatment of traveler's diarrhea. *Med Clin North Am.* 1999;83(4):945-73.

Day LJ. Ciprofloxacin use and misuse in the treatment of travelers' diarrhea. *Am J Med.* 2003;114(9):771-2.

Chapter

13 *Chronic Diarrhea* ▬▬▬▬▬

DEFINITION

Diarrhea means different things to different people (eg, increase in stool volume or weight, frequency, or fluidity of the stool). While for research purposes it is defined as a greater than 200.0 g of stool per day, clinically, chronic diarrhea is defined as a decrease in stool consistency of 4 or more weeks in duration.

EPIDEMIOLOGY

The prevalence rates for diarrhea depend upon the definition used and the population studied. Chronic diarrhea effects 5% of the population. It accounts for $350 million per year due to work loss alone. Its impact on quality of life has not been well studied.

ETIOLOGY

Chronic diarrhea may be caused by numerous diseases depending upon the socioeconomic status of the population. Infectious etiologies including chronic bacterial and parasitic infections are the predominant cause in the developing countries. IBS, IBD, and malabsorption syndrome, plus chronic infections in immune-compromised patients, are commonly encountered in the West.

PATHOGENESIS

Chronic diarrhea may occur due to systemic illnesses like hyperthyroidism, diabetes, vasculitis, tumors, Whipple's disease, IBD, tuberculosis, mastocytosis, and AIDS. Chronic infections frequently encountered include parasites like *Giardia, Entameba histolytica, Cyclospora, C. difficile,* and (in immune-compromised patients) *CMV, HIV, MAI complex, Microsporidia, Cryptosporidium,* and *Isospora belli.*

Osmotic diarrhea is frequently related to magnesium, phosphate, and carbohydrate malabsorption. Fatty diarrhea occurs due to malabsorption syndrome. Differential diagnosis of fatty diarrhea includes celiac sprue, short bowel syndrome, small bowel bacterial overgrowth (SBBO), mesenteric ischemia, as well as maldigestive processes (eg, pancreatic insufficiency and inadequate supply of bile acids).

Secretory diarrhea may occur due to laxative abuse, bacterial toxins, bile acid deficiency due to terminal ileum disease, IBD, vasculitis, medications, dysmotility, diabetic diarrhea, hyperthyroidism, and IBS. Neuroendocrine tumors (gastrinoma, VIPoma, somatostatinoma, carcinoid syndrome, and medullary carcinoma of the thyroid) are uncommon. Diarrhea may also occur as a result of other neoplasia like colon cancer, lymphoma and villous adenoma, and endocrine disorders like Addison's disease.

Inflammatory diarrhea occurs due to inflammatory bowel disease, ulcerative jejuno-ilietis, infections including *C. difficile colitis, tuberculosis, Yersinia,* viruses (*CMV, Herpes), amebiasi*s, ischemic colitis, radiation enteritis, lymphoma, and colon cancer.

CLINICAL FEATURES

History should include the specifics of the complaint including frequency, consistency and volume of stools or whether stool is greasy or malodorous. Ask for duration of symptoms, whether onset was gradual or sudden, history of urgency, incontinence, recent travels or outdoor picnics, risk factors for HIV infection, weight loss, any systemic symptoms (eg, fever, arthralgias, skin rash), any association with particular foods, and sexual history. History of medication use, especially those that may contain sorbitol or sugar-free products, is important. History of therapeutic interventions like antibiotics, radiation therapy, surgery, and chemotherapy should be sought.

Physical exam is usually not helpful but may provide findings of underlying disease like IBD, malabsorption syndrome, and Grave's disease. For example, mouth ulcers, skin rash or arthritis may be seen in inflammatory bowel disease; muscle wasting and anemia in malabsorption syndrome; and perianal irritation in fecal incontinence.

DIFFERENTIAL DIAGNOSIS

In general, chronic diarrhea is gradual except in cases of infections. A long history (greater than 1 year), straining with defecation, and absence of nocturnal defecation or weight loss suggests a functional etiology.

Chronic infections occur in patients who consume impure water. History of consumption of sugar-free foods may suggest the possibility of sorbitol-induced diarrhea, whereas a consumption of raw milk may point towards *Brainerd diarrhea*. Persistence of diarrhea during fasting suggests secretory diarrhea.

Associated abdominal pain is important in mesenteric ischemia, bowel obstruction, and IBS, while excessive flatus may point to a carbohydrate malabsorption. Fecal soiling suggests fecal incontinence, but may occur due to fecal impaction.

History of recent travel points to infectious diarrhea and chronic idiopathic secretary diarrhea. Weight loss is seen in malabsorption syndrome, pancreatic insufficiency, IBD, and malignancy.

Osmotic diarrhea is frequently seen in patients taking frequent antacids, sorbitol in diet products and medications, and those who exhibit lactose intolerance and laxative abuse.

Patients with inflammatory diarrhea frequently have fever, hematochezia, and abdominal pain.

Temporal association with the particular foods points towards food allergy. A history of anal intercourse should alert to the possibility of infectious proctitis.

Family history may provide clues for IBD, celiac disease, and multiple endocrine neoplasia.

While blood in stools suggests malignancy or IBD, oil particles in the stool point towards malabsorption syndrome. White or tan colored stools suggest cholestatic disorder.

INVESTIGATIONS

Diagnostic strategies depend upon the experience of the physician and the clinical presentation, since no studies have been done to outline any optimal strategy. A comprehensive history and physical examination along with a targeted investigation can achieve diagnosis in as many as 90% of the patients.

Initial Testing

Laboratory investigations include CBC, thyroid function tests, and a comprehensive metabolic profile including serum electrolytes, protein, and albumin. Exclude celiac sprue (see Chapter 68). Initial stool studies include testing for WBCs as well as for pathogens, occult blood, and Sudan III stain.

Depending upon age and clinical presentation, patients should undergo sigmoidoscopy or preferably colonoscopy. In some cases, an upper endoscopy may also be required.

Classification of Diarrhea

Based on baseline testing, the diarrhea may be classified as watery, inflammatory, or fatty. Watery diarrhea may further be classified into secretary or osmotic diarrhea. Further testing is targeted at the type of diarrhea.

Secretary vs Osmotic Diarrhea

Secretory diarrhea continues during fasting, where as osmotic diarrhea improves. The two types can be distinguished by calculating the osmotic gap in the stool. Osmotic gap of less than 50.0 mOsm/kg suggests secretory diarrhea, whereas a gap greater than 125.0 mOsm/kg points towards osmotic diarrhea.

Patients with normal osmotic gap and normal stool weight usually have irritable bowel syndrome or factitious diarrhea, whereas normal osmotic gap and increased stool weight point to laxative abuse or various secretory diarrhea.

Secretary Diarrhea

Work-up of secretary diarrhea includes stool cultures to exclude chronic infections, along with imaging of small and large bowel. A therapeutic trial of cholestyramine may be undertaken to exclude bile acid diarrhea. Further testing includes serum gastrin, calcitonin, VIP, somatostatin, TSH, protein electrophoresis, as well as immune-globulins. In addition, urinary 5-HIAA should be checked in order to exclude carcinoid syndrome.

Osmotic Diarrhea

Patients with osmotic diarrhea do not need further work-up if the cause can be identified by history (eg, sorbitol-diarrhea or lactose intolerance). Cause is investigated by a stool analysis for low pH (suggesting carbohydrate malabsorption), a screen for magnesium and laxatives, and a breath hydrogen test for lactose intolerance.

Inflammatory/Infectious Diarrhea

A work-up of inflammatory or infectious diarrhea includes testing of stools, as well as colonoscopy and ileoscopy. Stool investigations include testing for ova and parasites, bacterial cultures including *E. coli O157:H7* and *C. difficile* toxin. A small bowel series, a CT scan of the abdomen, and small bowel biopsy are also helpful. Patients may be tested for bacterial overgrowth or a therapeutic trial of antibiotics may be undertaken.

Fatty Diarrhea

Work-up should focus on fatty diarrhea in patients who present with greasy and malodorous stool and who are at risk for a fat malabsorption. Sudan III stain of stool detects clinically significant steatorrhea in 90% of patients. A 72-hour measurement of stool fat is the standard. An empiric trial of pancreatic enzymes supplementation may be undertaken for pancreatic insufficiency if there is no evidence of chronic pancreatitis on other studies.

Endoscopic Evaluation

It is a matter of frequent debate whether a sigmoidoscopy or colonoscopy should be the endoscopic method for evaluation of lower GI tract. I prefer a colonoscopy because it allows for visualization of the entire colon, permits an assessment of the terminal ileum, and gives us the ability to exclude lesions in right colon and terminal ileum (eg, *C. difficile* colitis, microcytic colitis, and Crohn's disease). An EGD with small bowel biopsy and aspiration for bacterial culture is helpful in select cases.

Imaging Studies

A small bowel series, mesenteric angiography, and CT scan may be helpful when no cause can be found.

TREATMENT

Treatment is directed at the underlying cause as well as providing symptomatic relief.

Empiric Therapy

Empiric therapy may be undertaken in situations where a diagnosis can be strongly suspected, as in an infectious organism identified in an outbreak, ileal resection in patient with possible bile-acid diarrhea, or a patient with known recurrence of small bowel bacterial overgrowth.

Symptomatic Therapy

Symptomatic treatment is undertaken when no definite therapy is available or no precise diagnosis can be made.

Options include loperamide, anticholinergics, antispasmodics, bismuth, fiber, and bile-acid binding resins. The improvement in diarrhea can be achieved by loperamide 4.0 mg initially followed by 2.0 mg q 4 to 6 hours PRN or Lomotil (diphenoxylate with atropine) 1 tablet 2 to 4 times per day.

Narcotics like morphine (2.0 to 20.0 mg qid), tincture opium (2 to 20 drops qid), or codeine (15.0 to 60.0 mg q PO 4 hours PRN) are effective in severe cases. Clonidine patch (0.1 to 0.2 mg/day for 7 days) and octreotide (50.0 mcg to 200.0 mcg SC 3 times a day) are useful in severe secretory diarrhea (eg, carcinoid tumor, dumping syndrome, and chemotherapy induced diarrhea) but may not be as well-tolerated. Oral dehydration solutions have a limited utility in chronic diarrhea.

Cholestyramine (4.0 g 1 to 4 times per day) is constipating in most diarrhea and is specific for a bile acid induced diarrhea. Antidiarrheal agents should be avoided in patients with *C. difficile* diarrhea.

COMMON CAUSES OF CHRONIC DIARRHEA

Irritable Bowel Syndrome

It presents with complaints of abdominal pain or discomfort plus alteration in bowel habit. It occurs more commonly in females and symptoms get worsened during stress. Presence of fever, large volume diarrhea, bloody stools, and nocturnal diarrhea suggest an organic pathology. A positive diagnosis of IBS can be made on clinical findings based upon ROME II criteria. Routine laboratory and endoscopic studies are normal. Lactose hydrogen breath test may be undertaken in select cases, although its utility is questionable. Use of biopsies during colonoscopy to exclude microscopic colitis is controversial. Serological studies to exclude celiac sprue has been advocated. Small bowel bacterial overgrowth may be the etiology in some of the patients and an empiric trial of antibiotics may be a reasonable option (see Chapter 74).

Inflammatory Bowel Disease

IBD comprises of Crohn's disease and ulcerative colitis and usually presents between the age of 15 and 40 years. While bloody diarrhea is the predominant feature in ulcerative colitis, diarrhea, abdominal pain, weight loss, and fever are seen in Crohn's disease. Physical exam may be normal or may reflect findings of weight loss, anemia and abdominal tenderness—especially in right lower quadrant in cases of Crohn's disease. Barium studies and CT scans are helpful in select cases. Endoscopic evaluation with a biopsy can help clinch the diagnosis (see Chapter 75).

Malabsorption Syndrome

This may occur due to maldigestion of nutrients or an impaired absorptive capacity. The malabsorption may be the result of congenital defects in small intestinal transport systems or may be acquired due to Crohn's disease, Whipple's disease, or celiac disease. Common disorders manifesting with malabsorption include lactose intolerance, chronic pancreatitis, Crohn's disease, celiac disease, and small bowel bacterial overgrowth. Patients frequently present with diarrhea along with weight loss and normal appetite. Stools may be voluminous. Flatulence may be increased. Labs show evidence of hypoalbuminemia; stool fat greater than 6.0 g/day; anemia; low serum iron, ferritin, and/or vitamin B_{12}; and prolonged prothrombin time. A majority of the patients with malabsorption have only mild symptoms that may mimic IBS. For example, iron deficiency anemia may be the sole manifestation of celiac sprue.

Chronic Infections

Whipple's disease, *Giardia, Cryptosporidium*, and *C. difficile* are associated with chronic diarrhea.

Brainerd diarrhea occurs in a sporadic or an epidemic form of prolonged diarrhea associated with patchy lymphocytic colonic inflammation that can last from months to years. It occurs following consumption of contaminated water or unpasteurized milk. A definite infectious etiology has not been established.

Some experts speculate that the onset of IBS is precipitated by an episode of bacterial infection in as many as 30% of the cases. Further speculation suggests that *Brainerd diarrhea* represents a severe form of infectious diarrhea-induced IBS.

PEARLS

○ Differential diagnosis depends upon the geographic region and socioeconomic status of the patient.

○ IBS and IBD in immune-competent hosts, and chronic infections in immune-compromised hosts, are common in the West.

○ Empiric therapy is undertaken when diagnosis is strongly suspected. Symptomatic treatment is undertaken when no definite treatment is available or no precise diagnosis can be made.

BIBLIOGRAPHY

Schiller LR. Diarrhea. *Med Clin North Am*. 2000;84(5):1259-74.

Chapter 14 *Constipation*

EPIDEMIOLOGY

Constipation is a very common digestive problem occurring in about 10 to 20% of the population. The prevalence of constipation rises with age, with a higher prevalence existing among elderly people. It is more common in females, nonwhites, and individuals with low socioeconomic status. Constipation in the elderly more accurately correlates with decreased caloric intake, and not with the reduction in fluid or fiber intake. It results in 2.5 million physician visits annually.

DEFINITION

Although classically defined as less than three bowel movements per week, constipation means different things to different people. As such, additional criteria have been used. Features like straining or feeling of incomplete evacuation, sensation of anorectal obstruction, use of manual physical maneuvers to facilitate defecation, or hard or lumpy stools on at least 25% of the bowel movements point to functional constipation.

The diagnosis of functional constipation requires the presence of any two of the above for at least 12 weeks, which need not be consecutive, over a 1 year period. Presence of loose stools, as well as the criteria for IBS, excludes the diagnosis of functional constipation. The diagnosis of functional constipation should be entertained after exclusion of organic disorders.

ETIOLOGY

Common causes for chronic constipation include neurogenic disorders (autonomic neuropathy, intestinal pseudo-obstruction, diabetes mellitus, multiple sclerosis, spinal cord injury, Parkinsonism);

IBS; and non-neurogenic disorders (hypothyroidism, hypercalcemia, hypocalcemia, pregnancy, porphyria, and scleroderma). Constipation may also occur as a side effect of numerous drugs including anticholinergics, antispasmodics, antidepressants, antipsychotics, iron, aluminum containing antacids, sucralfate, opiates, antihypertensives, and calcium channel blockers.

In patients complaining of infrequent defecation but normal colonic transit, misperception and high degree of psychosocial distress are the cause.

Among patients characterized as severe idiopathic chronic constipation, IBS is found to be the culprit in over 70% of the patients whereas pelvic floor dysfunction is seen in 13%.

CLINICAL FEATURES

Frequency of bowel movements should preferably be documented by a 2-week stool diary. Other important points of enquiry on history include medications, systemic and neurological disorders, recent change in bowel habit, abdominal pain, and bleeding. Physical exam, although usually not useful, is helpful if fissures, hemorrhoids, or a gaping anal opening are seen. Straining during the digital rectal examination helps assess contraction of puborectalis and external anal sphincter.

DIAGNOSIS

Routine Studies

CBC, comprehensive metabolic profile, and thyroid function tests should be checked and may provide important clues. A plain x-ray of the abdomen may provide evidence of large amount of stool in the colon.

Endoscopy vs Barium Enema

Flexible sigmoidoscopy or colonoscopy are undertaken based on clinical presentation and age of the patient. I prefer colonoscopy in most cases because it provides a greater degree of reassurance to the patient that there is no cancer. In addition, a clean colon after colonoscopy provides a better opportunity for bowel retraining. Some experts prefer a barium enema in young patients to assess the rectosigmoid diameters to exclude megarectum and megacolon.

Colonic Transit Studies

Colonic transit studies using markers help distinguish between normal and slow transit constipation, and may even provide clues about the region of slow transient. Prior to a transit study, patients should empty their colon using laxatives since they are not allowed to use laxatives during the study. A variety of protocols are used. The simplest test involves ingestion of markers on day 1 and an abdominal x-ray on fifth day. Presence of greater than 20% of markers remaining indicates slow transit. In another protocol, markers are ingested on three consecutive days and x-rays are taken on fourth and seventh days.

Colonic transit time greater than 72 hours is considered abnormal. A repeatedly normal study in a patient complaining of infrequent defecation suggests misinterpretation or misperception on the part of the patient.

In patients with normal colonic transit, a therapeutic trial should be undertaken and if there is no improvement, further testing should be undertaken.

Advanced Studies

If clinical presentation and the investigations suggest pelvic floor dysfunction, then anorectal manometry and balloon expulsion test, defecography, and EMG may be undertaken. Abnormality on one single test should be interpreted with caution since there is large overlap with the healthy population.

Dynamic magnetic resonance imaging defecography holds promise.

MANAGEMENT STRATEGY

Step 1

Initial management includes patient education regarding increase in fluid and fiber intake as well as attempting to defecate in the morning after breakfast. A daily intake of 20.0 to 35.0 g of fiber is recommended. Fiber supplements such as psyllium, methylcellulose, or calcium polycarbophil (2 to 4 tablets qid) with increased fluid intake enhance colonic transit. The dose of bulk laxatives should be increased slowly since they can cause gas and bloating. Encourage regular exercise.

Step 2

Patients not responding to bulk laxatives may be tried on other laxatives that are not usually harmful if taken two to three times per week under supervision. Stool softeners like docusate are of questionable benefit. Magnesium containing laxatives carry the risk of hypermagnesemia in patients with renal failure. Caution should be exercised with stimulant laxatives like bisacodyl (10.0 mg PO or suppository) and senna, as they may lead to electrolyte abnormalities and protein-losing enteropathy if used chronically. Castor oil is not routinely recommended for chronic basis. Lactulose or its cheaper alternative, sorbitol, may be used as osmotic laxatives.

Although tegaserod is approved for constipation-predominant IBS in females only, many experts recommend a therapeutic trial for patients with chronic constipation.

PEG solution (2 to 4 L every 1 to 2 weeks) is effective treatment especially in patients with severe constipation who are institutionalized or bedridden. Miralax is a powder preparation (17.0 g to 34.0 g qd) that does not contain electrolytes.

Step 3

Patients with severe constipation may benefit from bowel retraining which is initiated by first cleansing the colon completely by using an enema twice a day or drinking PEG solution (Golytely, NuLytely) until the cleansing is complete. Also, the administration of lactulose, sorbitol, or a solution containing polyethylene glycol (Miralax) titrated can be used to achieve at least one stool every other day.

Defecation should be attempted after breakfast in the morning. The patient should then take an enema or a glycerin suppository if there is no bowel movement after 2 days. In demented or bedridden patients with frequent fecal impaction, a regular regimen of enemas once or twice every week or polyethylene glycol solutions (2 to 4 L) every couple of weeks may be undertaken after initial cleansing out of the colon.

Step 4

Biofeedback is an effective treatment especially for patients with pelvic floor dysfunction. Pharmacological treatment to promote colonic motility has been disappointing. Metoclopramide and cisapride are ineffective. Misoprostol may be helpful in selective cases, but is avoided because of cost, tachyphylaxis, and a potential for miscarriage in pregnant women.

Step 5

Subtotal colectomy with ileorectal anastomosis may be indicated in patients with chronic severe constipation that is refractory to medical therapy. Slow colonic transit should be documented prior to surgery. Intestinal pseudo-obstruction should be excluded by radiological or manometric studies prior to surgery.

Since structural abnormalities like rectocele can be present without constipation, caution should be exercised before surgical repair and the results are better in patients who use vaginal maneuvers to facilitate defecation. Surgery is an effective treatment for Hirschsprung's disease.

PEARLS

O   Most of the patients characterized as severe refractory constipation actually have irritable bowel syndrome or some other more generalized disorder.

O   The management of refractory patients may be improved by investigating measures of anatomy and/or physiology: defecography, colon transit markers study, and anorectal manometry.

O   Abnormal results on a single imaging or manometric testing should be interpreted with caution since there is a huge overlap with healthy controls.

BIBLIOGRAPHY

Locke GR, Pemberton JH, Phillips SF. AGA technical review on constipation. *Gastroenterol.* 2000;119:1766-1778.

Wald A. Is chronic use of stimulant laxatives harmful to the colon? *J Clin Gastroenterol.* 2003;36(5):386-9.

Chapter
15 *Pruritus Ani*

CAUSES

It occurs due to a variety of local conditions including fecal seepage, poor anorectal hygiene, excessive or aggressive cleaning, and use of chemicals, soaps, ointments, or perfumes.

Frequently implicated systemic causes include dietary agents (caffeine, citrus, tomatoes, spices, beer, chocolate, cola drinks), obesity, tight fitting clothes, anorectal diseases, chronic diarrhea, pelvic radiotherapy, dermatological disorders (psoriasis, contact dermatitis, atopic dermatitis, Paget's disease), malignancy, perianal infections (perianal abscess or fistula), sexually transmitted diseases (anal warts, *Herpes, Gonorrhea, Candida*), parasitic infections (*Enterobius*), and diabetes.

It may be idiopathic in many cases and psychological factors have been implicated.

CLINICAL FEATURES AND DIAGNOSIS

Physical exam includes careful examination of perianal region as well as digital rectal exam along with biopsy of any suspicious lesions. Endoscopic evaluation of the colorectal region should preferably be carried out especially individuals above the age of 40 years in whom no etiology can be documented.

TREATMENT

Most patients only require conservative treatment and reassurance including improvement in hygiene, dietary manipulation, bulking agents like psyllium, treatment of underlying cause, and avoiding aggressive scratching or use of chemicals. Cleaning with premoistened toilet paper is helpful. Although no definite proof exist, elimination diets may be helpful.

A short course of 1% hydrocortisone cream twice daily for 1 to 2 weeks or local zinc oxide ointment may help. Oral antihistamines may be used at night to promote sleep while healing continues. Patients refractory to conservative measures may benefit from local injection of methylene blue under general anesthesia and the effect may last as long as 5 years.

PEARLS

○ Pruritus ani occurs due to numerous causes, and improvement in perianal hygiene provides relief in many cases.

○ Elimination diets may be helpful in select cases.

BIBLIOGRAPHY

Jones DJ. ABC of colorectal diseases. Pruritus ani. *BMJ*. 1992;5; 305(6853):575-7.

Mazier WP. Hemorrhoids, fissures, and pruritus ani. *Surg Clin North Am.* 1994;74(6):1277-92..

Chapter 16 *Chronic Rectal Pain Syndromes*

LEVATOR ANI SYNDROME

Levator ani syndrome or chronic rectal pain occurs in 5 to 10% of the population with female predominance. It is also know as pelvic tension myalgia. It is defined as an episodic rectal pain lasting for at least 20 minutes, sometimes as a constant dull-ache, over the previous 3 months in the absence of any organic causes. It is often precipitated by prolonged sitting or difficult/incomplete defecation.

Physical exam may be normal or tenderness of the levator ani muscles may be elicited as the examining finger moves from coccyx posteriorly to the pubis anteriorly during rectal exam. Role of anorectal manometry is controversial. Potential treatments include digital massage of levator ani muscles three to four times per week, sitz bath at 40° C, regularization of bowel habit, perineal strengthening exercises, muscle relaxants, and antidepressants.

Mechanical devices such as electrogalvanic stimulation through a rectal probe, acupuncture, and biofeedback have been used. Psychiatric evaluation may be needed in severe and refractory cases. Surgical division of puborectalis muscle is not recommended.

PROCTALAGLIA FUGAX

It is of uncertain etiology and occurs in 5 to 15% of the population. The issue of sex predominance is controversial. "Perfectionists" are at higher risk.

It is a chronic intermittent rectal pain that occurs all of a sudden, lasts for a few seconds to a few minutes with a maximum of 30 minutes, and then resolves spontaneously. Pain may be aching, gnawing, crampy, or stabbing with variable severity, and may occur any time of the day or night. Pain may wake the patient during sleep. Some patients, usually males, complain of pain during sexual intercourse. Patients are asymptomatic between the episodes.

Physical exam is normal. Diagnosis is made on clinical grounds and by exclusion of other pain syndromes. Because of the brief and infrequent nature of the pain, treatment consists of education and reassurance. Since anxiety and stress have been implicated, antidepressants and anxiolytics may be tried as appropriate. Long-term use of benzodiazepines should be avoided due to their addictive potential. Medications that have been used successfully include salbutamol inhaler, topical nitroglycerine 0.2% at onset of pain, oral clonidine, and diltiazem.

COCCYGODYNIA

Coccygodynia is a chronic rectal pain arising out of coccyx. It may be sharp or achy in character and may radiate to the buttocks. It may occur due to orthopedic causes, arthritis, or may be functional due to presumed injury during vaginal delivery. Pain can be reproduced upon manipulation of coccyx.

Treatment consist of moist heat application, analgesics, regularization of bowel habit and stool softeners as needed. Local injection of corticosteroids may be tried in patients who fail conservative therapy. Coccygectomy may be needed in severe and refractory cases.

PEARLS

○ Most functional rectal pain improves with reassurance and conservative measures.

BIBLIOGRAPHY

Wald A. Functional anorectal and pelvic pain. *Gastroenterol Clin North Am.* 2001;30(1):243-51.

Chapter
17 *Fecal Incontinence*

EPIDEMIOLOGY

Fecal incontinence is a common problem occurring in about 3% of the population, and is more common in the elderly. The prevalence is as high as 20% among patients greater than 65 years and living at home, which escalates to almost 50% in patients who are institutionalized. Women suffer from fecal incontinence several times more than men, most likely due to obstetric injury. Acute self-limiting incontinence may occur in healthy individuals during an episode of severe diarrhea. Though fecal incontinence is not a life-threatening symptom, it often causes significant psychosocial distress and impairs quality of life. The health care cost related to this problem runs into billions of dollars each year; approximately half a billion dollars is spent on adult diapers alone.

ETIOLOGY

Fecal incontinence may result from a loss of any of the continence maintenance functions. The broad mechanisms include anal sphincter weakness, impaired rectal or anal sensation, or decreased rectal compliance frequently accompanied by altered bowel habits (ie, constipation and/or diarrhea). Usually, more than one mechanism is involved.

Common causes of anal sphincter weakness include obstetric or surgical sphincter trauma and pudendal nerve injury. Local conditions such as rectal cancer, radiation enteritis, or fecal impaction need to be considered and excluded if necessary. Neurological disorders like multiple sclerosis and diabetes mellitus also impair continence mechanisms. Finally, immobility and inability to access the toilet, as well as psychological or behavioral problems like dementia and depression also contribute to fecal incontinence.

PATHOPHYSIOLOGY

Fecal incontinence may be classified into two broad categories based on pathophysiology. *Passive incontinence* occurs when there is a involuntary discharge of fecal matter and patient becomes aware of it after the fact. Patients have low resting anal pressures. In contrast, urge incontinence occurs when the discharge occurs despite the patient's active attempts to prevent it. These patients have reduced ability to produce squeeze pressure for any duration. Some experts define fecal spillage or soiling as a separate third category. This happens despite normal continent functions and occurs after incomplete defecation, or in cases of rectal prolapse, rectocele, or weak anal sphincter.

CLINICAL FEATURES

Staining, soiling, seepage, and leakage are terms used to reflect the nature and severity of incontinence. Soiling indicates more leakage than staining of underwear; soiling can be specified further in underwear, outer clothing, or furniture/bedding. Seepage refers to the leakage of small amounts of stool. Diagnostic clues include age of onset and duration of illness, precipitating factors (obstetrical, surgical, or back trauma), frequency and presence of nocturnal incontinence, and inability to distinguish between gas and stool.

In addition to a general physical examination, a comprehensive examination of the nervous system as well as the back followed by perianal inspection and digital rectal examination are key to establishing the etiology of fecal incontinence.

A comprehensive digital rectal examination includes assessment of sphincter tone both on resting and voluntary squeeze, length of anal canal, integrity of puborectalis sling, as well as any rectal mass or fecal impaction. Ano-cutaneous reflex, also known as anal wink sign, should be done by gently stroking the skin around the anus and observing a reflex contraction of the external anal sphincter.

INVESTIGATIONS

The diagnostic approach should be individualized based on whether the incontinence occurs only on liquid stools or regardless of the consistency of stools.

In patients with diarrhea, stool studies, as well as sigmoidoscopy or colonoscopy, should be considered. The stool studies should include examination for fecal leukocytes and infectious organisms; stool weight/volume and fat should also be measured if necessary. Measurements of colon transit may be helpful in refractory cases as some patients with incontinence have the 'worst of both worlds'— delayed colonic transit with a weak pelvic floor resulting in incontinence.

Anorectal Manometry

Anorectal manometry can measure resting anal pressure, squeeze pressure and its duration, recto-anal inhibitory reflex, threshold of rectal sensation, rectal compliance, and straining pressure.

Patients with anal sphincter defects may have reduced sphincter pressures. Internal anal sphincter dysfunction correlates with a decreased resting pressure, whereas external anal sphincter dysfunction manifests as decreased squeeze pressure. Rectal sensory threshold is measured by inflating a balloon in the rectum in a step-wise fashion up to a volume at which the sensation is first perceived or a desire to defecate is aroused.

Pudendal Nerve Latency

Pudendal nerve terminal latency correlates poorly with symptoms and does not predict success or lack thereof after surgical repair of anal sphincter defects.

Endosonography

Anal endosonography is useful to detect structural abnormalities of the anal sphincters as well as the rectal wall. It is less invasive, and when conducted by an experienced operator, it is generally reliable for detecting anal sphincter injury.

Miscellaneous

Role of defecography in evaluation of incontinence is limited; it is useful in selected patients (eg, in patients with a clinically suspected rectocele).

Since anal ultrasound can identify anal sphincter defects or thinning, anal EMG using concentric needle electrodes is useful only for identifying neurogenic or myopathic anal sphincter injury.

TREATMENT

Options include medical management, biofeedback, and surgery.

Improving Stool Consistency

Efforts should be made to improve the stool consistency and reduce the stool frequency by treating the cause of diarrhea. The stool consistency can be increased by using bulking agents like methylcellulose, antidiarrheal agents like loperamide or diphenoxylate (although loperamide is superior), and anticholinergic agents like hyoscyamine (NuLev 0.125 mg) taken before meals. Opiates (codeine 15.0 to 60.0 mg qid, morphine 2.0 to 20.0 mg qid, or tincture opium 2 to 20 drops qid) may be needed in difficult cases in addition to loperamide. Some experts recommend against their combined use.

Second line agents like clonidine (0.1 to 0.3 mg tid), octreotide (50.0 to 150.0 mcg SC tid), and cholestyramine (4.0 g bid to qid) are less effective and not as well tolerated.

Medical Management

Rectal suppository or enema may be helpful in patients with incomplete defecation followed by postdefecatory soiling.

Patients with overflow incontinence related to impaction, megarectum, or blunting of rectal sensation (diabetes, multiple sclerosis) may benefit from disimpaction, bowel cleansing, and habit retraining.

Patients with reservoir incontinence due to decreased compliance, inflammation, rectal surgery, or a tumor would benefit from low fiber diet, antidiarrheal agents, as well as treatment of inflammation.

Internal sphincter defects may be treated with antidiarrheal agents. Ten percent topical phenylephrine has been used. A disposable anal plug fits into the rectum and may be useful in patients with impaired sensation due to neurological disorders.

Patients with dementia or inability to access the toilet benefit from regular defecatory program.

Low doses of tricyclic antidepressants may be tried in idiopathic fecal incontinence. Direct sacral nerve electrical stimulation provides short-term relief in some patients.

Biofeedback

Biofeedback is frequently used to help improve rectal sensation in patients with impaired rectal sensation and structurally intact internal sphincter ring.

It is unlikely to help patients with cognitive problems, absence of rectal sensation, complete spinal cord lesions and major sphincter defects. While some studies suggest that up to 75 to 90% of carefully selected patients benefit from biofeedback therapy by either improving or resolving the problem, others have shown no superiority of biofeedback over conservative therapy including advice on diet, fluid, bowel training program, and use of antidiarrheal agents.

Surgery

Options include repair of the sphincter in patients with sphincter disruption, rectopexy for full thickness prolapse, and pelvic floor repair for neurogenic incontinence. However, in some cases, colostomy may be the only viable procedure. Except for treatment for rectal prolapse and acute sphincter disruption, the role of surgery is controversial because of questionable effectiveness and high complication rate.

Antegrade continent enema (ACE) procedure is frequently used in children with spina bifida. It allows antegrade colonic washout through an appendicostomy or button cecostomy device.

Newer Approaches

These include neosphincter by wrapping striated muscles surgically around the anal canal to increase the resting tone. Another option is synthetic sphincter device with an inflatable cuff that can be deflated for the purposes of defecation and is useful for patients with anal leakage. These devices are associated with considerable morbidity and not widely used.

A procon incontinence device consisting of a rectal balloon with a sensing device to alert the patient about impending bowel movement is being studied. Experience with sphincter bulking agents is limited.

Sacral nerve stimulation, which has been shown to help urinary incontinence has been reported to help some patients with fecal incontinence and is now approved for this indication in Europe.

PEARLS

○ Fecal incontinence is usually multifactorial disorder.

○ The role of surgery is limited to select patients.

○ Biofeedback therapy and modulation of bowel habits helps many patients.

BIBLIOGRAPHY

Bharucha AE. Fecal incontinence. *Gastroenterology*. 2003;124(6):1672-85.

NUTRITION

Chapter

18 *Malnutrition*

Malnutrition is widely prevalent amongst hospitalized patients with estimates ranging from 20 to 60%. It is often multifactorial.

PATHOGENESIS

Some contributing factors include reduced intake, which may, at times, be due to physician prescription or inappropriate cessation of food intake, decreased absorption, utilization, and/or increased losses and requirements. Physicians may overlook the problem in the majority of cases.

COMPLICATIONS OF MALNUTRITION

Malnutrition results in reduced bodily function, alteration in body chemistry and metabolism, reduced body mass, and deteriorating clinical outcomes.

It causes increased susceptibility to infection, poor healing, increased frequency of decubitus ulcers, bacterial overgrowth, and impaired cardiopulmonary function resulting in an increase in morbidity and mortality. Hospitalized veterans with plasma albumin concentration less than 2.0 g/dl have a mortality rate of 62%.

MARKERS OF NUTRITIONAL STATUS

While there are numerous markers that reflect severe malnutrition, there is no universally accepted standard for malnutrition in general. A global assessment using a combination of functional and biochemical parameters should be used.

One such global assessment scale utilizes history of weight loss in the prior month and over the preceding 6 months, dietary intake relative to normal, gastrointestinal (GI) symptoms greater than 2 weeks, functional capacity, primary metabolic needs, anthropometric findings of triceps skin-fold thickness, and muscle wasting.

History and physical examination provide clues to recent weight changes, as well as the presence of any nutritional deficiency. In general, patients with 60 to 80% of ideal body weight or serum albumin 2.1 to 3.0 g/dl may be considered moderately malnourished, whereas those with less than 60% of ideal body weight or serum albumin less than 2.1 g/dl are severely malnourished. Low albumin concentrations may reflect increased metabolic stress, systemic inflammatory response, or fluid overload due to a sickness and not necessarily malnutrition.

Weight Loss

A documented 10% weight loss over 6 months indicates malnourished state but is confounded by errors of recall. Unintentional weight loss during the preceding three months is a better indicator. Mild malnutrition results from less than 10% weight loss, moderate malnutrition from 10 to 20% weight loss, and severe malnutrition due to greater than 20% weight loss over the preceding 3 months.

Physical Examination

Temporal wasting, sunken supraclavicular fosse, decreased adipose stores, and thin, listless hair may be seen. Body fat can be assessed by triceps skin-fold thickness, while muscle mass is assessed by mid-arm muscle circumference. Functional tests like hand-grip are useful.

Biochemical Parameters

Serum albumin concentration is the most commonly used parameter and should be used in the context of serum albumin half-life of about 3 weeks. Prealbumin is a more reliable indicator since it has a shorter half-life of 2 to 3 days. Immune markers include total lymphocyte count (TLC) and delayed hypersensitivity testing. TLC of less than $1,000/mm^3$ or less than 5.0 mm skin induration on hypersensitivity testing suggests immune-compromised status. Routine assessment of these parameters for monitoring the nutritional therapy is controversial and probably not cost-effective.

GOALS OF NUTRITIONAL SUPPORT

The goal of nutritional support is to: provide nutrition to an otherwise healthy person who is unlikely to eat for greater than 10 to 14 days; prevent malnutrition, treat pre-existing malnutrition and its complications, as well as act as an adjunctive treatment of a systemic disorder by manipulating the composition of the nutrients (eg, immune-enhancing formula for critically ill subjects and branched chain amino-acids in liver disease). The last goal is the most ambitious and expensive, as well as the most controversial.

INDICATIONS

Nutritional support is indicated in individuals getting less than 75% of bodily needs. The timing of initiation depends upon pre-existing nutritional status, anticipated duration of food deprivation, as well as underlying metabolic stress. The threshold for initiating nutritional support is individualized based upon whether the patient is malnourished and/or catabolic.

Healthy Noncatabolic Subjects

In healthy noncatabolic subjects, enteral nutrition may be initiated in 7 to 10 days and when one suspects that insufficient volitional feeding will occur in 7 to 10 days, whereas parenteral nutritional may be initiated in 10 to 14 days. Parenteral nutrition for less than 5 days provides little benefit. Risks may also outweigh the benefits, especially in nutritionally replete subjects unable to eat for 10 to 14 days and in patients with severe cachexia due to metastatic cancer.

Choice of Route

If the gut works, use it. If the stomach is not accessible due to gastric outlet obstruction or gastroparesis, an enteral route should be chosen. Parenteral nutritional (PN) support may be required in cases of intestinal obstruction, maldigestion, malabsorption, or intestinal fistula.

Use peripheral parenteral nutrition (PPN) if anticipated duration is less than 10 days. Adopt a central parental nutrition route if the anticipated duration is greater than 10 days.

CALCULATION OF NUTRITIONAL NEEDS

Harris-Benedict Equation

Basal energy requirements are different in men and women. Based on the Harris-Benedict equation, the basal metabolic needs in men is 66+ (13.7 x weight in kg) + (5 x height in cm) – (6.8 x age in years). In women it is equal to 655.1 + (9.6 x weight) + (1.8 x height) – (4.7 x age). Different equations for the formula are provided by different texts, especially for women.

The ideal body weight formula should be used for obese patients. Although controversial, an additional stress factor of 20 to 100% has been advocated depending upon the severity and type of illness, but has the potential to increase the risk for complications.

Without the addition of stress factors, the Harris-Benedict equation calculates basal energy expenditure (BEE). BEE is a theoretical value, whereas a resting energy expenditure (REE) value represents the expenditure of a person at rest with minimal physical activity. REE is approximately 110 to 120% of BEE and correlates with approximately 25.0 K_{cal}/kg/day. This is the K_{cal} amount that the bedridden medical patient usually requires.

During sickness, frequently 30 to 35 calories/kg/day are administered. Healthy well-nourished individuals require 0.8 to 1.0 g protein/kg of ideal body weight per day. During sickness, the protein requirements vary from 1.1 to 1.5 g/kg/day, whereas highly stressed, critically ill patients (eg, those with severe burns) may require as high as 2.5 g/kg/day. It is controversial whether calories derived from protein (4 calories/g) should be included in the total calories provided. Metabolically stressed persons frequently burn proteins for energy.

Water

Water needs are roughly 1.0 mL/K_{cal} delivered or 30 mL/kg/day except in patients with fluid restriction. An additional 300 mL should be added for every 1° C rise in body temperature to account for insensible losses.

Monitoring Nutritional Therapy

Indirect calorimetry provides precise measurements of caloric needs but is cumbersome and not cost-effective. Adequacy of nutritional therapy can be determined by measuring nitrogen balance, but this does not affect outcome and is not usually done in practice.

PEARLS

○ Enteral nutrition is preferable to parenteral nutrition whenever possible. Note that enteral feeding has the potential for complications too and only standard formulas of enteral feeds may be cheaper than parenteral nutrition.

○ Low serum albumin concentration does not necessarily reflect a malnourished state since it can be affected by acute illness or other non-nutritional factors.

BIBLIOGRAPHY

Slomka J. Withholding nutrition at the end of life: clinical and ethical issues. *Cleve Clin J Med.* 2003;70(6):548-52.

Heys SD, Ogston KN. Peri-operative nutritional support: controversies and debates. *Int J Surg Investig.* 2000;2(2):107-15.

Chapter

19 *Enteral Nutrition* ▬▬▬

Enteral nutrition is better assimilated by the body. The only absolute contraindication to enteral feeding is intestinal obstruction. Options for access include oral, nasogastric or nasoenteric feeding tube, gastrostomy, or jejunostomy tube.

GASTRIC VS JEJUNAL FEEDING

If the anticipated period of enteral support exceeds 4 weeks, a gastrostomy or jejunostomy tube should be used. Feeding into the stomach is more physiologic, since unlike parenteral nutrition, the nutrients are absorbed into portal circulation with initial processing by the liver. It allows bolus feedings without the use of a pump and the infusion rate can be monitored by checking residual volumes.

Jejunal feeding through a nasoenteric tube or jejunostomy offers only a theoretic advantage of reduction of aspiration pneumonia since most aspiration pneumonia occurs due to aspiration of oropharyngeal secretions. An infusion pump is required since bolus feeding is not possible. Jejunal feeding is indicated when the feeding must be done distal to the ligament of Treitz, or in cases of gastric outlet obstruction or severe gastroparesis as manifested by high gastric residuals.

Issue of checking the residuals in case jejunal feeding is controversial and is based on "expert opinion" and not on evidence-based medicine. We do not recommend checking residuals in case of jejunal feeding especially in an otherwise asymptomatic patient tolerating the feed. A few experts suggest checking residuals intermittently in case of nasojejunal tubes or a jejunostomy converted from a gastrostomy. This is to ensure that the tube has not migrated back into the stomach. A large residual (greater than 10 to 30 mL) suggests the possibility of migration. Still others routinely check residuals, but do not intervene if patient is tolerating the feeding well.

CONTRAINDICATIONS

Contraindications to enteral nutrition include severe malabsorption, intestinal obstruction, perforation, peritonitis, paralytic ileus, shock, intractable vomiting, and some enteric fistulae. Other contraindications include an inability to establish enteral access, pseudo-obstruction, severe vomiting or diarrhea, severe malabsorption, or patient refusal.

SELECTION OF ENTERAL FORMULA

1. Once the enteral support route has been decided, the next step is to select an appropriate formula. Standard tube feeding formulas (eg, Ensure, Attain, Sustacal Basic, Osmolite, Isocal, Resource) are adequate for most patients and are usually lactose-free, gluten-free, isotonic, and contain intact protein along with variable amounts of medium chain triglycerides. They contain about 1.0 calorie/mL, and an intake of 1500 to 2000 mL provides full nutrition for the least cost in most cases. This 1500 to 2000 mL usually provides 100% RDI (recommended daily intake) for both vitamins and minerals.

2. Calorie dense formulas contain 1.5 to 2.0 calories/mL (EnsurePlus, ResourcePlus, SustacalPlus) and water is needed via tube flushes to avoid dehydration. Nutrient dense formulas contain extra amounts of protein or lipid.

3. Elemental formulas (Vivonex T.E.N. or and Tolerex) provide about 1.0 calorie/mL and contain free amino-acids, hydrolyzed carbohydrates, and small amounts of fats. Lipids provide 1 to 10% of total K_{cal} (depending upon choice of product).

4. Oligomeric or semielemental formulas (CriticareHN, Peptamen) contain 1.0 to 1.5 calories/mL, including proteins in the form of small peptides or free amino acids and carbohydrates as simple sugars and glucose polymers. Lipids in the form of medium and long-chain triglycerides provide 5 to 40% of total calories. It is controversial whether the use of oligomeric formulas reduces tube feeding induced diarrhea in critically ill patients.

5. Fiber may be included in various polymeric formulas like Ensure with fiber, Jevity, and Sustacal with fiber. The role of fiber supplementation in tube-feeding remains to be established.

6. Immune-modulating formulas contain omega 3-fatty acids, RNA and DNA, or glutamine and arginine, etc, in various com-

binations. They may be beneficial in select cases, although the data remains controversial.

7. Disease specific formulas for diabetes (Glucerna), pulmonary diseases (Pulmocare), liver diseases (HepaticAid), and renal dysfunction (AminAid, Suplena, Nepro) are available but are expensive and may not be cost-effective.

8. Low fat formulas may not be nutritionally complete.

TROUBLESHOOTING

Diarrhea

It is rarely caused by the formula itself and can be minimized by lowering the rate of infusion and using an isotonic formula or elemental formula:

1. Slowly advance tube feedings until tolerance is established.
2. Check for the possibility of antibiotic-induced diarrhea and small bowel bacterial overgrowth.
3. Avoid medications containing sorbital, antacids containing magnesium, and hypertonic preparations.
4. Switch from bolus to continuous feed. Do not bolus feed into the small bowel.
5. Warm the formula to room temperature.
6. Use isosmotic and lactose-free formula; use low fat formula in fat malabsorption. The use of elemental or semielemental formula in the critically ill, and concentrated formulas in volume-overloaded patients for the management of diarrhea, is controversial.
7. Use bulking agents such as fiber.

Tube Discomfort

This may be reduced by using small caliber polyurethane tubes.

Tube Clogging

Adequate tube caliber can reduce the incidence of tube clogging. Flushes following infusion of medication or formula should be undertaken. If the tube is clogged, using carbonated beverages, brushes, and pancreatic enzymes can be variably successful. Irrigation with 60 cc of warm water is superior to carbonated beverages. Gastrostomy tubes can also be cleared with a brush.

A daily administration of 3 to 5 cc of alcohol through the tube may help reduce tube deterioration. Since most clogging is due to proteinaceous precipitates, meat tenderizers have been recommended; however, there is potential for ulceration.

High Residuals

The approach to large gastric residual varies. There is poor correlation between the gastric-residual volume and clinical manifestations. Consideration for slowing or cessation of feeding should be undertaken once the gastric residual is greater than 200 mL. Exclude obstruction and add a prokinetic agent. Conversion from a gastrostomy to a jejunostomy tube may be needed.

As described above, we do not recommend checking residuals in case of jejunal feeding especially in an asymptomatic individual.

Nausea and Vomiting

If this occurs, reduce or suspend tube feeding, raise the patient's upper body (head and shoulders) to 45 degrees during feeding and 60 minutes after, switch to an isotonic formula, and try antiemetics and prokinetics.

DELIVERY OF ENTERAL NUTRITION

The appropriate formula should be started at 20 mL/hour and advanced to the goal rate within 48 to 72 hours. Goals are not often met in critically ill patients. Continuous tube feeding over 16 to 24 hours is preferred, at least initially. Alternately, in the case of gastric feeding, bolus feeds may be given at 200 to 400 mL every 2 to 4 hours depending on patient tolerance. Feeding tubes should be flushed every 4 to 8 hours with 100 mL of water to prevent clogging.

Most enteral formulas provide about 80 to 85% of fluid requirement and the remainder has to be made up as free water. Some nutritionists provide one half to one full can of water for each can of formula in patients without cardiac or renal problems and those without fluid restriction.

COMPLICATIONS OF ENTERAL NUTRITION

Complications of enteral feeding include diarrhea, intestinal ischemia, intestinal perforation, aspiration, lactobezoar, nasal colonization, sinusitis, tube clogging, and feeding into the lungs. Complications related to the formula include nausea, vomiting, diarrhea, gas cramps, constipation, bloating, glucose intolerance, and dehydration. Refeeding syndrome may occur both with enteral and parenteral nutrition, and may be life-threatening.

TRANSITION TO ORAL NUTRITION

Stop tube feeding 1 hour before and up to 1 hour after each meal. Tube feeding during the day is stopped once oral intake exceeds 50%

of the needs. Tube feeding is stopped completely once the patient is able to take in greater than 75% of his or her requirements orally.

PEARLS

- ○ Enteral nutrition is usually preferable to parenteral nutrition whenever possible.
- ○ The use of disease-specific and specialized formulas is controversial, and their routine use is not cost-effective.
- ○ Nutritional intervention is not always necessary, but nutritional assessment is essential.

BIBLIOGRAPHY

McClave SA, Chang WK. Complications of enteral access. *Gastrointest Endosc.* 2003;58(5):739-51.

McClave SA, Dryden GW. Critical care nutrition: reducing the risk of aspiration. *Semin Gastrointest Dis.* 2003;14(1):2-10.

Chapter

20 *Parenteral Nutrition* ▬▬

PN is used if enteral nutritional support is not a viable option. PPN is used if the anticipated duration of nutritional therapy is less than 10 days, otherwise central parenteral nutrition (CPN) is administered. The term "total parenteral nutrition" (TPN) is frequently used instead of CPN.

CENTRAL VENOUS ACCESS

A peripherally inserted central catheter (PICC) is sufficient for use up to 1 year, but carries a risk for phlebitis and thrombosis. For patients requiring long-term PN, a tunneled Hickman or Groshong catheter or subcutaneous implanted port is preferable.

CALCULATION OF THE FORMULA RECIPE

Total Caloric Needs

Calculate overall caloric needs by using the formula described in Chapter 18. Most hospitalized patients need 25.0 to 35.0 K_{cal}/kg of ideal body weight. Patients with severe stress (eg, burns) may benefit from 35.0 K_{cal}/kg or more.

Proteins

Usual protein requirements are 1.1 to 1.5 g/kg of ideal body weight in most and 1.5 to 2.0 g/kg in severely ill patients (eg, those with severe burns, trauma, etc). Whether calories derived from the proteins should be calculated toward the overall needs is controversial. Protein provide 4.0 K_{cal}/g.

Lipids

Fats should contribute at least 10%, and no more than 60%, of total caloric needs, and ideally between 20 and 30% of total calories. A 10% lipid emulsion yields 1.1 calories/mL, whereas a 20% emulsion yields 2.0 calories/mL. *Tip*: Using a 250 mL bottle of 20% emulsion (500 K_{cal}) for patients with body weight greater than 60.0 kg, and a 100 mL bottle for patients less than 60.0 kg, is adequate and cost-effective.

Carbohydrates

The remainder of the calories are provided by carbohydrates. Carbohydrates are administered as dextrose monohydrate which yields 3.4 K_{cal}/g and is available as 5 to 70% dextrose solutions. The maximum dextrose concentration to be infused is 35%. A minimum of 150.0 to 200.0 g/day of carbohydrate is essential to meet the needs of glycolytic tissues like RBCs, bone marrow, eyes, and brain.

Water

Water needs are roughly 1 mL/K_{cal} delivered or 30 mL/kg/day except in patients with fluid restriction. An additional 300 mL should be added for every 1° C rise in body temperature.

EXAMPLES OF A TYPICAL FORMULA RECIPE

A 2-L TPN solution containing 12 to 15% dextrose (816 to 1020 K_{cal}), 4% amino acids (80.0 g protein, 320 calories), plus 250 mL of 20% lipids (500 calories) is sufficient in most cases.

For patients with higher caloric needs, use 2 L of TPN containing 20 to 25% of dextrose (1360 to 1700 calories). Lipids may be increased to 500 mL of 20% emulsion (1000 calories). Five to 7% amino acids (100.0 g to 140.0 g of protein) may be used in patients with high protein requirements.

In cases of fluid restriction, decrease the volume and increase the concentration of amino acids and carbohydrates, keeping the amounts of lipids the same.

ADDITIVES TO THE TPN BAG

1. Add 100% recommended daily allowance (RDA) of multivitamins and trace elements daily. Standard trace element solutions contain four to seven elements. The most common ingredients are zinc, copper, chromium, and manganese. However, for long-term use, selenium is essential and is contained in the newer versions.

2. Electrolytes may be initially added as standard daily needs and further individualized based upon on chemistry profile. Phosphorus, potassium, and magnesium should be avoided in patients with renal failure initially if no laboratory values are available.

3. In patients with metabolic acidosis, acetate should be added at the expense of chloride. Bicarbonate is not added since it increases the pH of the solution, thereby decreasing the solubility of calcium phosphate, which can then precipitate out.

4. Older "standard" vitamin solutions do not contain vitamin K. It may be given as 10.0 mg once a week in patients not on Coumadin. Use of vitamin K in patients on anticoagulants like heparin or enoxaparin (Lovenox) is controversial.

5. Histamine-2 receptor antagonists and insulin are added to the TPN as needed.

Cimetidine and ranitidine may rarely cause an altered mental status. Switching from one H_2RA to another, with respect to their thrombocytopenic effect, is based on sparse anecdotal evidence.

CAUTIONS

1. Lipids are contra-indicated in hyperlipidemia (triglyceride >1000.0 mg/dl), in which case, only limited amounts are given to meet the needs of essential fatty acids.

2. Hypertriglyceridemia may occur as a cause as well as a result of acute pancreatitis. Lipids are safe to use in pancreatitis if the triglyceride levels are within normal limits. Although triglyceride levels of at least 1000.0 mg/dl are required to cause pancreatitis, most physicians reduce or discontinue lipid administration at a TG level of 500.0 to 750.0 mg/dl. In such cases, use lipids only to provide essential fatty acids (250 mL of 20% emulsion one to two times a week).

3. Many patients in the intensive care units are sedated using propofol (Diprivan) infusion. The drug is formulated as an oil-in-water emulsion containing 1.1 K_{cal}/mL. The TPN formula

therefore needs to be adjusted accordingly to account for these propofol-derived lipid-based calories. Most patients on constant propofol infusion do not require any additional lipid-derived calories in their TPN.

4. While massive doses of lipids can cause thrombocytopenia, the role of reduction in lipid dose in the presence of thrombocytopenia is controversial.

5. Excessive carbohydrate administration may result in hyperglycemia, fatty liver, as well as increased carbon dioxide and lactate production.

6. Role of excess lipids on immune function is controversial and limited data suggests that it may increase the risk for bacteremia.

7. Rarely, excess lipids have also been implicated in hypoxemia. Increased minute ventilation and azotemia may be caused by excess protein.

8. Patients receiving TPN frequently become hyperglycemic. Although tight glucose control is superior, efforts are usually directed at keeping blood glucose levels under 200.0 mg/dl.

COMPLICATIONS

Complications of parenteral nutrition include pneumothorax, hemothorax, catheter infections, septicemia, central venous thrombosis, nutrient excess or deficiency, metabolic bone disease, steatosis, and/or cholestasis and refeeding syndrome. Rarely nonalcoholic steatohepatitis (NASH) may occur. Some experts recommend using heparin in TPN bag (3000 to 6000 units/day) in order to avoid catheter-related venous thrombosis. However, heparin may cause osteoporosis. Some experts add 100 unit/kg/day of heparin to the TPN bag in bone marrow transplant patients in order to decrease the risk of veno-occlusive disease.

Refeeding Syndrome

This occurs in previously starved patients when high calorie, high glucose feedings are started abruptly leading to salt and volume overload and massive fluid and electrolyte shifts.

This results in an acute drop in serum potassium, phosphorus, and magnesium causing cardiac dysrhythmia, respiratory muscle dysfunction, hypotension, hyperosmolar nonketotic coma, congestive heart failure, respiratory depression and acidosis, neuromuscular dysfunction, renal failure, and even death.

Slow initiation of feeding with liberal amounts of electrolytes, conservative use of dextrose along with thiamine (in alcoholics) and close monitoring prevent this complication.

Micronutrient Deficiency States

Chromium deficiency causes peripheral neuropathy and glucose intolerance. Deficiency of selenium which is not contained in many standard trace elements, may cause cardiomyopathy, muscle pain, and tenderness. Zinc deficiency may cause diarrhea, dermatitis, T-cell dysfunction, hair loss, and impaired wound healing. Iron is not present in standard TPN solutions and iron deficiency anemia may occur in patients on long-term TPN.

INITIATING AND MONITORING TPN

Start at one-half to two-thirds of the required volume on the first day to allow the body time to adapt to glucose and fluid load. Initial volumes and concentrations vary depending upon how much volume and what kind of IV fluids the patient is already receiving. Advance as tolerated.

Monitor daily body weight, intake-output, and glucose finger sticks every 6 to 12 hours as indicated. Give 10% dextrose when TPN is stopped in the case of Type I diabetes. Stop TPN infusion if it becomes cloudy, layered, or precipitated. A gain of greater than 1.5 kg of body weight/week represents volume overload.

Frequency of laboratory tests for monitoring nutrition therapy is based not upon firm scientific data but on the physician's experience and preferences. A complete metabolic profile should be checked initially and then about once a week in hospitalized patients. A basic TPN panel consisting of Chem-7 (serum Na, K, CO_2, Cl, BUN, creatinine, glucose) plus serum magnesium and phosphorous may be done every day or every other day for 1 week, and then twice a week while gradually increasing the interval. CBC should be checked twice a week initially.

Periodic checking of serum albumin and prealbumin is controversial. Serum albumin may be checked at baseline and then once every 1 to 2 weeks to monitor therapy. Serum prealbumin has a shorter half-life and is better for monitoring. Lack of increase of serum prealbumin during nutritional support does not necessarily suggest inadequate nutritional therapy.

Serum triglyceride concentration should be checked at baseline and then periodically as indicated in patients with dyslipidemias and in cases of pancreatitis associated with elevated triglyceride level.

The utility of checking various labs at predetermined and fixed frequency versus on an as needed basis is controversial.

CONTINUOUS VS CYCLIC INFUSION

Initially TPN is infused over 24 hours, but may be done over as little as 10 to 12 hours depending on the patient's tolerance. Cyclic TPN results in reduced risk for hepatotoxicity and improved quality of life.

Check blood glucose 1 hour after stopping the infusion or if the patient is symptomatic after stopping the infusion. In cases of hypoglycemia, either increase the duration of infusion and/or taper the rate of infusion over the last 2 hours.

If hyperglycemia greater than 200.0 mg/dl is a problem, increase infusion time and add insulin, in addition to decreasing carbohydrates and increasing fat content.

SPECIFIC DISEASE STATES

Diabetes

Start with 150.0 to 200.0 g of dextrose initially. The goal is to maintain glucose level less than 200.0 mg/dl. Add a total of 15 units of insulin to the TPN bag if serum glucose is between 250.0 to 300.0 mg/dl, and 20 units if greater than 300.0 mg/dl. Also administer insulin according to sliding scale. The next day, further add two-thirds of the amount of insulin given as sliding scale the day before to the TPN bag. When hyperglycemia is controlled, advance the total dextrose in the TPN bag to the desired goal while adjusting insulin. The role of continuous infusion of insulin with TPN in critical care is evolving.

Respiratory Failure

High lipid, low carbohydrate formulas provide marginal benefit. Limit carbohydrates to 33% of total caloric needs. The best approach is to avoid overfeeding and to increase the time to wean off the ventilator.

Liver Failure

Use of branched-chain amino acids is controversial and most experts believe that the increased cost cannot be justified.

Renal Failure

Renal failure patients not on dialysis should receive 0.6 to 0.8 g/kg protein. In patients undergoing hemodialysis, proteins should be administered in the dose of 1.2 to 1.5 g/kg. Total caloric needs are unchanged. Do not add potassium, magnesium, and phosphorus to the first bag without checking laboratory values first.

Peritoneal Dialysis

Calculate the calories derived from dextrose in the dialysate, also for calculation of the overall nutritional support. Different dialysis bags have different dextrose concentrations. These patients need more protein as well.

Acute Pancreatitis

Twenty to 30% of calories can easily be given as lipids without causing significant pancreatic stimulation. In case serum triglyceride levels exceed 500.0 mg/dl, reduce lipid emulsion dose to 100 mL of 20% emulsion every day. Consider limiting the use of emulsion for providing only essential fatty acids if triglyceride levels exceed 700.0 mg/L (eg, 250 mL of 20% lipids one to two times per week). When in doubt, monitor serum triglyceride levels to see if the body can clear the triglycerides.

Chemotherapy or Radiation Therapy

The indications, as well as basal energy requirements, are the same. Benefits of nutrition support should be weighed against the risks as well as the outcome.

TRANSITION TO ENTERAL FEEDING

In the case of tube feedings, start full strength at 20 to 40 mL/hour and advance every 12 to 24 hours as tolerated over 2 to 3 days. In case of oral feeding, try small and frequent meals. If the patient can tolerate cyclic TPN, it may be administered only during the night in order to avoid suppressing appetite during the day. Once the patient can tolerate about half of the caloric needs reduce the TPN either to half the volume in case of 3-in-1 solutions, or discontinue the lipid emulsion if lipids are given separately. Discontinue TPN if the patient can tolerate about 75% of caloric needs.

If the goal is to wean a patient off TPN quickly, we usually recommend decreasing the current rate by 50% for 4 to 6 hours, then discontinuing TPN completely. A finger stick for glucose can be checked 1 hour later if there is concern for rebound hypoglycemia.

PERIPHERAL PARENTERAL NUTRITION

Although suboptimal, PPN can provide up to 2500 K_{cal}/day on a short-term basis. While the basic contents are similar to TPN, the concentrations are lower. A maximum of 3.5% amino acids and 10% dextrose may be given because of a risk for thrombosis and phlebitis due to high osmolality. However, some nutritionists push the upper limits to 4.25% amino acids and 11% dextrose. This pushes the limits of osmolar tolerance. Lipids may be used to make up the caloric deficit by providing 50% of the calories.

In case of patients not on fluid restriction, we usually use PPN solution involving 3 L of 5% dextrose and 3.5% amino acids, along with 250 mL of 20% lipids. This formula yields 1430 calories. Another option is a 2 L of PPN solution containing 10% dextrose (680 calories), 3.5% amino acids (70.0 g protein, 280 calories), plus 250 mL of 20% lipid emulsion (55.0 g fat, 500 calories), which is adequate in most cases. Lipids may be increased to 500 mL of 20% emulsion (1,000 calories, 110.0 g of fat) in case of high caloric requirements.

Add multivitamins, electrolytes, trace elements, as well as histamine-2 blockers and insulin, etc, as in TPN. Premixed commercial PPN formulas are available. Phlebitis is a major complication of PPN. Lipids protect against phlebitis and so they should be mixed 3 in 1 or piggybacked into the PPN line.

Hydrocortisone (5.0 mg/L) may be added to PPN solution for prevention of phlebitis. Some experts recommend heparin in solution (3000 to 6000 units) and nitroglycerine patch or ointment at the exit site.

PEARLS

O Refeeding syndrome may occur when parenteral nutrition or even enteral nutrition is started in previously starving subjects.

O Iron and vitamin K may not be present in many standard trace element and multivitamin solutions added to the TPN bag.

BIBLIOGRAPHY

Koretz RL, Lipman TO, Klein S. AGA technical review on parenteral nutrition. *Gastroenterol.* 2001;121:970-1001.

Buchman AL. *Practical Nutritional Support Techniques.* Thorofare, NJ: SLACK Incorporated; 2003.

ESOPHAGUS

Chapter 21 *Gastroesophageal Reflux Disease*

Gastroesophageal reflux (GER) is a normal phenomenon occurring in healthy individuals especially after meals. It is termed gastroesophageal reflux disease or GERD when the reflux occurs to the degree that it produces esophageal and/or extraesophageal symptoms or causes damage to the esophagus or other organs.

EPIDEMIOLOGY

Prevalence estimates vary depending upon the definition used. While uncommon in Asian countries, this is thought to be primarily a disease of the west. However, its prevalence is increasing even in the Eastern countries probably because of adoption of western diet and life styles. The prevalence of heartburn is 8% in Italy, 10% in Japan, 17% in Canada, and 20 to 25% in the United States. Heartburn occurs in 15 to 44% of Americans at least once a month, weekly in 20%, while about 7% of Americans have heartburn everyday. Only 5% of patients with heartburn seek medical attention, but this is rapidly changing because of the recognition of its potential seriousness and availability of effective medications for treatment. GERD occurs more in men and is uncommon in African Americans.

The prevalence of heartburn increases with age and increases dramatically after the age of 40. Complications of GERD are more frequent in white males and increase with age.

SOCIOECONOMIC IMPACT

GERD affects quality of life. Untreated patients have a quality of life worse than that seen in patients with untreated duodenal ulcer, angina pectoris, mild heart failure, and untreated hypertension.

PATHOGENESIS

In contrast to physiologic reflux episodes, pathologic reflux is associated with nocturnal symptoms and even complications. While the physiologic reflux episodes are short-lived, pathologic reflux may be prolonged.

The gastric refluxate causes damage to the tight junctions between the epithelial cells of the esophageal mucosa. This leads to widening of intercellular spaces and increased permeability of the mucosa allowing for increased acid penetration. The increased permeability allows contact of acid with the underlying nerves resulting in symptoms. At this point, the damage is only microscopic and may explain about 50% of GERD patients who have nonerosive reflux disease. In many patients, there is further disruption of intercellular junctions leading to cell damage and necrosis, inflammation, and endoscopically visible erosive esophagitis.

GER occurs due to numerous causes. The relative contribution of the various causes varies between different individuals.

Lower Esophageal Sphincter

The most important factor is the barrier function of the lower esophageal sphincter (LES). The LES is normally closed at rest and opens to facilitate the passage of the food and the salivary contents from the esophagus into the stomach in conjunction with swallowing. About 71% of reflux symptoms occur within 4 hours after a meal. Transient lower esophageal sphincter relaxations (TLESRs) cause reflux of the gastric contents throughout the day and night, especially after meals. In fact, these TLESRs are the major cause for GER in patients with nonerosive reflux disease. On the other hand, patients who have esophagitis have a tendency to have low LES pressures, making it easier for the gastric contents to be refluxed.

Esophageal Factors

These include gravity, peristaltic function of the esophagus, as well as the neutralization of the acid by salivary secretions. Both the salivary secretions as well as peristalsis of the esophagus are impaired during sleep and the protection by gravity is lost. This results in prolonging the exposure to the refluxate that occurs during sleep, eventually leading to greater esophageal damage.

Esophageal factors providing resistance to acid-induced damage include tight junctions, buffering action of blood flow, surface mucous, bicarbonate, and epidermal growth factors.

Gastric Factors

Delayed gastric emptying is present in about 5% of patients with GERD, and in up to 25% of those not responsive to therapy. Other factors include hiatal hernia, gastric outflow obstruction, pregnancy, and patients with restrictive bariatric surgery.

H. Pylori

The role of *H. pylori* (Hp) is controversial. An eradication of Hp in patients with duodenal ulcers results in the development of reflux symptoms in some studies. It is believed that chronic Hp infection leads to chronic gastritis in the body of the stomach, which then leads to hypochlorhydria—which affords protection against GERD. Patients with Hp infection and esophagitis heal more quickly with routine acid suppressive treatment than those without Hp infection. Some authors have reported lack of effect of Hp status on the healing of esophagitis.

Systemic Disorders

These include diabetes mellitus, scleroderma, and CREST syndrome. Patients with the connective tissue diseases show abnormal manometric findings including reduced amplitude of contractions in the esophagus as well as reduced pressure in the LES contributing to increased reflux. This results in a vicious cycle.

CLINICAL FEATURES

Patients typically complain of heartburn, a retrosternal burning sensation radiating to the neck that is usually postparandial. It may wake the patients at night. Some patients find it difficult to sleep unless they are in a recliner. The symptoms improve with antacids. Patients also may complain of regurgitation, which is an effortless return of gastric contents to the throat.

Atypical Manifestations

These include angina-like chest pain, water brash, asthma, globus sensation, dysphagia, odynophagia, pulmonary aspiration, hoarseness, frequent upper respiratory infections, halitosis, chronic cough, and chronic throat clearing. The mechanism may not just involve direct contact with the gastric contents, but also may involve vagally mediated neural reflexes.

In a majority of cases with airway symptoms and noncardiac chest pain, the typical symptom of heartburn is absent. Since there can be numerous causes for these symptoms, GERD frequently is diagnosed based on response to empiric acid suppressive therapy. GERD-associated, angina-like chest pain may mimic angina so much so that even the most astute physician may not be able to distinguish it from a pain of cardiac origin.

Odynophagia is uncommonly due to GERD and should raise suspicion of pill-induced or infectious esophagitis. Dysphagia is also uncommon, but its presence in a patient with GERD suggests the presence of severe esophagitis with either dysmotility, stricture, or adenocarcinoma complicating an underlying Barrett's esophagus (BE).

Thirty-five to 90% of patients with asthma have an abnormal esophageal pH profile, but this doesn't always reflect an underlying esophagitis. Abnormal esophageal acid exposure in asthmatics may in part be due to the use of bronchodilators; up to 40% of asthmatics in some studies have esophagitis. Asthma may occur due to aspiration of gastric contents into the air passages, as well as due to vagally mediated neural reflexes.

While GERD has been implicated in numerous extraesophageal problems, a cause-and-effect relationship has been difficult to establish in many instances. Symptom-index scores have been used to support a causal relationship; however, experts have questioned the validity of this approach.

Pediatric GERD

GERD is under-recognized in the pediatric population, especially during infancy. It occurs due to an underdeveloped LES that usually resolves by 1 to 2 years of age. The symptoms are nonspecific and include excessive fussiness, abnormal crying, aversion to food, inability to sleep, and even growth failure.

DIFFERENTIAL DIAGNOSIS

GERD may mimic or overlap with nonsteroid anti-inflammatory drug (NSAID)-induced gastropathy, peptic ulcer disease, infectious esophagitis, toxic esophagitis, nonulcer dyspepsia, chronic gallbladder disease, esophageal motility disorders, chronic pancreatitis, and irritable bowel syndrome (IBS). Since GERD is so widely prevalent, the diagnosis of GERD and many of these other entities is not mutually exclusive. For example, 20 to 60% of patients with duodenal ulcer have reflux symptoms.

DIAGNOSIS

Patients with typical symptoms do not need to have any diagnostic evaluation and may be treated empirically. Exceptions include patients with alarm symptoms like weight loss, bleeding, dysphagia, or odynophagia. A variety of diagnostic modalities are available and the diagnostic test should be tailored to answer a particular question.

1. EGD is indicated for patients with: a) atypical manifestations; b) those nonresponsive to acid-suppressive treatment; or c) patients with alarm symptoms such as dysphagia, odynophagia, bleeding, and weight loss. In addition, a one-time screening EGD is recommended for patients with longstanding heartburn (ie, greater than 5 to 10 years) to exclude BE (see Chapter 22). A routine EGD test is less likely to be of benefit for the simple diagnosis of GERD, since half of the patients will not show any endoscopically visible esophageal damage.

2. A barium swallow is an excellent test for patients with dysphagia and is more sensitive than an EGD. The sensitivity of barium swallow can be enhanced if a barium pill is administered along with the liquid barium. However, many physicians consider EGD to be a more cost-effective procedure, since it offers the therapeutic option of esophageal dilation at the same time. A barium swallow is not a sensitive enough test to detect mucosal lesions like esophagitis.

3. Twenty-four hour pH monitoring is recommended for patients with atypical symptoms, patients nonresponsive to treatment, and as part of preoperative evaluation prior to antireflux surgery. While a variety of parameters are measured during 24-hour pH monitoring, the total percentage time of esophageal pH below 4.0 is considered to be the most useful outcome measure. Twenty-four hour pH monitoring is also used for patients who have persistent reflux symptoms after the antireflux surgery. However, the equipment does not examine for alkaline reflux—the pathological significance of which is a matter of debate.

4. Impedance plethysmography can detect reflux episodes regardless of the pH. Putting this information together with the results of 24-hour pH monitoring can help the physician determine whether there are significant acidic or nonacidic reflux episodes allowing for correlation with the patient's symptoms.

5. Esophageal manometry is not useful for the diagnosis of GERD since most subjects have normal findings. Its main utility is in the preoperative evaluation prior to antireflux surgery. Patients with poor amplitude of contractions in the esophagus may undergo partial fundoplication (270 degrees) rather than the full wrap (360 degrees) as done in Nissen's fundoplication.

6. Provocative tests: The Bernstein test is a provocative test in which 0.1 N hydrochloric acid is infused into the esophagus,

alternating with normal saline as a placebo. Complaint of heartburn on infusion of acid suggests acid sensitive mucosa. Another test involves injection of edrophonium during manometry to potentiate esophageal contractions and provoke a painful episode. Both these tests have largely been abandoned.

7. Radionuclide scan: It is rarely used for demonstration of GER. It may be useful for demonstration of tracheal and pulmonary aspiration of gastric contents in patients with gastroparesis. Patients are fed a radionuclide-labeled meal and then images are taken after the meal as well as the next day. Evidence of radionuclide material in the pulmonary fields establishes the diagnosis of pulmonary aspiration.

HISTOLOGY

Biopsy may show thickening of the basal cell layer and elongation of the papillae of the epithelium. In addition, neutrophils, eosinophils, and distended pale balloon cells may be seen. Histologic findings should be sought in GERD patients with normal endoscopy. Notably excessive eosinophilia (ie, >15 to 20 eosinophils/high power field) is not typical of GERD, but suggests eosinophilic esophagitis, probably a food-allergy disease.

GRADING OF SEVERITY

Many classifications have been used to classify erosive esophagitis. A Los Angeles classification is the most widely used. Grade A implies one or more mucosal breaks no more than 5.0 mm; Grade B occurs when there are one or more mucosal erosions more than 5.0 mm, but not continuous between the tops of two folds; Grade C are mucosal erosions that are continuous in the top of two or more folds but involve less than 75% of the circumference; and Grade D occurs when erosive disease involves at least 75% of the esophageal circumference.

COMPLICATIONS

Complications include esophagitis, peptic stricture, BE, and cancer. About 50% of the patients diagnosed clinically with GERD have evidence of esophagitis on endoscopy and 10% of the patients have strictures. The prevalence of BE ranges between 5 to 10% in some series.

Patients with peptic stricture should receive aggressive acid suppressive treatment in addition to dilation of the esophagus. Surgery may rarely be required for the treatment of refractory strictures. Many patients have non-obstructive esophageal dysphagia and the management is controversial. Many of these patients respond to potent acid-suppression with or without esophageal dilation even if they do not have any significant heartburn.

MEDICAL TREATMENT

GERD is frequently a clinical diagnosis and empiric treatment is used in patients without evidence of alarm symptoms.

Uncomplicated GERD

A. While studies are lacking, lifestyle modifications may provide symptomatic relief in up to 25% of the cases. These include: 1) elevating the head end of the bed by using 4 to 6 inch blocks; 2) eating at least 3 hours before bedtime; 3) avoiding large fatty meals and bed-time snacks; 4) avoiding foods that precipitate reflux like chocolate and carbonated or caffeinated beverages; 5) quitting smoking and the excessive use of alcohol; and 6) avoiding tight clothes.

B. Acid neutralization by antacids, chewing gum, and alginic acid provide relief in many cases of intermittent heartburn. Their use for chronic heartburn on a regular basis is not cost-effective and may cause significant side effects.

C. Cisapride, a prokinetic, is effective in about 50% of GERD patients, but was withdrawn from US market because of serious side effects. Metoclopramide (Reglan) is rarely used except in cases of gastroparesis or regurgitation refractory to acid suppressant drugs because of its undesirable extrapyramidal side effects.

D. Acid suppression is the cornerstone of treatment and can be carried out using H_2 receptor antagonists (H_2RAs), which provide relief in about 50% of cases, or proton pump inhibitors (PPIs), which provide relief in 85 to 95% of the cases.

E. Cimetidine 400.0 mg bid, ranitidine 150.0 mg bid, nizatidine 150.0 mg bid, and famotidine 20.0 mg bid are effective in about half the cases. Higher doses exert a better response. In contrast to the treatment for peptic ulcer disease where a single total nighttime dose may be sufficient, divided doses are needed in GERD. Some experts recommend the use of a nighttime H_2RA, in addition to a morning dose of a PPI, to overcome the nocturnal acid breakthrough. H_2RAs may be taken on an as needed basis in patients with infrequent heartburn, especially when an episode is anticipated (eg, 1 hour before going for a big Thanksgiving meal). In general, twice a day doses of H_2RA are best given between breakfast and lunch and then at bedtime.

F. PPIs block the final step in the pathway to acid secretion and are more potent than H_2RAs for acid suppression, as well as for symptomatic relief and healing of esophagitis. The usual recommended doses of oral PPIs include omeprazole 20.0 mg/day, lansoprazole 30.0 mg/day, rabeprazole 20.0 mg/day, pantoprazole 40.0 mg/day, and esomeprazole 40.0 mg/day. The drugs are best given 30 to 45 minutes before breakfast, which is sufficient for most patients with GERD.

Some patients require twice a day dosing. In such cases, the second dose should be given 30 to 45 minutes before supper. In patients with exclusively nocturnal reflux symptoms without any significant day-time reflux, a single dose prior to supper may be administered. Patients with complications of GERD like stricture and BE should be treated with PPIs and not H_2RAs.

All PPIs are not the same pharmacologically and differences exist with the respect to their pharmacokinetic and pharmacodynamic parameters. Despite initial concerns for increased predisposition to cancer, no cancer cases have been reported to date. Maintenance therapy with PPIs is superior to therapy with H_2RAs or prokinetic agents.

Management of Nonresponders

Some patients will continue to suffer heartburn despite aggressive acid suppression therapy. Upon pH monitoring, they show little evidence of intraesophageal acid exposure. Impedance plethysmography, combined with pH monitoring, can help distinguish between nonacid GER vs no or minimal reflux. While the former may benefit from surgical treatment, the latter are termed as functional heartburn and may be treated with antidepressants and behavioral therapy as for other functional gastrointestinal (GI) disorders.

Refractory GERD

It is uncommon to see a patient with typical reflux symptoms that is refractory to PPI therapy. The only variable may be that the patient has not been treated enough because some patients may require twice a day dosing and few patients even higher three to four times per day. For reasons not fully understood, some patients may respond better to one brand of PPI versus another.

Differential diagnosis of refractory reflux symptoms on PPI therapy include an incorrect initial diagnosis like pill esophagitis, eosinophilic esophagitis, chest wall pain, dyspepsia, peptic ulcer disease, Zollinger-Ellison syndrome, and esophageal dysmotility. Alternatively, consideration should be given to failure because the patient is noncompliant or a rapid metabolizer of PPIs.

ROLE OF SURGERY

Surgery is an effective treatment for GERD and can be done laparoscopically. While many surgeons consider all GERD to be an indication for surgery, most gastroenterologists refer patients for surgery selectively. Preoperative evaluation includes EGD to exclude any other pathology, 24-hour pH monitoring to document pathological reflux and esophageal manometry to evaluate esophageal contractility. Some surgeons also like to have a barium swallow (and even a preoperative CT scan) to look for a hiatal hernia.

The effectiveness of surgery depends upon the expertise of the surgeon. Patients who do not respond well to PPI therapy are less likely to respond well to surgery.

A follow-up study of patients who had undergone a Nissen fundoplication indicated that as many as 63% of the patients were requiring some kind of medical therapy by the end of 10 years after the operation. The same study also showed an unexplained increase in mortality in the surgical group, presumably due to cardiovascular problems.

I generally offer surgery as an option to patients who are young with good esophageal function, those who are unable to afford the medications, those who are noncompliant, or those with regurgitant symptoms. Patients with functional heartburn, gastric dysmotility, or IBS may actually suffer worsening of symptoms after surgery.

NEWER ENDOSCOPIC TREATMENTS

The US Food & Drug Administration (FDA) has approved three endoscopic devices. The Bard Endocinch involves endoscopic suturing at the LES, thus, tightening it by pleating. The Stretta device uses radiofrequency injury of the LES and gastric cardia resulting in scarring of the region, thereby reducing the compliance and relaxation frequency of the LES. The Enteryx procedure involves injection of a liquid polymer into the LES that changes into a solid permanent implant that prevents GER.

While complications like perforations have been reported, there are no good long-term randomized controlled studies documenting their effectiveness and/or superiority to medical treatment. One short-term trial of sham procedure versus Stretta yielded equivocal benefits of the Stretta in terms of reduced heartburn and improved quality of life, but no reduction in acid reflux or medication usage at 6 months. Many experts suggest that these techniques are in their infancy and should only be offered to patients in the context of clinical trials.

PEARLS

- O EGD is an insensitive diagnostic test for GERD since half of the patients have nonerosive reflux disease. Sensitivity is enhanced by incorporating an esophageal biopsy.
- O A cardiac etiology for atypical chest pain should be excluded before consideration of more benign esophageal conditions like GERD.

BIBLIOGRAPHY

Orlando RC. Pathogenesis of gastroesophageal reflux disease. *Gastroenterol Clin North Am.* 2002;31(4 Suppl):S35-44.

Quigley EM. Factors that influence therapeutic outcomes in symptomatic gastroesophageal reflux disease. *Am J Gastroenterol.* 2003;98(3 Suppl):S24-30.

Chapter 22
Barrett's Esophagus

BE refers to the transformation of normal esophageal mucosa from stratified squamous epithelium to an abnormal columnar epithelium with intestinal metaplasia.

EPIDEMIOLOGY

The prevalence of BE among Caucasian adults during endoscopy is 1% for long segment BE (LSBE) where as 10 to 15% for short segment Barrett's esophagus (SSBE).

The mean age at diagnosis is 63 years. The disease is seen primarily in the West, more often in Caucasians with a 2- to 4-fold predominance for men. It is relatively uncommon in African Americans and Hispanics.

Patients with GERD symptoms are likely to have LSBE in 5 to 10% of the cases, whereas only 1% of those denying reflux symptoms will have BE on endoscopy. A recent study now suggests a much higher prevalence of BE in asymptomatic Caucasian male veterans presenting for a colonoscopy screening with 7% having LSBE and 17% having SSBE.

PATHOGENESIS

The metaplastic columnar epithelium of BE represents an adaptive response of the esophagus to the reflux induced injury. It occurs as a consequence of severe repetitive damage due to gastroesophageal reflux disease. Contrary to popular belief, the BE develops to its maximum length over a relatively short period, which may be less than 1 year and then does not extend further.

RISK FACTORS

Patients with Barrett's esophagus are more likely to have a hiatal hernia, poor LES pressures, and a greater duration of esophageal acid exposure. Genetics may also play in a role. Patients with Hp infection may be less likely to have BE compared to those without infection. In fact, some experts associate the declining incidence of Hp with the rising incidence of esophageal adenocarcinoma.

ENDOSCOPIC APPEARANCE

The metaplastic epithelium of BE appears salmon-colored, as opposed to the normal esophageal mucosa, which is pale. The LSBE implies that the metaplastic epithelium is equal to or greater than 3.0 cm, whereas a SSBE means less than 3.0 cm. Intestinal metaplasia of the cardia implies the presence of intestinal metaplasia just below the Z-line representing the normal squamo-columnar junction.

DIAGNOSIS

Diagnosis is based upon histological confirmation. Three different kinds of columnar epithelium (junctional, atrophic fundic, and specialized columnar epithelium) may be found as a result of metaplastic change; however, only the specialized intestinal metaplasia confers significantly increased malignant potential. The presence of goblet cells differentiates specialized intestinal metaplasia from gastric or fundic type of mucosa.

RISK FOR MALIGNANCY

Although the presence of BE increases the likelihood of developing esophageal adenocarcinoma by 25- to 125-fold over the general population, the absolute risk is low at 0.5% per year. Patients with BE appear to live just as long as people who do not have BE. The degree of risk for esophageal adenocarcinoma associated with SSBE is unknown, so the recommendations for surveillance for SSBE and LSBE are currently similar.

MANAGEMENT

Barrett's Without Dysplasia

The length of the metaplastic epithelium should be measured at endoscopy and four quadrant biopsies should be undertaken every 2.0 cm along the length. In addition, any nodules or ulcers, erosion, or strictures in the area need to be biopsied. Investigational endoscopic techniques to increase the yield for detection of dysplasia include chromoendoscopy, magnification endoscopy, endoscopic ultrasound, optical coherence tomography, and fluorescence endoscopy. In patients without evidence of dysplasia, a repeat endoscopy is carried out at 1 year. If no dysplasia is found at 1 year, a repeat endoscopy should be performed every 3 years.

Barrett's With Low-Grade Dysplasia

Patients should undergo aggressive acid suppression along with a repeat endoscopy at 6 months. Some experts perform another endoscopy at 12 months, after a 6 month endoscopy. If at least two endoscopies show a lack of progression, a surveillance EGD should be done every year.

Barrett's With High-Grade Dysplasia

A second opinion should be sought and diagnosis confirmed by another pathologist. Some experts recommend a repeat EGD in order to aggressively sample (biopsy) the BE to look for any focus of cancer missed on a previous EGD. Subsequent to confirmation, an esophagectomy is generally recommended because the risk for concurrent cancer may be as high as 30 to 40%. An alternate, but perhaps less desirable approach, is continued aggressive acid suppression plus a four-quadrant biopsy every 1.0 cm at three monthly intervals until cancer is identified. The recommendation for esophagectomy versus an intensive biopsy program should be tailored based on the mortality rate due to esophagectomy at one's particular institution, which can vary from 3 to 20%.

Use of ablative therapies like heater probe, Nd:YAG laser, argon laser, argon-plasma coagulation, cryotherapy, multipolar electrocoagulation, and photodynamic therapy are investigational. Results of endoscopic mucosal resection appear to be promising.

Intestinal Metaplasia of the Cardia

No surveillance is recommended for patients with intestinal metaplasia of the cardia.

SCREENING

Only a single screening endoscopy is required in patients with long-standing GERD especially white males who have had reflux symptoms for greater than 5 to 10 years. If this is negative for BE, the potential to develop it in the future are exceedingly low. The use of genetic markers like P53 abnormalities is investigational.

PEARLS

O Barrett's esophagus is primarily seen among Caucasians.

O Barrett's esophagus develops over a short period of time and repeated endoscopy for detection of development of Barrett's esophagus is not recommended.

O Although Barrett's esophagus increases the risk for transformation to cancer, the absolute risk is low.

BIBLIOGRAPHY

Spechler SJ. Barrett's esophagus and esophageal adenocarcinoma: pathogenesis, diagnosis, and therapy. *Med Clin North Am*. 2002; 86(6): 1423-45.

Gerson LB, Shetler K, Triadafilopoulos G. Prevalence of Barrett's esophagus in asymptomatic individuals. *Gastroenterology*. 2002;123(2):461-7.

Chapter

23 *Esophageal Cancer* ▬▬▬

EPIDEMIOLOGY

Esophageal cancer is the fastest growing cancer in the United States, although it is relatively uncommon compared to other cancers.

Adenocarcinoma (AC) is the most common form followed by squamous cell carcinoma (SCC) which comprises about 30 to 40% of esophageal malignancies. The incidence of SCC in the United States is about 3 to 5 per 100 000 persons. Whereas AC is predominately a disease of white males, SCC is more common among African Americans.

SCC tends to occur in the upper- and middle-third of the esophagus. AC is usually found in the distal third of the esophagus, as are the other rare forms of esophageal cancers like small cell carcinoma, choriocarcinoma, melanoma, sarcoma, and lymphoma.

RISK FACTORS

AC is mostly related to chronic heartburn and BE, whereas SCC is related to tobacco and alcohol use, and in rare cases, Plummer-Vinson syndrome, achalasia, tylosis, lye-ingestion, and human papilloma virus. Obese patients with heartburn are at an increased risk of esophageal cancer as compared to patients with heartburn alone. A definite relationship between drugs that lower the LES pressures and the development of AC has not been established.

PROTECTIVE FACTORS

There is a reduced incidence of cancer in patients who use aspirin routinely. Antireflux surgical procedures have no impact on the incidence of cancer. Similarly, avoiding foods that exacerbate acid reflux does not appear to impact the development of the cancer.

CLINICAL FEATURES

Patients usually present with dysphagia and, in some cases, may even have odynophagia. Onset of symptoms is gradual. Weight loss is present in majority of the cases. Patients may rarely complain of back pain, hematemesis, nausea, vomiting, or hoarseness. Hoarseness may occur due to involvement of laryngeal nerve.

DIAGNOSIS OF ESOPHAGEAL CANCER

Endoscopy and biopsy of the lesion establish the diagnosis. In many patients, a barium swallow has revealed a malignant stricture prior to referral to the gastroenterologist. A CT scan of the chest and abdomen are recommended as initial tests of choice for staging.

CANCER STAGING

Standard TNM (tumor-node-metastasis classification) is used. Combining all of the above, it is staged from Stages 0 to IV—Stage 0 means carcinoma in-situ with no lymph node involvement or metastasis, whereas Stage IV implies distant metastasis irrespective of T or N grading. Involvement of celiac lymph node is regarded as a distant metastasis making the tumor a Stage IV tumor. Accurate esophageal staging of cancer is important for management.

1. Endoscopic ultrasound (EUS) is accurate for the staging of esophageal cancer for T staging in approximately 90% of the cases, whereas it is accurate in 80% cases of lymph node staging. Lymph nodes greater than 1.0 cm in size seen on EUS are suspicious for cancer, and fine needle aspiration can be undertaken. The results are highly operator dependent and the expertise is not available in many medical centers. EUS cannot detect distant metastasis.

2. A CT scan is the most widely used staging modality and provides information about the tumor, as well as distant metastasis. It determines T-stage accurately in 60% of the cases. It is more helpful than EUS for detecting distant metastasis.

3. A PET scan is a functional test that is useful for detection of postoperative recurrence.

4. MRI has not been shown to be of help in the staging process.

TREATMENT

Early Cancer

Curative surgery is recommended for early stage disease including Stage I and Stage II-A. However, only half of patients who plan curative resection actually undergo this surgery because metastases are often found during the surgery. Laparoscopy-assisted esophagectomy has also been done. Mortality rate from the surgery is about 10%. One-year survival with esophagectomy is about 20%, whereas a 5-year survival is 5%. There is no role for chemotherapy or radiation therapy in early esophageal cancer.

Locally Advanced Cancer

For Stage II-B and III, a multimodality approach including chemotherapy, radiation therapy, and surgery offers the best hope, since surgery alone will cure less than 10% of these patients. However, the treatment is aggressive and expensive with a high incidence of side effects. Patients in poor health may not be able to withstand this approach and may elect to undergo palliative management.

Metastatic Disease

Patients with Stage IV disease (distant metastasis) can only be offered palliative treatment. Radiation, chemotherapy, and endoscopic methods are available. Esophageal dilation offers only a short-term relief of dysphagia. Usually stents are used for palliation for dysphagia and are particularly useful for midesophageal cancer. The complications of stents include esophageal perforation, severe pain, bleeding, and compression of trachea or bronchus. Late complications may be stent migration or fistula formation. Mortality rate from stent placement is less than 2%.

Laser therapy is another option. Argon plasma coagulation (APC) is less expensive than laser treatment, but it is equally effective. Photodynamic therapy is also used and is safe and well-tolerated. Injection of absolute alcohol into the tumor is inexpensive, but risks perforation and chemical mediastinitis.

There are no good studies comparing stents to other modalities for palliation of esophageal cancer.

ENDOSCOPIC CURATIVE THERAPY

Since early esophageal cancers can sometimes be detected, endoscopic therapy such as endoscopic mucosal resection (EMR) offers hope. Using this technique, pieces of mucosa of about 1.0 cm in diameter at a time can be removed down to the level of deep submucosa. EMR can cure superficial cancers in about 94% of the cases.

CANCER SCREENING

Routine cancer screening is not recommended. Some experts suggest performing a one time EGD in patients who are above the age of 40 and have long-time heartburn greater than 5 to 10 years, especially among white males. The data to support that is lacking.

CANCER SURVEILLANCE

Surveillance is recommended in patients with BE (see Chapter 22).

PEARLS

○ Adenocarcinoma occurs mainly in Caucasians and is related to longstanding GERD and BE. Squamous cell carcinoma occurs predominantly among African Americans and the risk is increased by alcohol and smoking.

○ Mass screening for esophageal cancer is not recommended.

BIBLIOGRAPHY

Spechler SJ. Barrett's esophagus and esophageal adenocarcinoma: pathogenesis, diagnosis, and therapy. *Med Clin North Am.* 2002;86(6): 1423-45.

Chapter

24 *Gas-Bloat Syndrome* ▬▬▬

EPIDEMIOLOGY

Gas-bloat syndrome occurs in 25 to 50% patients after the fundoplication surgery.

PATHOGENESIS

A natural consequence of a tight wrap to prevent acid reflux is that the tightened valve does not allow for upward expulsion of air either, thus preventing belching. This results in symptoms caused by an accumulation of swallowed gas in the stomach.

Gas-bloat syndrome may also occur in patients who are learning to use their esophagus for speech after laryngectomy for cancer, etc. This new form of speech involves sucking air into esophagus, and then expelling it immediately in the form of words. Increased aerophagia into the stomach may lead to gas-bloat in such patients.

CLINICAL FEATURES

Patients feel full of gas and bloated, especially after a meal. They develop discomfort because of their inability to belch and get rid of that gas. Not only do they develop abdominal cramps, but may also pass large amounts of flatus resulting in socially embarrassing situations.

TREATMENT

Symptoms resolve over time in most cases although revision surgery may rarely be needed to correct the problem. Patients should eat slowly, as well as avoid chewing gum and carbonated beverages.

PEARLS

○ Gas-bloat syndrome is a common disorder after Nissen's fundoplication and with reassurance, symptoms resolve over time.

BIBLIOGRAPHY

Waring JP. Postfundoplication complications. Prevention and management. *Gastroenterol Clin North Am.* 1999;28(4):1007-19.

Chapter 25   *Schatzki's Ring*

Schatzki's Ring is a ring-like mucosal abnormality occurring at gastroesophageal junction. It seen in about 10% of barium studies and is the underlying cause of symptoms in about 15 to 20% of patients presenting with dysphagia.

PATHOGENESIS

Rings may be congenital or acquired. Although a narrowing of 13.0 mm or less of esophageal lumen is required for manifesting as dysphagia, symptoms can occur with rings as wide as 18.0 mm in cases of patients with is a superimposed esophageal dysmotility.

CLINICAL FEATURES

Patients typically present with intermittent dysphagia to solids only. There is no associated weight loss.

DIAGNOSIS

Barium swallow with barium pill is the test of choice; endoscopy is less sensitive. However, proceeding to endoscopy without an imaging study in patients with dysphagia without alarm symptoms may be more cost-effective.

DIFFERENTIAL DIAGNOSIS

Consider peptic stricture and eosinophilic esophagitis especially in patients not responding to first line therapy.

TREATMENT

First line options include dilation with a large diameter bougie at least 50 F (preferably 56 F or greater) or disruption of the ring by biopsy forceps. Patients with rings refractory to above treatments may benefit from pneumatic balloon dilation, intralesional steroid injection (triamcinolone or Kenalog 40.0 mg/mL), surgery, and electrocautery incision. Since GERD has been implicated in the pathogenesis, acid suppressive treatment is recommended.

COURSE

Majority of the patients will develop recurrence of rings within 2 to 5 years and require repeated dilation.

PEARLS

- ○ Schatzki's ring is frequently an incidental finding and does not cause symptoms in most cases.
- ○ Although uncommon, rings with as high as an 18.0-mm diameter may cause dysphagia.

BIBLIOGRAPHY

Chotiprasidhi P, Minocha A. Effectiveness of single dilation with Maloney dilator versus endoscopic rupture of Schatzki's Ring using biopsy forceps. *Dig Dis Sci*. 2000;45(2):281-4.

Jalil S, Castell DO. Schatzki's ring: a benign cause of dysphagia in adults. *J Clin Gastroenterol*. 2002;35(4):295-8.

Chapter

26 *Infectious Esophagitis* ▬▬▬

EPIDIEMOLOGY

It usually occurs in immune-compromised individuals, especially those with HIV infection or receiving immunosuppressive agents, and occasionally in patients with longstanding diabetes mellitus. On rare occasions, infectious esophagitis may be seen in healthy adults also.

PATHOGENESIS

In addition to the above, risk for candida esophagitis is increased among patients receiving corticosteroids, antibiotics, or acid suppressive agents; alcoholics; those with achlorhydria secondary to gastroduodenal surgery or gastric atrophy; and patients with scleroderma.

The most common organisms involved are *Candida, Cytomegalovirus (CMV),* and *Herpes simplex.* Frequently, more than one organism may be involved.

CLINICAL MANIFESTATIONS

Patients typically complain of dysphagia or odynophagia, retrosternal chest pain, nausea, and vomiting. Absence of oropharyngeal lesions like thrush does not exclude the possibility of esophageal candidiasis.

DIAGNOSIS

Endoscopy

Endoscopy is required for precise diagnosis. White mucosal plaque like lesions are seen in candidiasis. Combined cytology and biopsy of lesions may be superior to either alone for diagnosis of *Candida* although endoscopic appearance is classic.

Esophageal erosions or ulcers are seen in viral esophagitis with typical biopsy findings. The diagnosis of viral infection may be difficult in patients with superimposed *Candida*.

Lesions in *Herpes* infection are initially small vesicles that coalesce to form circumscribed ulcers. The ulcer may be small, but may be as much as 2.0 cm in diameter with raised yellow edges. In contrast, *CMV* ulcers are small or serpiginous, may be shallow or deep, and may coalesce to form large ulcers. Both infections may be present simultaneously. *Herpes* is best diagnosed when the biopsies are taken from the margin of the ulcer, whereas *CMV* is best diagnosed when the biopsies are taken from the center of the ulcer. Eight biopsies should be undertaken to get optimal yield.

Histopathology

Biopsies show intracytoplasmic inclusion bodies as well as intranuclear inclusion bodies in *CMV* infection. Multinucleated giant cells with ballooning degeneration of squamous cells and ground glass nuclei are seen in *Herpes simplex* virus infection.

Role of Serology and Cultures

Serology and cultures for viruses are frequently done, but are probably not very helpful since many patients have already been exposed to these infections.

DIFFERENTIAL DIAGNOSIS

Differential diagnosis includes idiopathic ulcers in patients with HIV. The direct infection of the ulcer by HIV is controversial. HIV-like particles can be identified in the biopsies. These ulcers respond to prednisone 40.0 mg/day PO until symptoms improve, then tapering by 10.0 mg/week.

Uncommon causes of viral esophagitis include *Epstein Barr virus, Varicella zoster virus,* and *human papilloma virus.*

Bacterial esophagitis is rare and may occur in neutropenic patients. Tuberculosis infection of esophagus due to Mycobacterium avium-intracellulare (MAI) occurs usually as part of disseminated disease. Tissue stains and cultures for MAI may be undertaken in select cases.

MANAGEMENT

Candida Esophagitis

In an immune-compromised host, an empiric diagnosis of candida esophagitis may be made, and treatment can be started empirically with fluconazole (200.0 mg PO bolus and then 100.0 to 200.0 mg/day PO for 2 weeks). Treatment is continued if symptoms improve, otherwise an endoscopy is performed. Other options include nystatin swish and swallow (dose 500 000 units 5 times/day for 2 weeks), although many experts advise against its use. Ketoconazole is not recommended because of unpredictable absorption. Patients with granulocytopenia may need amphotericin-B.

Viral Esophagitis

Herpes esophagitis occurring in conjunction with oropharyngeal esophagitis may not require treatment. *CMV* esophagitis is treated with ganciclovir. Alternate option is Foscarnet but is more expensive and is used in patients resistant to ganciclovir or in granulocytopenic patients. Maintenance therapy for *CMV* esophagitis in immune-compromised patients is often recommended.

PEARLS

- ○ Infectious esophagitis can occur in non-AIDS patients especially in patients with diabetes or taking corticosteroids. Rarely, it may be seen in healthy subjects.
- ○ Patients with suspected Candida esophagitis may be started on treatment empirically, and EGD undertaken only if there is no response.

REFERENCES

Mulhall BP, Wong RK. Infectious esophagitis. *Current Treatment Options Gastroenterology*. 2003;6(1):55-70.

Chapter 27   *Pill Esophagitis*

Pill esophagitis implies esophageal injury due to direct contact of the medication with the esophageal mucosa. Over 75 medications have been reported to cause pill-induced esophagitis.

PATHOGENESIS

Injury occurs due to a prolonged and direct contact of the caustic medication with the esophageal mucosa. Factors promoting prolonged retention of medication in the esophagus include lack of adequate fluid along with drug ingestion, prolonged period of recumbency, ingestion of medication immediately prior to sleep, age greater than 70, and cardiac disease. There is no correlation with esophageal dysmotility.

In some cases, injury occurs as a result of medication-induced changes in esophageal pH. For example, doxycycline, tetracycline, vitamin C, and iron have a pH of less than 3, which is acidic when mixed in water. On the other hand, medications like potassium and quinidine do not affect the pH. Local hyperosmolality due to the pills may be another important factor.

MEDICATIONS IMPLICATED

Tetracycline is the commonest culprit especially doxycycline. In addition to NSAIDs especially aspirin, other medications include potassium, quinidine, iron, and aspirin. Alendronate-induced esophagitis is being increasingly seen.

CLINICAL FEATURES

Patients without prior history of esophageal disease present with sudden onset of chest pain and/or odynophagia. Typically, it is seen amongst teenagers taking tetracycline for acne or elderly patients taking multiple medications.

DIAGNOSIS

History is fairly typical in majority of cases. EGD is recommended in patients with severe, atypical symptoms or if other diagnosis are possible. Barium swallow is less sensitive; however, it helps to exclude extrinsic compression as a possible cause.

Endoscopically, there is a discrete ulcer with normal surrounding mucosa. Multiple small ulcers may be seen. Occasionally the lesion may be circumferencial or nodular suggesting malignancy. The presence of midesophageal stricture suggests NSAIDs as the cause. Biopsies are helpful to exclude infectious causes and malignancy. Absence of esophageal findings during the symptomatic phase excludes the diagnosis of pill esophagitis.

DIFFERENTIAL DIAGNOSIS

This includes reflux esophagitis, infectious esophagitis, and cancer.

TREATMENT

Most cases resolve without treatment. Histamine-2 receptor antagonists, PPIs, sucralfate, and local anesthetic agents are frequently prescribed, but there are no studies to substantiate their use. I use sucralfate slurry with viscous lidocaine four times a day to promote healing, plus twice-a-day PPIs to prevent any reflux-induced exacerbation of injury. Rarely, intravenous fluids or short-term parenteral nutrition may be required for those unable to eat or drink.

PREVENTION

Prevention of recurrent injury is key to the management. If the offending medication cannot be discontinued, a liquid preparation should be used if possible. Tablet forms are better than capsule formulations. Patients should take their medications in an upright position, and should maintain the position for at least 30 minutes. A small sip of water prior to ingestion of medication followed by a glass of water after taking the drug is helpful.

COMPLICATIONS

Esophageal stricture occurs rarely upon healing and dilatation may be needed.

PEARLS

○ Patients should take pills with a glass of water and while remaining upright for 30 minutes thereafter.
○ Treatment of pill-esophagitis is largely symptomatic and prevention is key to management.

BIBLIOGRAPHY

Minocha A, Greenbaum DS. Pill-Esophagitis caused by nonsteroidal anti-inflammatory drugs. *Am J Gastroenterol.* 1991;86:1086-9.
Kikendall JW. Pill esophagitis. *J Clin Gastroenterol.* 1999;28(4):298-305.

Chapter
28 *Caustic Ingestion*

EPIDEMIOLOGY

Caustic ingestion usually occurs in children. It may occur in adults as a result of underlying psychosis, alcoholism, or attempted suicide. These ingestions cause significant injury in over 5000 cases each year in the United States. Ingestion is generally accidental in children and intentional in teenagers and adults.

CAUSTICS INVOLVED

Sodium and potassium hydroxide are the most commonly involved. These are contained in drain cleaners and household cleaning products or small batteries. Sometimes the term "lye" ingestion is used to imply sodium or potassium hydroxide containing products.

Liquid household bleach is the most common culprit but does not cause severe esophageal injury in most subjects. Concentrated acids in toilet bowl or swimming pool cleaners and battery fluid are involved less frequently.

PATHOGENESIS

Alkaline injury is seen more often in the esophagus than the stomach. Liquid preparations are more likely to cause extensive damage compared to solids like small batteries. The larynx, as well as air passages, may be involved. Injury can extend rapidly through the esophageal wall. Liquefaction necrosis continues for 3 to 4 days, followed by progressive thinning of the wall of the esophagus due to sloughing and granulation tissue, as well as fibrosis. Complete healing takes 1 to 3 months.

Neutralization of the alkali by the acid in stomach results in reduced injury to the stomach. The duodenum is involved in less than one-third of the cases. Ingestion of small batteries (eg, watch batteries) is dangerous because of the potential damage due to the release of alkaline discharge or local electrical current, as well as necrosis due to direct pressure from the battery. This can result in burns and perforation within a few hours.

Acid ingestion causes coagulation necrosis. In contrast to alkali, acids cause less esophageal but more severe gastric injury. Patients usually ingest only small amounts of acid because it tends to be painful as compared to the alkaline solutions. In addition, acid travels through the esophagus quicker than the viscous alkaline solutions.

PATHOLOGY

The esophageal injury is classified on the basis of its severity. First degree injury involves a superficial mucosal damage manifesting as erythema, edema, and hemorrhage. Grade II-A is characterized by superficial noncircumferential ulcers and bleeding, whereas Grade II-B has deep or circumferential ulcers. Deep ulcers with black discoloration are seen in Grade III injury. Grade III-A shows focal necrosis in contrast to Grade III-B, which shows extensive necrosis.

CLINICAL MANIFESTATIONS

The spectrum of clinical manifestations varies widely. Absence of oropharyngeal lesions does not exclude esophageal or gastric injury. Similarly, early signs and symptoms do not predict the extent or severity of injury.

Patients may complain of oropharyngeal pain, dysphagia, odynophagia, retrosternal chest pain, epigastric pain, nausea, vomiting, hematemesis, and hypersalivation. Severe chest or back pain suggests the possibility of esophageal perforation. Patients with injury to the air passages may complain of hoarseness, stridor, and dyspnea. In extreme cases, patients may have fever, tachycardia, and hypotension. Gastric perforation may occur as late as 48 hours.

MANAGEMENT

Early management includes hospitalization, NPO, intravenous fluid and blood products as needed, and x-rays of the neck, chest, and abdomen. Laryngoscopy should be performed in patients with any hoarseness or respiratory symptoms. Emetics like ipecac are contraindicated. Use of neutralizing substances is controversial and is not routinely recommended.

Nasogastric Tube

A nasogastric tube should not be placed for lavage since such a placement can cause retching and increase the potential for perforation. A thin-bore flexible nasogastric tube may be placed endoscopically or under fluoroscopy for the purpose of medications as well as nutritional support.

Tracheotomy

Patients with glottic edema should not undergo endotracheal intubation, but should undergo tracheotomy. On the other hand, endotracheal intubation prior to endoscopy should be performed in noncooperative patients, or patients with respiratory difficulty.

Endoscopy

Endoscopy should be performed within first 24 to 48 hours to assess damage and to decide on management options. Some experts suggest waiting 48 to 72 hours in order to better assess the damage. EGD should not be performed if the patient is unstable, in respiratory distress or has severe glottic edema.

Post-EGD Management

Over half the patients with history of caustic ingestion do not show evidence of esophageal or gastric damage and can be safely discharged to home assuming that any underlying psychological factors have been addressed. Patients with Grade I and II-A should receive a liquid diet that can be advanced to regular diet within next 24 to 48 hours.

Patients with Grade II-B and III may be fed via nasogastric tube after 24 hours with oral feeding initiated after 48 hours (if patient is able to swallow saliva).

Corticosteroids and Antibiotics

The role of corticosteroids and antibiotics is controversial; most experts recommend against their use unless specifically indicated. For example, steroids may be administered to patients with impending airway compromise.

Surgery

Role of early surgery in Grade II-B and III injury in the absence of perforation is controversial and is usually not recommended by most physicians. Patients with Grade III-B injury frequently require esophageal resection because of complications.

Follow-Up

The issue of the timing of esophageal dilation has not been subjected to randomized controlled trials and as such continues to be a matter of debate. I do not recommend routine use of early esophageal dilation. In addition, prophylactic esophageal stents to maintain luminal patency are not recommended.

I recommend a barium swallow at 2 to 3 weeks in patients with significant esophageal injury, supplemented by a chest CT in select cases. Patients with circumferencial injury on initial EGD should receive prophylactic dilatation starting at about 3 weeks—even in the absence of the complaint of dysphagia.

COMPLICATIONS

1. Patients with II-B and III injury are at high-risk for perforation.
2. About 30 to 40% of patients develop strictures especially in cases of Grade II-B and III injury. The stricture may manifest within a few weeks to a few years, although the peak incidence is at about 2 months. Multiple sessions of dilatation in a gradually increasing fashion are required to dilate these strictures.
3. Vomiting, abdominal distention, and early satiety suggest pyloric stenosis.
4. There is an increase in the risk for esophageal squamous carcinoma by 1000-fold and it occurs at the site of previous stricture. Risk for gastric cancer is not changed.

PROGNOSIS

Grades I and II-A resolve without any problems or long-term sequelae, whereas Grades II-B and III-A develop strictures in most cases. There is a 65% early mortality rate in patients with Grade III-B. Overall mortality rate from caustic ingestion varies from 1 to 2%.

SURVEILLANCE

Patients with history of caustic stricture should undergo a surveillance endoscopy every 1 to 3 years beginning 15 to 20 years after the ingestion.

PEARLS

- ○ No significant injury is seen on endoscopy in the majority of the patients with a history of caustic injury.
- ○ EGD should be performed within 24 to 48 hours of ingestion to assess the damage and decide on management options.

BIBLIOGRAPHY

Trowers E, Thomas C Jr, Silverstein FE. Chemical- and radiation-induced esophageal injury. *Gastrointest Endosc Clin N Am.* 1994;4(4):657-75.

Jaillard S. Extensive corrosive injuries of the upper airways and gastrointestinal tract. *J Thorac Cardiovasc Surg.* 2002;123(1):186-8.

STOMACH AND DUODENUM

Chapter
29 *Gastritis*

Gastritis is a very nebulous term meaning different things to different people. Patients and clinicians frequently refer to gastritis as the presence of dyspeptic symptoms, whereas endoscopists go by endoscopic evidence of inflammation. On the other hand, pathologists rely on histopathological features. The correlation between endoscopic and histologic findings is poor.

ACUTE GASTRITIS

Acute gastritis may be acute hemorrhagic gastritis, erosive gastritis, or acute neutrophilic gastritis. Acute hemorrhagic gastritis occurs as a result of a chemical injury due to alcohol, nonsteroidal anti-inflammatory drugs (NSAIDs), corticosteroids, and in response to major physical stress like head trauma, surgery, sepsis, burns, and hypothermia. Acute neutrophilic gastritis is associated with *H. pylori* (Hp) infection.

CLASSIFICATION OF GASTRITIS

Gastritis may broadly be classified into nonatrophic form, atrophic form, and specialized forms. The nonatrophic form is usually related to Hp. The atrophic form is associated with autoimmune diseases and environmental factors. The specialized forms include chemical or radiation-induced, lymphocytic, noninfectious granulomatous, eosinophilic, and other infectious gastritis.

1. *Nonatrophic chronic gastritis* is also known as Type B gastritis. This is related to the presence of inflammation in the gastric antrum more than in the corpus. It is associated with Hp infec-

tion. Its relationship to dyspeptic symptoms is controversial. Eradication of Hp does not relieve symptoms of nonulcer dyspepsia. At best, 9% of patients undergoing such a treatment may have improvement of symptoms.

2. *Atrophic gastritis* is comprised of autoimmune metaplastic atrophic gastritis and environmental metaplastic atrophic gastritis (multifocal atrophic gastritis). Autoimmune gastritis is confined to the fundus and corpus. It is characterized by severe diffuse atrophy of acidophilic glands and is associated with achlorhydria, anti-intrinsic factor antibodies, antiparietal cell antibodies, hypergastrinemia, anemia related to iron deficiency, and malabsorption of vitamin B_{12}. It is associated with increased risk for gastric malignancy. In multifocal atrophic gastritis, the inflammation is similar in antrum and corpus; it is usually seen in the presence of Hp infection.

3. *Reactive gastritis* is caused by chemical irritants such as alcohol, NSAIDs, and bile. It usually involves antrum.

4. *Lymphocytic gastritis* is characterized by dense infiltration of lymphocytes in the gastric body and antrum. It is associated with celiac disease, as well as lymphocytic colitis. Proton pump inhibitors (PPIs) are helpful in some patients. A gluten-free diet will result in improvement in patients with celiac disease.

5. *Viral gastritis* is usually caused by *Cytomegalovirus (CMV)* and is generally seen among the immune-suppressed patients like those with AIDS or who have undergone organ transplantation. Treatment is ganciclovir; however, relapses are common after withdrawal of medication. *Herpes simplex* infection may also be seen on occasion.

6. *Bacterial gastritis* may be caused by bacteria other than Hp (eg, *Streptococcus, Staphylococcus, Klebsiella*, and *E. coli*). While frequently seen in the gastric lumen, these organisms cause problems only in the presence of severe ischemia or immune- suppression. Phlegmonous gastritis occurs when these organisms cause purulent necrosis of the gastric wall. Emphysematous gastritis occurs when the pathologic organism is a gas-forming organism.

7. *Fungal gastritis* rarely causes gastritis by itself, although colonization of gastric ulcers by *Candida* may be seen. However, severe necotrizing gastritis may be caused by opportunistic fungi especially in immune-suppressed patients.

8. *Parasitic gastritis* is rare and may occur due to *Strongyloides* and *Cryptosporidium*, etc.

9. *Granulomatous gastritis* occurs due to infections or toxins (eg, tuberculosis, syphilis, histoplasmosis) and noninfectious causes (eg, sarcoidosis, Crohn's disease, and Wegner's granulomatosis). Mycobacterium infection may occur in the presence of AIDS or in patients with disseminated tuberculosis. Syphilitic gastritis occurs in the second and third stages of syphilis.

10. *Eosinophilic gastritis* is marked by extensive eosinophilic infiltration of the antrum more than the body or fundus. It may occur due to hypersensitivity to medications or some foods or as a result of parasitic infection. Patients may present with abdominal pain, nausea, and vomiting. Stools should be tested for infectious pathogens. No cause is found in most cases. Treatment with corticosteroids provides relief.

11. *Gastric Antral Vascular Ectasia* (GAVE), also known as watermelon stomach, is predominately seen in females in association with achlorhydria and gastric atrophy. Patients have acute and chronic gastrointestinal (GI) bleeding leading to anemia. Endoscopically, longitudinal columns of continuous blood vessels across the antrum are seen converging onto the pylorus. Histology is pathognomic and is characterized by vascular ectasia, spindle cell proliferation, and fibrohyalinosis. Most patients respond to local treatment with Nd:YAG laser or Argon plasma coagulation. Surgery in the form of antrectomy is the last resort.

12. *Portal hypertensive gastropathy* is seen in patients with liver disease. A mosaic pattern of mucosa is seen predominantly in the fundus and body. Treatment includes nonselective beta-blockers (propranolol or nadolol), transjugular intrahepatic portosyetemic shunts (TIPS), or portal decompression surgery. Local therapy with lasers or Argon plasma coagulation may worsen the situation.

PEARLS

○ Gastritis is a nebulous term and means different things to different people.

○ *H. pylori* is a common cause of gastritis, but its relationship to causing dyspeptic symptoms is controversial.

BIBLIOGRAPHY

Faraji EI, Frank BB. Multifocal atrophic gastritis and gastric carcinoma. *Gastroenterol Clin North Am.* 2002;31(2):499-516.

Stolte M, Meining A. The updated Sydney system: classification and grad-
    ing of gastritis as the basis of diagnosis and treatment. *Can J
    Gastroenterol.* 2001;15(9):591-8.

Cave DR. Chronic gastritis and Helicobacter pylori. *Semin Gastrointest Dis.*
    2001;12(3):196-202.

Chapter

30 *Peptic Ulcer Disease*

EPIDEMIOLOGY

Peptic ulcer disease accounts for approximately $6 billion per year
to the health care system in the United States. Although the incidence
has been declining, duodenal ulcer accounts for approximately
200 000 to 400 000 cases each year. The spectrum of natural history
varies from spontaneous resolution without any symptoms to complications leading to endoscopic or surgical interventions and even mortality.

PATHOGENESIS

Despite the recent surge in knowledge implicating Hp in the
pathogenesis of the majority of gastroduodenal ulcers, the old dictum
"no acid, no ulcer" still applies. Patients with duodenal ulcers secrete
more gastric acid. Patients who develop complications from the ulcers
are more likely to develop ulcer complications in the future. The ulcer
occurs when virulence of pathogenic factors overwhelms the body
defenses.

The pathogenic factors include increased gastric acid secretion,
low sodium bicarbonate, gastric metaplasia, smoking, and NSAIDs.
The components of defenses against ulcer formation include mucus,
mucosal blood flow, intercellular junctions, and epithelial renewal, as
well as repair.

Ulcer size effects the healing rate. Large ulcers take longer to heal.
The healing rate is approximately 3.0 mm/week for gastric ulcers.
Healing is slower in cases of elderly subjects, alcoholics, simultaneous
occurrence of duodenal and gastric ulcers, as well as stressful life situations.

Most ulcers can be accounted for by Hp infection and NSAID use. Other causes include Zollinger-Ellison syndrome, *Helicobacter heilmannii*, and viral infections like *Herpes* and *CMV*.

Hp-Induced Ulceration

Hp causes antral gastritis leading to loss of the D cells that release somatostatin. This reduction of somatostatin leads to decreased inhibition of antral G cells resulting in increased gastric acid secretion. Hp also leads to gastric metaplasia of the duodenum thus contributing to duodenal ulcers. In addition, the Hp secretes enzymes and cytotoxins that have the potential to disrupt the protective mechanisms.

NSAID-Induced Ulceration

NSAIDs cause ulceration by their local and systemic effects by inhibiting prostaglandins. Approximately 10% of long-term NSAID users may develop duodenal ulcers. Risk factors for significant NSAID ulceration include age older than 65, a history of peptic ulcer disease, a history of upper GI bleed, use of more than one NSAID concomitantly, use of anticoagulants, and severe comorbidity—especially congestive heart failure. COX-2 inhibitors have somewhat less ulcerogenic effect but are not devoid of gastrotoxicity.

CLINICAL FEATURES

Duodenal ulcer typically causes epigastric pain 2 to 3 hours after a meal. Pain improves with food and as a result, patients tend to eat more and may become overweight. The gastric ulcers on the other hand cause pain soon after eating and as such patients are afraid to eat and lose weight. These distinctions between duodenal and gastric ulcers, while classic, are neither sensitive nor specific.

Symptoms of complicated ulcer disease include upper GI bleeding, vomiting due to gastric outlet obstruction, acute abdomen due to perforation, and pancreatitis due to penetrating ulcer.

DIAGNOSIS

UGI Series and Endoscopy

Findings on history and physical examination are neither sensitive nor specific, and only 15 to 25% of the patients suspected to have ulcer-like symptoms are actually found to have ulcers upon endoscopy. Therefore, for precise diagnosis, either upper GI series or endoscopy is required. EGD is preferred because it is more sensitive for small lesions and also allows for the taking of biopsies.

Hp Testing

All patients with peptic ulcer disease should undergo testing for Hp. During endoscopy, biopsies can be taken and a rapid urease test (RUT) can be performed. Biopsy specimens can also be examined under microscope after staining them with hemotoxylin and eosin (H&E) or special stains. A urea breath test (UBT), as well as a stool antigen Hp test, can be performed in patients not undergoing endoscopy. A false negative RUT, urea breath test, and stool test may be seen in patients taking PPIs, antibiotics, or in cases of acute upper GI hemorrhage. Serology is useful for initial diagnosis, but cannot be used to document eradication of Hp after therapy.

TREATMENT

The treatment of peptic ulcer disease is 2-fold:
1. To heal the ulcer.
2. To prevent the ulcer recurrence.

While dietary changes are not routinely recommended, cessation of NSAIDs and smoking is strongly advised. Antacids containing aluminum and magnesium hydroxide are effective, but the side effects preclude their routine use. Histamine-2 receptor antagonists (H_2RAs) like cimetidine (400.0 mg bid), ranitidine (150.0 mg bid), famotidine (20.0 mg bid), and nizatidine (150.0 mg bid) produce a healing rate of 70 to 80% at 4 weeks and 85 to 95% after 8 weeks of therapy for duodenal ulcers. They may be administered as split dose or a single night-time dose.

Sucralfate heals by promoting angiogenesis and granulation tissue formation. It should be administered 30 to 60 minutes before meals since a pH less than 3.5 promotes a binding of the drug to the ulcer.

PPIs like omeprazole (20.0 mg qd), lansoprazole (30.0 mg qd), pantoprazole (40.0 mg qd), rabeprazole (20.0 mg qd), and esomeprazole (40.0 mg qd) result in an 80 to 100% healing rate for duodenal ulcers at 4 weeks. The superiority of PPIs over H_2RAs for healing of gastric ulcers is modest however. The effectiveness of PPIs may be diminished by concomitant use of H_2RAs.

Healing rates using moderate to high doses of antacids are equal to H_2RAs. Misoprostol is effective in healing duodenal ulcers but has significant side effects without any superiority over acid-suppressive agents; as such, it is not used for this purpose.

Prevention of Recurrence of Hp-Related Ulcers

Patients testing positive for Hp should undergo eradication of Hp using a 10 to 14 day course of at least three drugs. Most regimens have either metronidazole and/or clarithromycin. Resistance to metronida-

zole is high—approaching as much as 50%. The addition of a high
dose (twice-a-day dose) of PPIs to metronidazole-based regimen over-
comes this resistance. Dose-packs improve compliance.

Numerous regimens have been advocated. The classic therapy
includes use of metronidazole, tetracycline, and Pepto-Bismol. It is
also available as Helidac dosepack. Amoxicillin may be substituted
for tetracycline, but it is less effective. PrevPac (clarithromycin, amoxicillin, and lansoprazole) is an example of a clarithromycin-based regimen available as dose-pack (see Chapter 32).

Prevention of Recurrence of NSAID-Induced Ulcers

Patients with NSAID-induced ulcers should preferably cease the
use of the drug. If that is not feasible, patients can be treated with
misoprostol or a PPI for maintenance. The drawback of misoprostol
therapy is that it causes diarrhea in 20 to 30% of the patients.
Combination dose-packs containing NSAID, along with prophylactic
medication, include Prevacid NapraPac (naproxen with lansoprazole), and Arthrotec (diclofenac plus misoprostol).

Another option is to use COX-2 inhibitors, which have lesser, but
not zero, gastrotoxic potential. Patients with history of complicated
ulcers may benefit from COX-2 inhibitor plus ulcer prophylaxis with
PPI or misoprostol.

Maintenance

Maintenance therapy is indicated in high-risk patients in whom
Hp eradication is unsuccessful or in those who have non-Hp, non-
NSAID ulcers. These include complicated ulcers, recurrent ulcers,
refractory ulcers, or giant ulcers. Alternate causes for ulcers should be
sought including the exclusion of Zollinger-Ellison syndrome and *H.
heilmannii*.

H_2RAs are effective in reducing the recurrence of duodenal ulcer
to 25% over a 12 month period, compared to 60 to 90% for placebo.
The dose for the H_2RA is half of the dose used for healing. For example, the ranitidine healing dose is 300.0 mg/day, whereas for maintenance 150.0 mg/day is used. All H_2RAs have similar effectiveness.
PPIs may be used for maintenance in case H_2RAs fail or if there are
giant and/or refractory ulcers. Because of the risk for rebound acid
secretion upon cessation of PPIs, stepping down to a full dose of
H_2RAs may be an appropriate caution.

Follow-Up Endoscopy

Follow-up endoscopy is not required in uncomplicated duodenal
ulcer disease unless there is a persistence of symptoms or a recurrence. While a follow-up endoscopy for gastric ulcers is recommend-

ed to document healing and exclude the presence of cancer, it is probably not needed if adequate sampling of biopsies have been done during initial endoscopy. A repeat endoscopy should be considered in patients with high risk for ulcers including Asians and Latinos, those with and absence of history of NSAIDs, those with concomitant duodenal and gastric ulcers, and those with giant ulcers greater than 2.0 cm.

ULCER PROPHYLAXIS

Patients with non-Hp, non-NSAID ulcers benefit from long term prophylaxis using a single daily nighttime dose of H_2RA (ranitidine 150.0 mg or famotidine 20.0 mg qhs). NSAIDs cause serious complications only in a small fraction of NSAID users. Hence, NSAID prophylaxis is advised for those older than 65, cases of severe comorbidity like CHF, those with previous history of ulcers or upper GI bleed, and those using anticoagulants and corticosteroids. Both misoprostol and PPIs are effective.

Stress ulcer prophylaxis is indicated for patients with severe burns, head trauma, mechanical ventilation, sepsis, renal failure, and coagulopathy. Intravenous H_2RAs are usually used. Sucralfate is equally effective. PPIs may be superior to H_2RAs but their exact role remains to be established.

PEARLS

- ○ Most patients with ulcer-like symptoms do not have ulcers.
- ○ Treatment of ulcer involves therapy to heal the ulcer and to prevent its recurrence.
- ○ Only a small fraction of NSAID users require NSAID prophylaxis.

REFERENCE

Hawkey CJ, Langman MJ. Non-steroidal anti-inflammatory drugs: overall risks and management. Complementary roles for COX-2 inhibitors and proton pump inhibitors. *Gut*. 2003 Apr;52(4):600-8.

Cappell MS. Gastric and duodenal ulcers during pregnancy. *Gastroenterol Clin North Am*. 2003;32(1):263-308.

Yang YX, Lewis JD. Prevention and treatment of stress ulcers in critically ill patients. *Semin Gastrointest Dis*. 2003;14(1):11-9.

Chapter
31 *Functional Dyspepsia* ▰▰▰▰▰

Functional dyspepsia is defined as presence of dyspeptic symptoms for at least 12 weeks (which may not be consecutive in a 12 month period) characterized by upper abdominal discomfort or pain without any evidence of organic disease on endoscopy or without any disturbance of or association with bowel function.

EPIDEMIOLOGY

The prevalence of functional dyspepsia varies from 10 to 20%.

PATHOGENESIS

Gastroparesis is seen in 30 to 80% of these patients; however, there is poor correlation with symptoms. Gastric compliance is lower as compared to healthy controls. There is enhanced visceral hypersensitivity lowering the pain threshold.

The role of Hp infection remains controversial. The onset of dyspeptic symptoms may be preceded by a bout of flu-like infection in some patients. There is increased incidence of psychopathology like anxiety, neuroticism, and depression in patients with nonulcer dyspepsia compared to duodenal ulcer.

DIAGNOSIS

The diagnosis is made by the typical clinical features and exclusion of other causes of dyspepsia by appropriate investigations. Less than 25% of patients with ulcer-like symptoms are actually found to have an ulcer on endoscopy.

TREATMENT

Treatment is frequently as difficult as it is for other functional disorders. It includes explanation, education, as well as management of psychosocial factors and dietary modification. Medications that may cause and contribute to dyspeptic symptoms (eg, NSAIDs or antibiotics) should be substituted or discontinued if possible. Similarly, caffeine and excessive alcohol should be avoided.

If symptoms persist despite simple dietary or medication modifications, patient should undergo empiric trial with drug therapy (eg, antisecretory [PPI] or prokinetic therapy). PPIs have been shown to be superior to placebo for symptom relief, whereas H$_2$RAs and sucralfate provide inconsistent relief. Stop the empiric trial of PPI at 4 weeks if the symptoms resolve. If the symptoms persist, switch to alternate therapy.

Prokinetics like cisapride have been shown to be of benefit; however cisapride is only available on a restricted basis in the United States. Metoclopramide has extrapyramidal side-effects that make its use less desirable. Domperidone (10.0 to 30.0 mg PO qid) is available as an orphan drug in compound pharmacies only.

Although not approved by the US Food & Drug Administration (FDA) for the purpose, some experts employ a therapeutic trial of tegaserod (Zelnorm 6.0 mg bid) based on its pharmacological properties.

The role of Hp eradication in Hp-infected patients remains controversial. The drawbacks of such a treatment include questionable or limited benefit; antibiotic side-effects; emergence of resistant strains; as well as a possible unmasking or worsening of symptoms of gastroesophageal reflux disease (GERD).

Antidepressants have been tried with some success. A combination of peppermint and caraway oil is superior to placebo. Bismuth subsalicylate (Pepto-Bismol) has not been adequately studied, although it is frequently used. Limited data suggests benefit from sumatriptan and buspirone. Hypnotherapy has been shown to be beneficial in randomized control trials. Additional options include stress management, relaxation training, as well as behavioral and psychotherapy.

PEARLS

- ○ Over half of the patients with dyspeptic symptoms have functional dyspepsia.
- ○ Eradication of *H. pylori* as a treatment of functional dyspepsia is controversial.

BIBLIOGRAPHY

Moayyedi P, Soo S, Deeks J, Forman D, Harris A, Innes M, Delaney B. Systematic review: Antacids, H2-receptor antagonists, prokinetics, bismuth and sucralfate therapy for non-ulcer dyspepsia. *Aliment Pharmacol Ther*. 2003;17(10):1215-27.

Stanghellini V, De Ponti F, De Giorgio R, Barbara G, Tosetti C, Corinaldesi R. New developments in the treatment of functional dyspepsia. *Drugs*. 2003;63(9):869-92.

Chapter
32 *Helicobacter Pylori* ▮▮▮▮▮

Although *Helicobacter pylori* organisms, commonly referred to as *H. pylori* (Hp), have been observed on gastric biopsies for about a century, the true significance came to light only after Warren and Marshall described its association with chronic gastritis and peptic ulcer disease.

ORGANISM

Hp is a spiral shaped microaerophilic, Gram-negative organism. The bacteria produces a urease enzyme that is essential for its colonization and survival. Its urease activity, motility, and ability to adhere to gastric epithelium allow it to survive the harsh gastric environment.

EPIDEMIOLOGY

It is the most common bacterial infection occurring worldwide in humans of all ages and both sexes. Approximately 50% of the world's population is affected, with the prevalence being higher in developing countries. The prevalence is the highest amongst non-Whites. The prevalence is higher amongst individuals of lower socioeconomic status, reflected by the higher density of housing, number of siblings, the sharing of beds, and a lack of running water. However, the difference between races cannot be accounted for solely by the differences in socioeconomic status.

Most infections are acquired during childhood. Although the route of transmission is unknown, person-to-person transmission through fecal-oral or oral-oral transmission are the most likely mechanisms. Iatrogenic infection may occur as the result of suboptimal disinfection of gastric devices, endoscopies, or accessories. Humans are the major reservoir of infection.

DISEASE ASSOCIATIONS

In addition to its association with peptic ulcer disease and gastritis, Hp has also been linked to anorexia of aging, autoimmune thrombocytopenic purpura, stroke, urticaria, coronary artery disease, hyperammonemia, hypertension, iron deficiency anemia, migraine, Raynaud's phenomenon, and sudden infant death syndrome (SIDS).

However, the data linking Hp with non-GI conditions is weak. Hp is protective against GERD. Its role in NSAID-induced gastric injury is controversial.

RISK FOR MALIGNANCY

There is a 3- to 6-fold increase in gastric malignancy in patients infected with Hp. Whether or not the eradication of Hp results in reduction in the risk of malignancy remains to be established. There is a strong association between gastric lymphoma (MALToma) and Hp infection.

Association between Hp and colon polyps/cancer remains controversial. An association between Hp infection and pancreatic cancer has also been suggested.

DIAGNOSIS

Indications for Testing

Since Hp infection is very common in the general population, testing for this organism should only be undertaken if you plan to treat. It should be performed in patients who have peptic ulcer disease, past history of documented peptic ulcer, or gastric mucosa-associated lymphoid tissue (MALT) lymphoma. Even though Hp is associated with most cases of peptic ulcer disease, an empiric treatment is not advisable and a confirmation of infection should be obtained prior to undertaking treatment.

Asymptomatic patients without prior history of peptic ulcer disease should not be tested for Hp, except in patients with family history of Hp infection or fear of gastric cancer—especially in patients of Japanese or Chinese descent in whom the prevalence of gastric cancer is increased.

Testing for Hp is not recommended for prevention of atrophic gastritis in patients on long-term PPIs or in patients with nonulcer dyspepsia.

Methods of Testing

1. *Urease test*: In patients undergoing endoscopy, the test of choice is an RUT on endoscopic biopsy specimen. Urease tests may be false negative in patients taking PPIs and in patients with recent or active bleeding. As such, the patient should not take PPIs for at least 2 weeks prior to testing. The sensitivity and specificity of a biopsy urease test varies from 90 to 100%.

2. *Histology:* If the urease test is negative, histology should be studied or serology may by undertaken. When biopsies are undertaken for histology, multiple biopsies should be taken from antrum, as well as the body, because of variation in the density of Hp in different areas. Brush cytology of the stomach may be undertaken in patients in whom gastric biopsy is contraindicated; the specificity and sensitivity rates vary from 95 to 98%. Culture and sensitivity for Hp can be undertaken on the biopsy specimen, although routine culture is not recommended.

3. *Urea breath test:* A UBT is best done to document for eradication of infection, although stool antigen testing is being increasingly used. False positive results are uncommon for UBT, but a false negative test may occur in patients taking PPIs or when there is a presence of blood in stomach due GI bleeding.

4. *Hp serology:* It detects IgG or IgA antibodies. It is a noninvasive method suitable for screening for Hp in a primary care practice. The accuracy rates vary from 80 to 98%. Serology should not be done in patients to document eradication after treatment since antibodies persist for a long time after the Hp has been eradicated.

5. ^{13}C *Bicarbonate test:* This has been approved as a noninvasive tool and involves measuring two serum specimens, 1 hour before and 1 hour after the ingestion of a ^{13}C-labeled urea-rich meal. A significant rise in postparandial serum ^{13}C bicarbonate level suggests presence of Hp infection. The sensitivity and specificity is about 95%.

6. *Stool antigen:* It is a noninvasive method and its sensitivity and specificity, as well as its limitations, are comparable to UBT.

7. *PCR test for Hp:* It is useful in research labs.

Testing Strategy

In patients undergoing an endoscopy, the presence of Hp can be documented by doing an RUT on an endoscopic biopsy specimen—if the patient is not taking a PPI and there is no evidence of bleeding. If a biopsy is not performed in cases of a recently bleeding gastroduodenal ulcer, the patient's blood sample may be tested for Hp serology, or, alternatively, a UBT or Hp stool test may be undertaken. A UBT or stool test may be false negative in cases of the presence of blood in the stomach and concomitant PPI use. As such, patients should be off PPI for at least 10 to 14 days prior to testing. A serological test is the preferred screening test in patients with a past history of peptic ulcer.

TREATMENT

Hp is a resistant organism and multiple drugs have to be used simultaneously in order to eradicate it. Multiple drug regimens have been studied; in general, a triple drug regimen for 10 to 14 days is recommended, although an ideal therapeutic regimen has not been identified. Dosepacks like PrevPac and Helidac improve compliance.

Treatment regimens

1. The classic regimen of metronidazole 250.0 mg qid, Pepto-Bismol 2 tablets qid, and tetracycline 500.0 mg qid for 2 weeks carries the problems of poor compliance and drug resistance. Such a regimen is commercially available as Helidac. Amoxicillin should be used instead of tetracycline in children, but is less effective. The problem of resistance to metronidazole can be overcome if a twice a day dose of a PPI is added to the regimen, converting it to a four-drug regimen.

2. A twice-a-day regimen of clarithromycin 500.0 mg bid, amoxicillin 1.0 g bid, and a PPI bid is likely to have the highest compliance rate with the least chances for resistance. This regimen is commercially available as PrevPac. In patients allergic to amoxicillin, metronidazole may be used instead of amoxicillin. However, one must realize that metronidazole resistance is high and can lower the effectiveness of the treatment.

3. Dual drug regimens using a PPI and an antibiotic like amoxicillin or clarithromycin have been studied but the eradication rates are low.

Failure of Treatment

For patients who fail the first course of Hp treatment, a quadruple drug therapy may be undertaken using a PPI bid in combination with of Pepto-Bismol 2 tablets qid, tetracycline 500.0 mg qid, and metronidazole 500.0 mg qid for 14 days. A combination of lansoprazole 30.0 bid, amoxicillin 1.0 g bid, and levofloxacin 200.0 mg bid has been shown to eradicate Hp in 69% of patients who had failed a previous clarithromycin-based regimen. Another effective combination is PPI bid, rifabutin (300.0 mg qd), and amoxicillin (1.0 g bid).

In case of metronidazole resistant patients, a quadruple therapy consisting of 2 weeks of omeprazole 20.0 mg bid, amoxicillin 1.0 g bid, bismuth subcitrate 240.0 mg bid, plus either clarithromycin 500.0 mg bid or furazolidone 200.0 mg bid has been used.

Resistance to Therapy

Metronidazole resistance rates vary from 20 to 50% in the United States, whereas clarithromycin resistance is 10 to 12%. Resistance to amoxicillin and tetracycline is rare. Although culture and sensitivity of Hp is not generally recommended, it may be undertaken in patients with refractory disease. Adverse reactions associated with Hp eradication regimens are usually mild, and less than 10% patients stop treatment prematurely due to side effects.

REINFECTION

The reinfection of Hp following the eradication is rare and is less than 5% per year.

PEARLS

- ❍ Hp eradication is unlikely to relieve symptoms of nonulcer dyspepsia.
- ❍ Although Hp is the most common cause of peptic ulcers, eradication treatment should not be given empirically but only after documentation of presence of Hp infection.
- ❍ Hp serology is good for screening only but not for documentation of eradication after therapy.
- ❍ Dose-packs like PrevPac and Helidac improve compliance.

BIBLIOGRAPHY

Sanders MK, Peura DA. Helicobacter pylori-Associated Diseases. *Curr Gastroenterol Rep*. 2002;4(6):448-54.

Versalovic J. Helicobacter pylori. Pathology and diagnostic strategies. *Am J Clin Pathol*. 2003;119(3):403-12.

Chapter
33 *Gastroparesis* ▰▰▰▰▰

Gastroparesis means delayed gastric emptying of solids and liquids, although clinically it refers to delayed solid gastric emptying in an appropriate clinical setting. A new term—gastropathy—has been proposed, encompassing disordered emptying (either delayed or rapid) and involving upper and/or lower stomach.

EPIDEMIOLOGY

Although widespread, the prevalence, as well as age and sex distribution of gastroparesis, is unknown. There are approximately 50 000 patients with severe symptomatic and drug refractory gastroparesis in the United States. As many as 27 to 40% of diabetic patients have a delayed gastric emptying; however, not all patients with delayed gastric emptying have symptoms.

PATHOPHYSIOLOGY

The stomach is essentially made up of two chambers: upper and lower. The upper chamber, through fundic contraction, is responsible for liquid emptying, whereas the lower stomach empties solids by myoelectric activity. These two pumps function in a cooperative arrangement. Both the enteric nervous system (ENS) and the autonomic nervous system (ANS) play an important role in the gastric emptying. Thus a variety of structural or neuromuscular injuries can result in gastroparesis.

CAUSES

The majority of the cases are idiopathic and are usually preceded by a viral illness. Delayed or disordered gastric emptying may be seen in systemic disorders like scleroderma, as well as other connective tissue disorders, endocrine disorders (diabetes and thyroid dysfunction), neurological disorders (multiple sclerosis, Parkinsonism), anorexia nervosa and bulimia, chronic liver or renal failure, pancreatitis, medications, TPN, bone marrow transplantation, paraneoplastic syndromes, or abnormal gastric pacemaker activity due to ENS damage.

Gastroparesis can also be associated with previous gastric surgery, particularly if the neural innervation of the stomach is disrupted.

DIFFERENTIAL DIAGNOSIS

Disordered gastric emptying, usually defined as delayed gastric emptying of solids, can also be seen in some patients who empty the stomach rapidly. This is classically seen in patients postgastric surgery who may have rapid "dumping" from the stomach into the small intestine. However, rapid gastric emptying has been described in a number of other disorders including diabetes mellitus as a manifestation of diabetic ANS dysfunction sometimes labeled as a diabetic "gastropathy."

CLINICAL FEATURES

Patients present with nausea, vomiting, abdominal distension, early satiety, and sometimes weight loss. Initial assessment should focus just not on the GI system but also look out for systemic disorders that may contribute to possible gastroparesis.

DIAGNOSIS

Upper endoscopy and/or upper GI barium study are useful to exclude any structural disorder. A 4-hour radionuclide solid gastric emptying, using only four measurements, is the standard. The percent fraction of the remaining radionuclide-labeled meal determines the presence, as well as the severity, of gastroparesis—clinically normal being less than 6% remaining at 4 hours. Results between 6 to 10% represent a gray zone.

Abnormal parameters for "rapid emptying" remain to be established. Based on preliminary data, a 1 hour value of <37% remaining (from the standardized meal) can be used to define rapid emptying, with a sensitivity of about 80%.

Ultrasound of the stomach has also been used for diagnosis. Electrogastrography (EGG) helps detect abnormalities of gastric electrical rhythm. Gastric manometry may be useful in select cases and is usually used in research settings. A UBT has been used in research protocols.

TREATMENT

Modification of lifestyle, including small frequent meals and ingestion of low fat meals, is the first step. Medical therapy is effective in as many as 60% of the patients.

Metoclopramide, a central and peripheral dopamine antagonistic is useful, but its utility is limited by its high incidence of central nervous system (CNS) side effects. Domperidone (10.0 to 30.0 mg PO qid) is similar to metoclopramide except that it has primarily peripheral dopamine antagonistic actions and as such is devoid of extrapyramidal CNS side effects. However it is available only as an orphan drug in the United States.

Erythromycin is effective in improving gastric emptying, but suffers from the problem of tachyphylaxis. Cisapride, an effective promotility agent, is available on compassionate use basis in the US. Bethanecol is a nonspecific cholinergic agonist, but it's utility is limited by its side effects.

Botulinum toxin injection into the pyloric sphincter has been used in cases where outflow resistance due to pylorospasm has been suspected to be the cause as in diabetes mellitus. Several investigational drugs, including motilin agonists, are being investigated for the treatment of gastroparesis.

Electroacupuncture has been shown to help the symptoms in some patients. Results from surgery are disappointing. Gastric electrical stimulation (GES) has been approved by the FDA for drug-refractory gastroparesis.

GES results in the improvement of gastric emptying, maintenance or improvement of nutritional status and reduced healthcare cost. In addition to the complications associated with endoscopy and surgery, the most common complication of GES device is pocket infection, which occurs in less than 10% of the cases.

PEARLS

- ❍ Gastroparesis may be occult. Consider it in any patient with refractory upper gut symptoms.
- ❍ Gastric electrical stimulation has been shown to help many patients with gastroparesis, and is currently approved as an FDA humanitarian use device.

BIBLIOGRAPHY

Abell TL, Minocha A. Gastroparesis and the gastric pacemaker: a revolutionary treatment for an old disease. *J Miss State Med Assoc.* 2002;43(12):369-75.

Talley NJ. Diabetic gastropathy and prokinetics. *Am J Gastroenterol.* 2003;98(2):264-71.

Chapter

34 *Gastric Polyps*

EPIDEMIOLOGY

Gastric polyps are usually an incidental finding when an upper GI series or EGD is performed for an unrelated reason. Overall, gastric polyps occur in about 1% of the gastroscopies performed. They are usually found in patients above the age of 60.

PATHOLOGY

Histologically, they are usually hyperplastic in about 75% of the cases. Adenomas are seen in less than 10%. The remainder are inflammatory polyps, carcinoids, Brunner's gland hypertrophy, and juvenile polyps, etc.

PATHOGENESIS

Pathogenesis of gastric polyps remains to be established. Factors that have been implicated include gastric acidity, coffee, tea, bile reflux, Hp, and acid suppression with PPIs.

CLINICAL FEATURES

Clinical manifestations are rare and include occult GI bleeding, abdominal pain, and gastric outlet obstruction.

CANCER RISK

Risk for malignancy is less than 10% with adenomas and about 2% with hyperplastic polyps. Malignant transformation tends to occur in polyps greater than 2.0 cm in size. While gastroduodenal polyps occur in majority of the patients with familial adenomatous polyposis, the malignant potential for gastric polyps is rare.

MANAGEMENT STRATEGIES

In case a patient has multiple gastric polyps, the larger ones should be excised while a sample biopsy should be taken from the smaller ones.

Peutz-Jeghers Syndrome

Juvenile polyps are seen in Peutz-Jeghers syndrome. There is an increased risk for malignancy and as such endoscopic surveillance (EGD q 2 to 3 years) is recommended. Management includes biopsies of all polyps as well as excision of all polyps greater than 1.0 cm for histological examination. Multiple endoscopies may be required for complete removal if multiple polyps are present.

H. Pylori Infection

Patients who are Hp positive and have small hyperplastic polyps may show regression of polyps after Hp eradication. However, polyps greater than 1.0 cm should always be removed.

Gastric Adenoma

While endoscopic surveillance for gastric adenomas is recommended, there are no guidelines for the interval. We perform surveillance for gastric adenoma at one year and subsequently every 3 years. The interval is reduced to every 1 to 2 years if there is family history of gastric cancer. The finding of gastric adenoma should also prompt a colonoscopic evaluation unless already done.

Fundic Gland Polyps

Sporadic fundic gland polyps (FGP) are usually less than 10 in number in the general population. Sporadic fundic gland polyposis is defined as greater than 10 polyps, and in some patients, the number may be as high as 50 or more. PPIs can also lead to polyps in the stomach, while Hp appears to be protective against FGP. In familial adenomatous polyposis (FAP), the number of polyps is in dozens to hundreds.

No surveillance is needed in sporadic FGP. In case FAP or attenuated FAP is suspected based on the EGD findings, a colonoscopy is indicated unless already done. If a diagnosis of FAP is made, the surveillance plan is as outlined in Chapter 81.

Large Polyp

If there is a large sessile polyp that can not be removed endoscopically and the biopsies show adenoma, surgery is advisable. Surgery should be also considered even if it is not adenoma, since the polyp may be mixed and the focus of adenoma may be missed.

Malignant Polyp

Patients with advanced or poorly differentiated malignant polyps require surgery. Surgery may be avoided in case of a polyp with a small focus of malignancy that is moderately to well differentiated and confined to the mucosa. Frequent follow-up should be undertaken in such cases.

PEARLS

- ○ Gastric polyps are usually an incidental finding on EGD or upper GI series.
- ○ Surveillance EGD for gastric adenoma is recommended.

BIBLIOGRAPHY

Oberhuber G, Stolte M. Gastric polyps: an update of their pathology and biological significance. *Virchows Arch.* 2000;437(6):581-90.

Chapter

35 *Gastric Cancer*

EPIDEMIOLOGY

Gastric cancer is a major cause of cancer related mortality in many parts of the world. The highest rates of gastric cancer occur in Costa Rica and Japan, whereas the lowest incidences are in the United States and India. African Americans, Hispanics, and Native Americans are twice as likely to develop gastric cancer than Whites.

Overall the incidence of gastric cancer is declining globally. The decrease is a reflection of the decline in cancer of the distal stomach, body, and antrum. However, cancers of the proximal stomach and gastroesophageal (GE) junction have actually been increasing.

Men suffer from gastric cancer almost twice as much as the women. It rarely occurs before the age of 40. Most of the malignant neoplasms of the stomach are adenocarcinoma (AC).

RISK FACTORS

These include chronic atrophic gastritis, intestinal metaplasia, pernicious anemia, benign gastric ulcer disease, partial gastrectomy, Hp infection, gastric adenoma, immune-deficiency syndrome, Barrett's esophagus (BE), family history of gastric cancer, hypertrophic gastropathy (including Menetrier's disease), low consumption of fruits and vegetables, and high consumption of salty, smoked, or poorly preserved foods.

BE increases the risk for cancer of the GE junction and proximal stomach. Obesity increases the risk for cancer of gastric cardia and GE junction. Epstein-Barr virus infection is also involved in carcinogenesis.

Whether smoking is a causative factor or is a marker for some other unknown carcinogen is controversial. The role of alcohol abuse has not been established. Genetic risk factors include family history of gastric cancer, blood type A, and hereditary nonpolyposis colon cancer syndrome (HNPCC).

PATHOGENESIS

The transformation of hyperplastic gastric polyps into cancer is rare. Initiating factors like chronic Hp infection, pernicious anemia, high salt diet, etc, lead to chronic atrophic gastritis and intestinal metaplasia. Chronic gastritis produces epithelial cell damage with increased free radical generation.

Atrophic gastritis also results in reduced acid secretion, which in turn leads to hypergastrinemia, causing a stimulation of gastric epithelial proliferative processes. The increased cellular proliferation causes increased generation of free radicals and decreased levels of protective factors like vitamin C contributing to carcinogenesis in a susceptible individual.

PATHOLOGY

The lesion may be as a small polyp, superficial plaque, depression, or ulceration. Most cancers in the United States are diagnosed in the advanced stage and are seen as polypoidal or fungating masses with ulceration.

Histologically, gastric cancer is usually adenocarcinoma. Early gastric cancer is defined as adenocarcinoma confined to the gastric mucosa or submucosa regardless of whether the regional lymph nodes are involved or not. These are usually seen amongst high-risk populations during screening for gastric cancer and carry a survival rate of 85 to 90% over 5 years after resection.

CLINICAL FEATURES

Because of nonspecific symptoms, gastric cancer in the United States is usually metastatic at the time of diagnosis. Patients complain of weight loss and vague abdominal pain that may become severe and constant. A cancer of the GE junction may lead to pseudoachalasia syndrome. Nausea, vomiting, heme-occult positive stools, hematemesis, and iron deficiency anemia may be seen. Uncommon presentations include feculent emesis due to gastrocolic fistula, ascites, jaundice, and massive GI bleed.

Physical exam may reveal epigastric fullness or mass. A periumbilical lymph node (Sister Mary Joseph's node) or left supraclavicular adenopathy (Virchow's node) may be evident.

EXTRAGASTROINTESTINAL MANIFESTATIONS

Paraneoplastic manifestations include diffuse seborrhic keratosis, acanthosis nigricans, microangiopathic hemolytic anemia, membranous nephropathy, hemolytic anemia, hypercoagulable states, and polyarteritis nodosa.

DIAGNOSTIC

A double-contrast upper GI series (or preferably an endoscopy) should be undertaken promptly, especially in patients with dyspeptic symptoms and older than 45 or in young patients with alarm symptoms or no response to empiric therapy for dyspepsia. Histologic confirmation of a benign appearing ulcer is essential since about 5% of them are actually malignant. Use of at least seven biopsies from a mass or ulcer lesion has a sensitivity of 98%.

The diffuse gastric cancer known as linitis plastica presents with a nondistensible stomach on barium study, as well as on an endoscopy, although the mucosa may otherwise look normal. Superficial biopsies may be negative in such cases. Biopsy of suspicious appearing lesions in the liver on CT scan should be performed.

While repeat endoscopy at 8 to 12 weeks to document healing of a gastric ulcer is still recommended, its cost-effectiveness remains to be established. Serological markers have no role in diagnosis.

TUMOR STAGING

The tumor-node-metastasis (TNM) classification is used. A dynamic CT scan has accuracy rates varying between 50 and 60%. However, it is not good for an assessment of tumor depth or lymph node involvement. While an endoscopic ultrasound (EUS) is more accurate, its effect on survival and outcome remains to be established. EUS is not useful for distant metastasis. Laparoscopy may be superior to EUS and CT because it provides direct visualization. The choice of modality depends upon the local expertise. Patients with good performance status require laparotomy unless documented to be unresectable by imaging studies.

TREATMENT

Patients who are good surgical candidates should undergo surgery for curative or palliative purposes. All patients who are positive for Hp should also undergo Hp eradication. Total gastrectomy is performed for early gastric cancers located in the upper third of the stomach. Patients with early gastric cancer in the lower two-thirds of the stomach may undergo subtotal gastrectomy. The use of preoperative chemotherapy to down-stage a localized unresectable cancer is investigational. Laparoscopic gastric resection is being done in some centers.

Endoscopic mucosal resection (EMR) is performed for early gastric cancer at select centers for elevated lesions less than 2.0 cm in size, depressed lesions less than 1.0 cm in size without ulceration, and those without lymph node metastasis. EMR is contraindicated in patients with lesions greater than 3.0 cm in diameter and those with deep submucosal or lymphatic invasion.

Palliative options for unresectable cancers include resection, surgical bypass, radiation therapy, chemotherapy, chemoradiation therapy, and endoscopic stent placement. A combination chemotherapeutic regimen including 5FU is used for metastatic gastric cancer. In elderly and sick patients, 5FU with leucovorin alone may be given. The role of intraperitoneal chemotherapy is controversial. Patients with peritoneal carcinomatosis may benefit from systemic or intraperitoneal chemotherapy.

PROGNOSIS

Survival rate for early-treated gastric cancer is about 90% at 5 years and about 80 to 85% at 10 years. Late recurrences or metachronous cancers may occur in about 5% of the cases.

SCREENING

The role of screening for gastric cancer continues to be a matter of debate. While helpful in areas where the incidence of gastric cancer is high (as in Japan), it is not cost-effective in the United States.

Screening in Special Situations

1. There is no role for screening EGD in patients with Hp infection, even when chronic atrophic gastritis with intestinal metaplasia is present.

2. A single endoscopy for screening may be performed in patients with pernicious anemia; however, no surveillance is recommended.

3. The risk of cancer in patients with subtotal gastric resection for gastric ulcer is low; as such, no screening is recommended.

4. Surveillance is recommended for patients with gastric adenomas (see Chapter 34).

5. Patients with familial adenomatous polyposis should undergo upper endoscopy for gastroduodenal polyps initially and then every 3 years. Multiple biopsies should be obtained from ampulla even if it appears normal endoscopically. If no adenoma is detected, repeat exam should be undertaken in 3 years. On the other hand, if a periampullary adenoma is found, surveillance endoscopy and biopsy should be performed every 1 to 3 years.

6. No screening is recommended for patients with hereditary nonpolyposis colon cancer (HNPCC), unless patients have a family history of gastric cancer or reside in a high-risk geographic region.

7. Screening endoscopy for BE is recommended but is of doubtful benefit in detecting gastric cancer.

GASTRIC LYMPHOMA

As many as 3% of gastric neoplasms are primary gastric lymphomas. The stomach is the most common extra-nodal site of lymphoma comprising 10% of the overall lymphomas. Lymphoma arising from the mucosa is known as mucosa associated lymphoid tissue tumor or MALToma or MALT lymphoma. Although MALTomas arise primarily in the stomach, they can also occur in the small and large intestine.

CLINICAL FEATURES AND DIAGNOSIS

Symptoms include epigastric discomfort, weight loss, anorexia, nausea, vomiting, and GI bleeding. Diagnosis is made by endoscopic biopsies; superficial biopsies may be negative. Immune-stains are done to establish monoclonality. Flow cytometry is used at select centers.

TREATMENT

Anti-Hp therapy should be undertaken for patients with localized mucosal and nonbulky disease without the presence of metastasis or lymphadenopathy or diffused large B-cell lymphoma. Complete remission as a result of Hp therapy occurs in as many as 50 to 70% of the patients and is more likely in patients whose tumor is superficially located in the distal stomach.

Patients who undergo remission following anti-Hp therapy should undergo long- term follow-up with histologic surveillance. Staging by endoscopic ultrasound helps predict the response to anti-Hp therapy. In patients with an incomplete response to Hp therapy or relapse following therapy, chemotherapy, radiation therapy, and surgery should be considered.

PEARLS

○ Most gastric cancer in the United States is detected in advanced stages.

○ Mass screening for early detection of gastric cancer is not cost-effective in the United States.

○ The majority of patients with MALT lymphoma respond to Hp eradication therapy.

BIBLIOGRAPHY

Hohenberger P, Gretschel S. Gastric cancer. *Lancet*. 2003;26;362(9380):305-15.

Ahmad A, Govil Y, Frank BB. Gastric mucosa-associated lymphoid tissue lymphoma. *Am J Gastroenterol*. 2003;98(5):975-86.

LIVER

Chapter
36 *Hepatitis A*

EPIDEMIOLOGY

Hepatitis A (HAV) is an RNA virus. There are approximately 125 000 to 200 000 infections annually year in the United States resulting in about 100 deaths each year. About a quarter to one-third of the cases occur in children.

PATHOGENESIS

HAV is usually transmitted by fecal-oral route, and is particularly prevalent where poor sanitation standards exist. Transmission by intravenous drug use and by blood is rare.

People at risk for developing HAV infection include people living or traveling to areas where sanitation standards are low, children in daycare centers, and homosexual men. Fecal or oral transmission may also include acquisition of the virus by eating raw shellfish from sewage-contaminated waters. Natural disasters that disrupt sanitation systems (eg, floods) can result in large epidemics.

DIAGNOSIS

The serologic diagnosis is established by the presence of anti-HAV-IgM fraction in a patient with signs and symptoms of acute hepatitis. A positive anti-HAV (total) with a negative anti-HAV-IgM fraction indicates immunity either from prior infection or from immunization.

CLINICAL FEATURES

The incubation period for HAV is 2 to 6 weeks. The virus is excreted in stools from about 10 days before and 2 to 3 weeks after the onset of acute illness. The sickness is acute and is usually self-limited. The severity varies from asymptomatic unapparent infection to fulminant liver failure.

Patients who get infected at less than 6 years of age have mild non-specific symptoms and rarely develop jaundice. In contrast, adults acquiring infection develop more severe form of hepatitis.

The spectrum of symptoms varies and includes malaise, anorexia, fever, nausea, vomiting, abdominal discomfort, itching, dark urine, and pale stools. Extrahepatic manifestations like skin rash and arthralgias are uncommon.

Serum alanine aminotransferase (ALT) and aspartate aminotransferase (AST) may exceed 1000 IU/L. Serum bilirubin and alkaline phosphatase may be elevated.

Course

The disease usually is self-limited. The virus disappears from the body in about 6 months. Chronic hepatitis or carrier-state does not occur. Atypical manifestations include relapsing hepatitis without progression and cholestatic hepatitis with jaundice and pruritus. HAV may trigger autoimmune hepatitis (AIH) in some patients.

TREATMENT

Treatment is largely supportive.

PREVENTION

Use of pooled gammaglobulin results in preventing infection in 90% of exposed subjects. Passive pre-exposure immune prophylaxis is recommended for subjects going on a single trip to an endemic area, whereas candidates for postexposure prophylaxis include household and daycare contacts of cases and subjects exposed in local outbreaks (raw shellfish, food handlers).

HAV vaccine should be offered to travelers 1 month before going to an endemic area, children and adults living in endemic areas, those who engage in high-risk behavior including homosexual men and intravenous drug users, as well as patients with chronic liver disease. A booster dose should follow the initial dose at 6 to 18 months. Universal vaccination is not recommended.

PEARLS

- ○ Hepatitis A is transmitted via fecal-oral route.
- ○ Acute hepatitis A can not be distinguished from other causes of acute hepatitis on clinical grounds alone.

○ Both active and passive immunization against hepatitis A are
effective.

BIBLIOGRAPHY

Rosenthal P. Cost-effectiveness of hepatitis A vaccination in children, adolescents, and adults. *Hepatology*. 2003;37(1):44-51.

Chapter
37 *Hepatitis B*

EPIDEMIOLOGY

There are about 350 million people worldwide with chronic hepatitis B (HBV) infection. The prevalence is high in Asia and Africa,
whereas it is low in the United States. About 250,000 patients die of
HBV-related causes each year.

Of all the cases of acute viral hepatitis, HBV accounts for 40 to 50%.
HAV is the next common with 30 to 40%. In contrast, hepatitis C
(HCV) is the most common cause of chronic viral hepatitis, with only
15% of the chronic viral hepatitis due to HBV in the United States. The
peak prevalence of HBV is between the ages of 20 to 30.

PATHOGENESIS

Risk factors for acute HBV include heterosexual contact with acute
cases or carriers. Those with multiple sex partners are implicated in
41% of the cases, whereas homosexual activity accounts for only 9%.
Intravenous drug use is seen in 15%, household contacts in 2%, and
occupational hazards account for 1% of the cases. The source for acute
HBV may be unknown in about one-third of cases.

CLINICAL FEATURES

The incubation period for HBV varies from 45 to 180 days (average
of 60 to 90 days). Spectrum of presentation varies. Symptoms are
indistinguishable from any other acute hepatitis. Some people have
anicteric flu-like symptoms including anorexia, malaise, fever, and
mild abdominal discomfort. Among adults, icteric hepatitis occurs in
30 to 50% of cases. Progression to chronic infection occurs in 90% cases

of infants, 25 to 50% for infections acquired as toddlers, and less than 5% among adults.

SEROLOGICAL DIAGNOSIS

Diagnosis is established by assessment of antigen-antibody systems in addition to HBV viral titers. The three antigen-antibody systems include hepatitis B surface antigen (HBsAg) and antibody (HBsAb), hepatitis E antigen (HBeAg), and antibody (HBeAb), as well as hepatitis B core antibody (HBcAb) IgM and IgG.

Presence of HBsAg indicates a current acute or chronic infection and its disappearance indicates the resolution of the infection. The presence of HBsAb indicates immunity either due to immunization or as a result of infection. Recent acute infection or occasional reactivation of chronic infection is suggested by IgM form of HBcAb. In contrast, HBcAb (IgG) suggests remote infection. The presence of HBeAg and/or HBV DNA greater than 105 viral copies/mL indicates active viral replication and high infectivity.

Acute Hepatitis B

The typical serological response in acute HBV includes presence of HBsAg at 4 weeks and resolution by 24 weeks. At about 6 weeks after infection, IgM HBcAb appears and disappears by 32 weeks, but IgG HBcAb persists. At about 32 weeks HBsAb appears. HBeAg is present from 2 to 10 weeks, and thereafter HBeAb appears. Thus, patients with acute infection have positive HBsAg, HBcAb (IgM), HbeAg, as well as HBV DNA.

Chronic Hepatitis

In patients who progress to chronic HBV, the HBsAg fails to resolve. In addition HBeAg may persist for months to years. During all this time, the HBcAb (total) is present, although IgM resolves by about 32 to 36 weeks after exposure.

Acute vs Chronic Infection

Those who fail to clear the HBsAg by 6 months are considered chronic. The presence of HBsAg confirms the infection but does not distinguish between acute and chronic infection, which can only be distinguished by testing for HBcAb IgM. HBV core IgM is usually detectable up to 6 to 8 months and always indicates a recent infection or reactivation of chronic infection.

Immunization vs Prior Infection With Immunity

Prior infection with immunity is suggested by the presence of HBsAb and HBcAb (IgG). Subjects with HBV vaccination are positive only for HBV surface antibody.

Resolved Infection vs Chronic Infection and Carrier State

Presence of HBcAb (IgG) with HBsAb in the absence of HBsAg suggests resolved infection; presence of HBcAb (IgG) with HBsAg implies chronic infection or inactive carrier state.

Isolated HBcAb may sometimes be present. In HBsAg negative patients, presence of HBcAb without HBsAb may indicate prior infection with loss of detectable HBsAb, or an occult HBV infection with an undetectable HBsAg but positive HBV DNA. False positive HBcAb may rarely occur.

Effect of Precore Mutation

These patients are unable to make HBeAg. Thus, serological markers in chronic hepatitis are marked by the presence of HBsAg, HBeAb and viral titers greater than 10^5 copies/mL in the absence of HBeAg. Thus, patients are positive for HBeAb but negative for HBeAg despite active viral replication. In contrast, chronic infection with wild-type HBV is characterized by a positive HBeAg, while HBeAb is negative. Patients infected with precore mutants are less likely to clear virus with antiviral therapy.

SEQUELAE

Recovery

Acute hepatitis results in total recovery in 95% of the adult patients, while only a minority go on to chronic disease. Immune-suppressed patients have a greater risk of developing chronic infection.

Reactivation of Acute Hepatitis

Causes of acute hepatitis in patients with chronic HBV infection include spontaneous reactivation of HBV, flare-up due to a transient period of immune-suppression (eg, chemotherapy, induction by antiviral therapy), superimposed infection with another virus including hepatitis D, and other etiology of hepatitis including alcohol and medications.

Asymptomatic Carrier State vs Chronic Hepatitis

Patients with persistent infection may develop an asymptomatic carrier state or chronic hepatitis. Chronic HBV with active viral replication is marked by HbsAg and BeAg with viral DNA titers greater than 10^5 copies/mL, while chronic HBV without active viral replication is marked by the presence of HBsAg and HBeAb with viral DNA titers less than 10^5 copies/mL.

An inactive carrier state is defined as persistence of HBsAg for greater than 6 months associated with normal liver enzyme levels, low (<10^4 copies/mL) or undetectable HBV DNA and little to no necroinflammatory activity on a liver biopsy. Some consider the threshold to be less than 10^5 copies/mL. Chronic hepatitis is characterized by elevated liver enzyme levels, high (>10^5 copies/mL) HBV DNA, and necroinflammatory changes on liver biopsy. A viral load between 10^4 and 10^5 copies/mL falls into a gray zone. In precore mutant infections, viral loads of >10^4 copies/mL are considered significant.

Seroconversion

Five to 10% of chronic hepatitis cases seroconvert each year from HBeAg (positive) to HBeAb (positive). Seroconversion is associated with an improvement in liver enzymes and conversion of an active to inactive carrier state (ie, a replicative phase to low or nonreplicative state) where HBeAg is absent and HBsAg continues to be present with absent or low levels of HBV DNA along with the presence of HBeAb. There is minimal or low level of activity on liver biopsy.

TREATMENT

Indications

Treatment is indicated for patients with persistent elevation in liver enzymes, positive markers for viral replication including HBsAg, HBeAg, HBV viral DNA, as well as a presence of active inflammation in the liver biopsy.

No specific treatment for acute HBV is required and management is generally supportive. Patients with fulminant hepatic failure should be managed at a liver transplantation center.

Treatment options

Treatment options for chronic HBV include interferon, lamuvidine, and adefovir.

INTERFERON

The advantages include a high response rate in selected patients and a short duration of treatment. Disadvantages include parenteral administration, poor tolerance, and a lack of response when treating precore mutant infection. Interferon-alpha is administered in the doses of 5 MU daily or 10 MU three times weekly for 4 to 6 months.

Patients develop flu-like symptoms in the first few weeks, which improve with continued therapy.

HBeAg seroconversion occurs in 30 to 40% and HBsAg seroconversion in 5 to 10% of treated patients. HBsAg seroconversion may occur during therapy; however, it usually occurs years after completion of treatment. Platelets and neutrophil count should be monitored during interferon therapy and dose adjustments made as needed.

A flare up of hepatitis due to immune system activation occurs about 4 to 8 weeks into therapy, but treatment should be continued unless there is a clinical or biochemical decompensation. Patients with child's Class B and C cirrhosis should not be treated with interferon because of the possibility of the flare up leading to decompensation.

LAMIVUDINE

Advantages of lamuvidine 100.0 mg/day include oral administration, minimal side effects, and potential for use in decompensated cirrhosis. Lamuvidine is preferable over interferon in patients with decompensated liver disease, immune-suppressed patients such as organ transplantation or HIV infection, and patients with HBeAg negative chronic HBV.

The disadvantages include drug resistance. About 20 to 40% of the patients treated for 1 to 2 years develop a YMDD mutation, resulting in reappearance of HBV DNA sometimes associated with increases in ALT levels. Patients who develop YMDD mutants should be considered candidates for adefovir therapy.

Ninety percent of the patients treated with lamuvidine have some improvement in HBV DNA levels. These may even become negative in a small fraction of patients. Most patients also have improvement in liver enzymes. Unlike interferon, the flare-up of the disease during treatment is uncommon. Twenty to 30% of patients have a seroconversion of HBeAg after 1 to 2 years of treatment. Although seroconversion of HBsAg is unusual during treatment, it may occur during long-term follow up after HBeAg seroconversion is achieved and treatment is completed.

ADEFOVIR

Adefovir (10.0 mg/day) is the latest drug approved for HBV. Its advantages include oral administration, excellent tolerance, and its effectiveness in decompensated cirrhosis and in patients infected with lamivudine-resistant strains. Its advantage over lamivudine is the rarity of resistant strains emerging during therapy. The dose needs to be adjusted according to renal function.

Response to Treatment

Factors predicting high response rate include high ALT levels, low HBV DNA level, short duration of disease, and female gender. Poor response to treatment is seen in patients with chronic long-standing infections since childhood, infection with precore mutants, and those with HIV or immune suppression.

PROGNOSIS

There is 15 to 25% rate of premature mortality from chronic liver disease due to HBV. Chronic hepatitis can lead to cirrhosis, hepato-cellular carcinoma (HCC), and death. Risk of HCC is increased especially in patients with liver cirrhosis, older than 40, and those with a family history of liver cancer. Asymptomatic carriers are also at risk for development of HCC even in the absence of cirrhosis.

PREVENTION OF TRANSMISSION

The prevention of HBV includes behavioral modification to prevent disease transmission, passive immunoprophylaxis and active immunization. Routine vaccination is recommended in all infants, all unvaccinated children up to the age of 12 years, and adults in high-risk groups.

Active Immunization

Vaccination for HBV is highly effective and immunity develops in 95% of the cases. There is no need to check for HBV surface antibody except in patients with immune-deficiency or high-risk patients such as those with chronic liver disease.

Passive Immune-Prophylaxis

Indications for passive immune-prophylaxis with hepatitis B immunoglobulin (HBIG) include neonates born to HBV surface antigen positive mothers, subjects after needle stick exposure, and after liver transplantation in patients who are HBsAg-positive prior to transplantation.

Passive immune-prophylaxis also should be given to household and sexual contacts of acute HBV patients if they have not been vaccinated before.

Postexposure Immune-Prophylaxis

A combination of HBIG and HBV vaccine is recommended for sexual contacts of acutely infected individuals and neonates of HBsAg-positive mothers identified during pregnancy. In these circumstances, HBIG and the first dose of the vaccine can be given at the same time.

Preventing Perinatal HBV Transmission

HBsAg testing is performed in all pregnant women. Prevention of perinatal transmission of HBV is undertaken by administration of HBIG and HBV vaccination to the infected mother's newborn starting within 12 hours of birth. Both can be given at the same time but at a different site. HBV vaccination is administered at 0, 1, and 6 months. HBsAb and HBsAg should be checked at 12 months.

Screening Recommendations

Screening for HBV is recommended for all pregnant women, homosexual men, intravenous drug users; persons born in hyperendemic areas, dialysis patients; HIV-infected individuals; family members, household members, and sexual contacts of HBV-infected persons.

PEARLS

- ○ Universal childhood vaccination is recommended.
- ○ Acute hepatitis B does not require specific treatment.
- ○ About 1 to 5% of adult patients with acute HBV infection develop chronic hepatitis B.
- ○ Presence of HBsAg as seen in chronic hepatitis or carrier state carries an increased risk of hepatocellular carcinoma even without presence of cirrhosis.

BIBLIOGRAPHY

Fattovich G. Natural history and prognosis of hepatitis B. *Semin Liver Dis.* 2003;23(1):47-58.

Chapter

38 *Hepatitis C*

EPIDEMIOLOGY

Approximately 170 million people are infected with hepatitis C (HCV) worldwide, whereas in the United States 3 to 4 million people are infected. Although the number of new cases in the United States is declining, the number of chronic cases is increasing, resulting in greater morbidity and mortality as time goes on. HCV is responsible for about 40% of all cases of chronic liver disease resulting in 10 000 to 20 000 deaths per year. This number is expected to triple in the next 10 to 20 years if no intervention is taken. It is the most common indication for liver transplantation in the United States.

NATURAL HISTORY OF HEPATITIS C

Acute HCV leads to chronic hepatitis in about 75 to 85% of the patients, while about 20% go on to develop cirrhosis. Risk factors for progression of liver disease in chronic hepatitis are the duration of infection, alcohol intake greater than 50.0 g per day, male gender, and coinfection with HBV or HIV.

Once chronic infection is established, the body cannot usually clear the virus spontaneously. The progression of acute to chronic hepatitis occurs over a period of 10 to 20 years. Of the patients who develop cirrhosis, the annual rate of decompensation is 6% and HCC occurs in 4% per year.

Transmission

The most common risk factor is intravenous drug abuse, which is responsible for 60% of the cases. Sexual transmission occurs in 2 to 15% and is seen almost exclusively in people with high-risk sexual behavior and sexually transmitted diseases. Other factors include blood transfusion prior to screening guidelines (10%); occupational exposure (4%); and unknown reasons in about 10% of the cases. Occupational exposure of HCV is inefficient. There is a 1.8% incidence of infection following needle stick exposure from a HCV positive source. Nosocomial, iatrogenic, or perinatal spread is less than 1%.

Household transmission of HCV is rare and may occur as a result of percutaneous or mucosal exposure to blood through sharing of contaminated personal articles like razors or toothbrushes.

Sexual transmission in a stable monogamous heterosexual relationship is low. HCV is not spread by kissing, hugging, sneezing, coughing, sharing of food or water, utensils, drinking glasses, or casual contact. Patients should not be excluded from work, school, play, or child care/daycare settings.

Perinatal transmission of HCV occurs only in those women who are positive for HCV RNA and not just the HCV antibody. The rate of infection is 6% and may be up to 17% if the woman is coinfected with HIV.

CLINICAL FEATURES

Incubation period varies from 2 weeks to 22 weeks. Patients rarely present as acute hepatitis. The infection is usually asymptomatic or has nonspecific flu-like symptoms with mild to moderate elevation of serum transaminase levels. Right upper abdominal discomfort may be present. Most patients are detected through routine testing of blood at the time of:

1. Blood donation.
2. Complications of end stage liver disease.
3. Extrahepatic manifestations. Suspect HCV on the basis of risk factors and not the symptoms.

Extrahepatic manifestations include mixed cryoglobulinemia in 10 to 25% of the cases; glomerulonephritis; and dermatological manifestations including porphyria cutanea tarda, lichen planus, and cutaneous narcotizing vasculitis. Diabetes and depression occur more often in HCV-infected individuals.

DIAGNOSIS

Screening Tests

Serum transaminases may be normal in about 30% of the patients with chronic infection. ELISA test (third generation) is used for detection of HCV antibodies and its sensitivity and specificity exceeds 99%. A positive HCV antibody test suggests past exposure or current infection with the HCV virus unless proven otherwise. It is usually diagnostic of HCV in patients with abnormal liver enzymes and presence of risk factors.

Average duration before appearance of HCV antibody after infection is about 4 to 6 weeks. A false positive HCV antibody result may be seen in AIH, hypergammaglobulinemia, and patients with normal liver enzymes with no risk factors for HCV.

False negative test may be seen in immune-suppressed patients like organ transplant recipients and chronic dialysis patients. Measurement of HCV RNA in serum should be used to confirm current infection in questionable cases.

HCV RNA test should be used in children until the age of 18 months for the purposes of assessing perinatal exposure since maternally derived HCV antibody will be found in the baby.

HCV RNA and Genotype

HCV RNA quantitative test is used to determine the viral load and is useful for monitoring the patients during therapy. A HCV-genotype should be tested for deciding on treatment options. Genotype 1 is the most common in the United States occurring in about 75% of the patients. Genotype 1 is also the most difficult to eradicate. Genotypes

2 and 3 are seen in greater proportion in Europe and India, whereas in the Middle East, genotype 4 is predominant.

Role of Liver Biopsy

Liver biopsy is not a requirement for establishing the diagnosis; however, it provides information regarding the degree of inflammation, tissue damage, and presence or absence of cirrhosis. The degree of inflammation and fibrosis/cirrhosis helps determine the prognosis, the need for treatment, as well as helping to exclude other causes for liver disease.

Twenty-five to 30% of patients with chronic HCV have normal liver enzymes. In such patients, the risk of progression of the disease is lower, and as such, the role of liver biopsy and treatment is controversial.

Approach to Accidental Needle Stick

The patient should be immediately tested for HCV antibody and liver enzyme levels to get a baseline. A repeat HCV antibody should be tested in 8 to 12 weeks. An alternative option is to check HCV RNA in 3 to 6 weeks and if negative, to test at 12 weeks again. Documented acute infections that are asymptomatic can probably be treated in order to prevent chronic infection. Symptomatic acute infections have a higher spontaneous clearance rate and should be observed for 12 to 24 weeks prior to instituting antiviral therapy.

Approach to Infants Born to HCV-Positive Mothers

Children born to mothers with HCV should be tested for the HCV antibody at the age of 18 months. Infected children should be evaluated for chronic liver disease. Antiviral therapy should not be administered at an early age as spontaneous clearance of viremia is often seen.

TREATMENT

Indications

Treatment of chronic HCV should be individualized based on patient's age, histologic severity of the disease, comorbid conditions, and effectiveness of available therapies. Patients with persistently elevated ALT, detectable HCV RNA levels, liver biopsy changes showing portal or bridging fibrosis, and inflammation and piecemeal necrosis at moderate levels are excellent candidates for treatment.

Implications of Therapy

Current combination therapy including interferon and ribavirin is expensive and has many side effects. Do not rush to start the therapy.

Ways to improve compliance include addressing psychological issues prior to starting therapy, educating the patient that it is a long-term commitment, explaining side effects, and addressing the side effects promptly. Patients should strictly abstain from alcohol or use of any other illicit substances and should be vaccinated against HAV and HBV unless they already have immunity.

Current Therapy

Two forms of pegylated interferon are available. Pegylated interferon alpha-2b (Peg-Intron) and pegylated interferon alpha-2a (Pegasys). Peg-Intron dose is based on body weight ranging from 50.0 to 150.0 mcg/kg/week, whereas the Pegasys dose is fixed at 180.0 mcg/week.

Ribavirin is administered at 1200.0 mg/day PO if body weight is equal or greater than 75.0 kg and 1000.0 mg/day PO if body weight is less than 75.0 kg. Patients weighing greater than 105.0 kg receive 1400.0 mg/day. Ribavirin is a pregnancy category X drug and couples must not plan conception during the treatment and for 6 months after treatment. A pregnancy test should be undertaken in women of child-bearing potential before initiating the therapy, every month during therapy and 6 months thereafter. Couples should use two reliable means of contraception. Effective contraception should be used even if the male partner is the one undergoing antiviral therapy.

Therapeutic Strategy

Once combination therapy is started, quantitative HCV RNA should be obtained at 3 months. Patients who exhibit a drop in a viral load >2 logs are considered early viral responders and have a high likelihood of sustained viral clearance. Patients who fail to reach this landmark are unlikely to clear the virus with continued therapy. At 6 months of therapy, a qualitative HCV RNA test should be obtained. If a positive result predicts a low likelihood of viral clearance, discontinuation of therapy should be considered.

Among the responders, therapy should be stopped at 6 months in genotype 2 or 3, but should be continued for a period of 1 year in patients with genotype 1. Patients with advanced fibrosis or cirrhosis may benefit from 1 year of therapy if infected with genotype 2 or 3 or if viral clearance is not achieved in the first 6 months of therapy.

Response to Therapy

Combination therapy with pegylated interferon and ribavirin results in 50 to 60% of sustained response for all patients, and greater than 80% response in patients with genotype 2 or 3. Favorable factors associated with sustained response to therapy include genotype 2 or

3, HCV RNA level less than 2 million copies/mL, the female gender, and those younger than 40.

Sustained Responders vs Relapsers

Sustained response is defined as the absence of HCV RNA 6 months after the completion of therapy. Once sustained response to HCV is obtained, patients continue to be HCV RNA negative in blood and liver for 5 to 10 years after therapy. Patients who clear the HCV RNA during therapy, but develop viremia after the discontinuation of therapy, are called relapsers.

Side Effects of Therapy

The side effects of ribavirin include hemolytic anemia, birth defects, cough, dyspnea, rash, pruritus, insomnia, and anorexia. Side effects of interferon include flu-like symptoms including headache, fatigue, myalgia, arthralgias, nausea, depression, insomnia, alopecia, leukopenia, thrombocytopenia, hypothyroidism, and retinopathy.

Monitoring Therapy

Pretreatment evaluation includes assessment for baseline fundoscopic exam, liver enzymes, quantitative HCV RNA titer and genotype, TSH, CBC, prothrombin time, serum ANA, pregnancy test, HBV and HIV testing, liver ultrasound, and liver biopsy. An EKG should be done on patients with pre-existing cardiac abnormalities. A pregnancy test should be done, and therapy should not be initiated unless a negative pregnancy test has been obtained. Patients should be monitored for anemia, bone marrow toxicity, pulmonary disorders, pancreatitis, and psychiatric dysfunction.

At 2 and 4 weeks after starting therapy, check a CBC. Perform a pregnancy test, as well as CBC every month during treatment. Serum TSH levels should be undertaken at baseline and at 6 and 12 months of therapy. Fundoscopic exam should be done periodically on an as needed basis.

Quantitative HCV RNA should be performed at 3 months and HCV-qualitative test at 6 months to assess response to therapy. Six months after completion of therapy, a HCV qualitative test should be done to assess for sustained response.

Special Considerations

Treatment should be offered to patients with extrahepatic manifestations of HCV, an anticipated long life span (eg, those younger than 40), and to reduce the risk of potential transmission, such as health care workers who perform invasive procedures, regardless of the results of liver biopsy.

Patients with concurrent hemochromatosis should receive phlebotomy treatment prior to HCV treatment.

About 30% of HIV infected patients also suffer from HCV infection; the progression to cirrhosis in such cases is accelerated. The combination treatment should be considered for patients with relatively preserved immune function and compensated liver disease. Treatment in coinfected patients should be for 1 year regardless of genotype.

Who Should Not Be Treated

People who should not be treated include those with: decompensated cirrhosis, significant psychiatry history or current major depression, active alcoholism or substance abuse, underlying autoimmune disease, uncorrected thyroid disease and significant coronary artery disease, and renal transplantation. Pregnant and nursing mothers, patients less than 18 years of age, or those older than 70 years should also not be treated. Treatment is also not given in cases of WBC less than $3000/mm^3$, platelet count less than $60\,000/mm^3$, and hemoglobin less than $11.0\ g/dl$.

Ribavirin is contraindicated in end-stage kidney disease. Pegylated interferon may be administered to patients undergoing dialysis in reduced doses with close monitoring of therapy.

Patients with Normal Liver Enzymes

Patients who choose not to undergo biopsy or therapy should have liver enzyme testing every year. If the liver enzymes become abnormal, a liver biopsy should be undertaken. Many experts perform liver biopsy in all patients even with normal liver enzymes because 15 to 30% of these patients may have significant changes in the biopsy. The treatment of such patients is controversial.

Follow-Up of Mild Changes on Liver Biopsy

For those patients whose initial liver biopsy shows early stage disease and who were not treated, a repeat liver biopsy that looks for histologic progression may be undertaken in a period of 3 to 5 years.

Screening for HCC

Patients who develop liver cirrhosis as a result of HCV are at an increased risk for developing hepatocellular carcinoma at the rate of 1.4 to 4% per year. Repeat screening with alpha-fetoprotein and a liver ultrasound every 6 months is recommended in such patients. Some experts prefer a CT scan for screening of these patients. These screening strategies are not based on scientific data but on "expert opinion." The benefit of screening has not been established.

Liver Transplantation

Patients with liver cirrhosis due to HCV, including those with hepatocellular carcinoma, should be considered for liver transplantation and should be referred to a liver transplantation center for evaluation if their Child's Pugh score is 8 or greater. Post-transplant viremia occurs in all cases of HCV patients and histologic changes in the allograft can be seen. However, survival is generally good for the first 5 to 8 years after transplantation.

Vaccination

No vaccine is available for HCV.

HCV SCREENING

Screening for HCV is recommended for patients with increased risk for infection including those with history of intravenous drug abuse, who received clotting factors made before 1987, who received blood or organs before July 1992, patients on chronic hemodialysis, patients with evidence of liver disease, or those with evidence of extrahepatic manifestations of HCV.

PREVENTION

Avoiding the risk factors is key to prevention since no vaccination is available.

Sexual Practice

Safe sexual practices are advised for individuals with multiple sex partners. In patients with a stable, monogamous long-term relationship, a change in sexual practices is probably not needed. The decision to use condoms should be left to the infected individual and his or her partner. However, the testing of the sexual partner for HCV infection is advised.

Perinatal Prevention

The perinatal transmission is not associated with the method of delivery and there is no transmission during breastfeeding. There is no need to determine mode of delivery based on a HCV infection. There is no need to avoid pregnancy or breastfeeding. Bottle feeding should be considered if nipples are cracked or bleeding.

PEARLS

○ Most patients with acute hepatitis go on to chronic hepatitis and 20 to 25% go on to cirrhosis.

○ Risk of transmission of hepatitis C via sexual and household exposure is low.

○ Ribavirin is a pregnancy category-X drug and both the patient and his or her sexual partner must not plan on conception during therapy or 6 months after therapy by using two reliable means of contraception.

BIBLIOGRAPHY

Russo MW, Fried MW. Side effects of therapy for chronic HCV. *Gastroenterology*. 2003;124(6):1711-9.

Flamm SL. Chronic HCV virus infection. *JAMA*. 2003;289(18):2413-7.

Chapter
39 *Hepatitis D and E* ▬▬▬▬

HEPATITIS D

Hepatitis D (HDV) is a defective virus that cannot cause disease on its own and can only become pathogenic in the presence of HBV surface antigen. It may occur as an acute coinfection with HBV in a person who was previously healthy or as a super-infection during the course of chronic HBV. Intravenous users are at the highest risk for developing HDV.

Diagnosis

It is diagnosed by detecting HDV antibody and HDV antigen in the serum, which indicates ongoing viral replication. Since this incompetent virus is unable to cause disease in the absence of HBV surface antigen, there is no need for ordering HDV antibody testing in individuals without HBV infection.

HEPATITIS E

Hepatitis E (HEV) is an RNA virus transmitted by via fecal-oral route. As such, it occurs in regions of the world where sanitation standards are poor. It may rarely be seen in the United States, except in patients with recent travel to an endemic area.

Incubation period is 14 to 45 days. Clinical manifestations are the same as in any other acute hepatitis illness. Serum bilirubin and transaminases are elevated. HEV IgG and IgM antibody tests are available from reference laboratories, and can be used to establish the diagnosis in patients with acute non-A, non-B, and non-C hepatitis. Infection is usually acute and clears within a few months. HEV does not cause chronic infection or a carrier state. There is an increased risk of fulminant hepatitis in women who acquire HEV during pregnancy.

PEARLS

○ Hepatitis D is a defective virus and can occur only in the presence of hepatitis B surface antigen.

○ Hepatitis E may lead to fulminant hepatic failure in pregnant females.

BIBLIOGRAPHY

Hyams KC. New perspectives on hepatitis E. *Curr Gastroenterol Rep.* 2002;4(4):302-7.

Chapter 40 *Primary Biliary Cirrhosis*

EPIDEMIOLOGY

Primary biliary cirrhosis (PBC) is a chronic cholestatic liver disease that usually occurs in middle age women. Prevalence estimates vary between 40 and 150 per million.

PATHOGENESIS

PBC is presumed to be an autoimmune disorder. Genetic susceptibility, infections and environmental factors have been implicated. About 50% of the patients are detected in the asymptomatic stage. The hallmark is a granulomatous destruction of the bile ducts with progressive fibrosis and cirrhosis.

CLINICAL FEATURES

Fatigue is present in 70% of the cases. Other symptoms include right upper quadrant abdominal pain, pruritus, portal hypertension with ascites or variceal bleeding, osteoporosis, xanthomata, fat soluble vitamin malabsorption, osteomalacia, and recurrent urinary tract infections.

Associated conditions include hypothyroidism, Sicca syndrome (xerophthalmia, xerostomia, dysphagia, and dyspareunia), CREST syndrome, Raynaud's syndrome, celiac disease, and ulcerative colitis (UC).

DIAGNOSIS

Diagnosis is made by a cholestatic pattern of liver enzymes with an elevated alkaline phosphatase (AP), gammaglutamyl transpeptidase (GGT), along with serum antimitochondrial antibody (AMA), which is positive in over 95% of the cases. Serums ALT/AST are minimally elevated early in course of the disease. Serum ANA and serum smooth muscle antibody (SMA) may be elevated in about one-third of the cases. Less commonly, some patients may be AMA negative with high titers of antinuclear antibody (ANA) or SMA. Serum IgM levels are elevated. Patients with AMA-negative PBC may have elevated IgG but normal IgM levels.

Cholesterol is usually elevated with predominance of HDL fraction, and most experts believe that risk for heart disease is not increased in most patients despite elevated total cholesterol levels.

Imaging Studies

An ultrasound of the liver and biliary system must be done to exclude biliary obstruction, but they are typically normal.

Role of Liver Biopsy

Liver biopsy is not essential in patients with classic biochemical and immunological parameters. Patients with AMA positive, but normal alkaline phosphatase, should have annual liver enzyme testing. Patients with persistent alkaline phosphatase elevation but AMA negative and normal ultrasound should undergo further work-up, including ERCP and liver biopsy, to exclude other causes of cholestasis.

Histology

PBC is divided into four stages. Stage I shows portal hepatitis with inflammatory destruction of bile ducts. Granulomas may be absent. Periportal hepatitis and bile duct proliferation is seen in Stage II, whereas bridging fibrosis manifests in Stage III. Stage IV is classified as cirrhosis. More than one stage can be present at a given time.

PROGRESSION

The progression of PBC is variable, but it is usually a slowly progressive disease. Most asymptomatic patients develop symptoms in 2 to 4 years. Median survival for symptomatic patients is 7 to 10 years, whereas in asymptomatic cases it is 16 years.

TREATMENT

Ursodeoxycholic acid (13.0 to 15.0 mg/kg/d) results in improvement of biochemical parameters including decline in serum cholesterol. It has modest effect on pruritus and the progression of portal hypertension. It is most effective when used in early stages of the disease, where it delays progression to fibrosis. Treatment does not improve fatigue or osteoporosis. Immune-suppressive therapy is not recommended.

Cholestyramine (4.0 to 16.0 g/day) is useful for pruritus but should be taken 2 hours apart from any other medications. Rifampin (150.0 mg PO bid to tid) is effective in some cases, but can be associated with hepatotoxicity. Naltrexone (25.0 to 50.0 mg PO tid) may help in refractory pruritus.

Regular exercise, smoking cessation, plus calcium and vitamin D supplementation is recommended. Consider hormone replacement therapy in postmenopausal patients, preferably using the transdermal route to minimize worsening of cholestasis. Bisphosphonates are recommended in patients with osteoporosis. Fat soluble vitamin supplementation is needed for fat soluble vitamin deficiency.

Liver transplantation is indicated in cases of uncontrolled pruritus, severe osteoporosis and liver failure. PBC may recur in the transplanted liver.

MONITORING

Serum TSH should be measured initially and periodically thereafter. Patients should undergo EGD at the time of diagnosis for screening of varices and then every 3 years until found. Bone mineral density should be measured at time of initial diagnosis and then every 2 years.

CANCER RISK

There is an increased risk for hepatocellular carcinoma. The potential for increase in cancer of the breast is controversial.

PEARLS

○ Primary biliary cirrhosis usually occurs in middle-aged females and 95% of them are positive for AMA.

○ Biliary obstruction must always be excluded in patients suspected of PBC.

BIBLIOGRAPHY

Talwalkar JA, Lindor KD. Primary biliary cirrhosis. *Lancet*. 2003;362(9377):53-61.

Chapter 41 *Primary Sclerosing Cholangitis*

Primary sclerosing cholangitis (PSC) is a chronic progressive cholestatic liver disease.

EPIDEMIOLOGY

It is estimated to occur in 1 to 6 per 100 000 population, and occurs predominantly in men. About 80 to 90% of patients with PSC have UC; however, only about 4% of UC patients develop PSC. The risk of PSC is also increased in Crohn's disease.

PATHOGENESIS

The etiology is multifactorial including genetic predisposition, autoimmune dysfunction, infection, and ischemic injury to the hepatobiliary system. PSC may occur after colectomy for UC, while UC may present for the first time after liver transplantation for PSC.

CLINICAL FEATURES

Most patients are asymptomatic at the time of diagnosis. Symptoms may include fatigue, pruritus, recurrent episodes of fever, chills, night sweats, and right upper quadrant pain. There is increased risk for metabolic bone disease and fractures.

DIAGNOSIS

Laboratory Studies

Liver chemistries reveal cholestatic pattern with the elevation of serum alkaline phosphatase and bilirubin that may fluctuate. Serum AMA is negative. Serum ANA, SMA, and perinuclear antineutrophil cytoplasmic antibody (pANCA) may be positive in 75% of the patients, but are not diagnostic. Similarly, serum IgM and IgG may be elevated.

Imaging Studies

Ultrasound may be normal or may show abnormalities of bile ducts. MRCP may be an alternative to ERCP for the diagnosis of PSC. A CT scan may identify any hepatobiliary malignancy.

Endoscopy

Diagnosis requires an ERCP that shows multifocal strictures and dilations of intrahepatic and extrahepatic bile ducts. About 90% of the patients have both intrahepatic and extrahepatic biliary strictures whereas only 2% have exclusively extrahepatic biliary strictures. If a dominant stricture is identified, brushings should be performed to exclude malignancy.

ERCP may be normal in patients with small duct PSC. These patients have biochemical and histological features similar to PSC, but a better prognosis. Small duct PSC can evolve into a full-blown PSC.

Liver Biopsy

Liver biopsy is not diagnostic; however, prophylactic antibiotics like ciprofloxacin or ampicillin/sulbactam (Unasyn) should be given prior to the procedure. Fibrosis and obliteration of small bile ducts with onion skin appearance is seen. Biopsy findings are usually non-specific and may mimic PBC.

DIFFERENTIAL DIAGNOSIS

It includes PBC, bacterial cholangitis, prior biliary surgery, medications, and AIDS cholangiopathy. Sclerosing pancreato-cholangitis should be considered in patients with pancreatitis but without ulcerative colitis. Such patients have chronic pancreatitis with associated exocrine pancreatic deficiency.

TREATMENT

General Management

Patients with mild pruritus may be treated with warm baths, antihistamines, or phenobarbital, whereas moderate to severe pruritus should be treated with cholestyramine or ursodeoxycholic acid. Ursodeoxycholic acid does not alter the natural course of the disease.

Patients should be screened for fat-soluble vitamin deficiencies and supplementation should be undertaken as necessary. Bone density should be checked at diagnosis and treatment of metabolic bone disease undertaken as necessary.

Endoscopic Therapy

Patients with dominant extrahepatic biliary strictures benefit from endoscopic therapy; however, an ERCP should be performed by a highly experienced endoscopist to exclude cholangiocarcinoma. Surgical therapy for biliary system obstruction should be avoided. Radiological-guided balloon dilatation of strictures or stent placements may also be an option.

Cholelithiasis

Stones in the gallbladder and biliary system may be seen in 30% of patients; however, asymptomatic gallstones are not treated.

Cholangitis

Because of the risk for cholangitis, prophylactic antibiotics should be used prior to any biliary procedure or liver biopsy. Cholangitis, if present, should be treated with antibiotics like ciprofloxacin (500.0 mg IV bid) or ampicillin/sulbactam (Unasyn 2.0 to 3.0 g IV q 6 hours) for 1 week in addition to the relief of biliary obstruction as appropriate placement.

Specific Treatment

Liver transplantation is the treatment of choice. It is curative in 80% of the patients, since recurrence may occur in up to 20% of cases. In some cases, UC may become aggressive after liver transplantation despite immunosuppressive therapy.

Immunosuppressive and anti-inflammatory agents like D-penicillamine, corticosteroids, methotrexate, azathioprine, ursodeoxycholic acid, and tacrolimus do not alter the course of PSC.

Management of Ulcerative Colitis

Proctocolectomy does not improve clinical manifestations or alter the course of PSC and as such should be only undertaken if indicated for UC.

RISK FOR MALIGNANCY

There is increased risk for cholangiocarcinoma. Lifetime risk is 15%, especially in patients with inflammatory bowel disease (IBD) and liver cirrhosis. Cholangiocarcinoma in patients with PSC carries only 10% survival rate over a period of 2 years, and the results of liver transplantation have been disappointing.

Because of increased risk for colon cancer, a surveillance colonoscopy should be undertaken once a diagnosis of UC is established, and at periodic intervals afterwards. Annual surveillance colonoscopy is recommended in patients who have undergone liver transplantation for PSC.

PROGNOSIS

Median survival after diagnosis is 12 years without transplantation. It is worse for patients who are symptomatic at the time of diagnosis. PSC-specific Mayo model predicts survival.

There is a 80 to 90% 5-year survival rate after liver transplantation performed for advanced liver disease. PSC can recur following liver transplantation in up to 20% of cases but is not associated with reduced patient survival.

PEARLS

○ Primary sclerosing cholangitis usually develops in association with inflammatory bowel disease; however, less than 5% of patients with inflammatory bowel disease develop primary sclerosing cholangitis.

○ Liver transplantation is the only effective cure for primary sclerosing cholangitis.

BIBLIOGRAPHY

Chapman RW. The management of primary sclerosing cholangitis. *Curr Gastroenterol Rep.* 2003;5(1):9-17.

42 *Alcoholic Liver Disease*

EPIDEMIOLOGY

Alcoholism is responsible for over half the liver-related mortality in the United States. In addition, it accounts for $3 billion per year in health care costs. The clinical spectrum varies from fatty liver, alcoholic hepatitis, to cirrhosis.

PATHOGENESIS

Fatty liver occurs as a result of a short-term period of alcohol abuse, usually after binge drinking. It is asymptomatic and reversible if abstinence is practiced. While fatty liver is common amongst most people who do binge drinking, advanced liver disease occurs in only a small fraction of patients.

The risk factors for advanced alcoholic liver disease include excessive alcohol consumption of 60.0 to 80.0 g/day for several years. The threshold is lower for women—as low as half of a man's threshold. Women in general are more predisposed to the development of advanced disease even after taking into account the weight adjustment for the dose of alcohol use. This may be related to the relative deficiency of gastric alcohol dehydrogenase, as well as hormonal effects.

Alcoholic hepatitis may occur alone or in patients with liver cirrhosis. Genetic factors have also been implicated. Toxic mediators for liver damage include acetaldehyde (a metabolite of alcohol) and increased oxidative stress.

FATTY LIVER

Patients are usually asymptomatic or may complain of nonspecific symptoms of malaise, fatigue, lethargy, abdominal discomfort, anorexia, and nausea. Hepatomegaly is frequently present; however, the stigmata of chronic liver disease are absent. Except for mild elevations of liver enzymes with predominantly AST and serum bilirubin, the remainder of the laboratory studies is normal.

The diagnosis is usually clinical and biopsy is not required. Biopsy may be undertaken in select cases to determine if advanced liver disease is present. Typically, micro- or macrovesicular steatosis is seen.

Wilson's disease should be excluded in young individuals since it may also show steatosis. Because most patients who habitually drink alcohol do not develop significant liver disease, alcoholic liver disease should be considered a diagnosis of exclusion and other causes of liver disease should be excluded.

Abstinence is the only effective treatment and the condition reverses upon abstinence. About 25% of the patients who continue to abuse alcohol develop advanced alcoholic liver disease.

ALCOHOLIC HEPATITIS

Epidemiology

It occurs in patients with prolonged alcohol use of 60.0 to 80.0 g/day (six to eight drinks per day). Risk factors for viral hepatitis, as well as drug induced and metabolic injury, should be elicited to exclude other diagnoses.

Clinical Features

Patients may be asymptomatic or may present with nonspecific symptoms or symptoms of liver failure. These include fatigue, generalized weakness, anorexia, nausea, vomiting, abdominal discomfort, and in some cases, weight loss. Physical examination shows tachycardia, fever, and hepatosplenomegaly. Prominent abdominal collateral veins, gynecomastia, hypogonadism, palmar erythema, and spider angiomas may be seen. Portal hypertension may supervene in severe cases and patients may have gastrointestinal (GI) bleeding, ascites, and encephalopathy even in the absence of cirrhosis. Patients frequently have concomitant infection such as pneumonia, cellulitis, or spontaneous bacterial peritonitis.

Investigations

Liver enzymes reflect alcoholic patterns with an AST/ALT ratio of greater than 2.0, although a ratio of less than 1.0 may be seen in alcoholic patients in ambulatory settings. Total elevation of AST/ALT is less than 400 IU/L. Alkaline phosphatase may be mildly elevated. Other laboratory results may show macrocytic anemia, leukocytosis, thrombocytopenia, hyperglycemia hyperuricemia, hypertriglyceridemia, ketosis, hypoalbuminemia, and hyperbilirubinemia. Macrocytosis suggests chronic alcohol use assuming hemolysis has been excluded. PT/INR may be elevated.

Diagnosis

It is based upon clinical and laboratory features. Biopsy may be needed to exclude the coexisting or alternate etiologies. For example, many patients have high iron stores, low to low normal ceruloplasmin, and high titers of autoimmune markers; biopsy may be needed to exclude these diagnoses.

Fever, leukocytosis, and leukemoid reaction may be present even in the absence of infection; however, evidence of infection should be sought aggressively.

There is a high prevalence rate of HCV antibody positivity and HCV RNA levels should be measured to confirm HCV infection. Nonalcoholic fatty liver disease (NAFLD) cannot be differentiated from alcoholic hepatitis based on liver biopsy results.

Treatment

Abstinence is the cornerstone of treatment. Clinical and biochemical recovery may take as long as 6 months in patients who have abstained from further drinking.

Patients are frequently malnourished and a diet consisting of 30 to 35 K_{cal}/kg plus 1.1 to 1.4 g/kg of protein should be provided. Vegetable proteins are preferred. The complications such as hepatic encephalopathy, bleeding varices, ascites, hepatorenal syndrome, and infections like spontaneous bacterial peritonitis are treated appropriately.

Most cases of encephalopathy do not require protein restriction; in severe encephalopathy, branched-chain amino acid administration may be considered, although this is controversial.

The role of corticosteroids is controversial, although some benefit may be obtained in patients with severe alcoholic hepatitis. Active GI bleeding or infection usually precludes their use. Recent data suggests that pentoxifylline (Trental) 400.0 mg tid may be of benefit.

Prognosis

Patients may deteriorate despite abstinence. Patients who continue to drink have a 5-year survival of less than 30%.

ALCOHOLIC CIRRHOSIS

About 20% of the patients with prolonged alcohol abuse go on to develop liver cirrhosis.

Clinical Features

The clinical picture depends upon whether hepatic decompensation is present or not. Patients with compensated liver disease who abstain from alcohol may have minimal to no symptoms. Patients who continue to drink or those with decompensated liver disease may complain of fatigue, weakness, weight loss, and anorexia. In addition, the manifestations may reflect complications of chronic liver disease including GI bleeding, ascites, encephalopathy, hepatorenal syndrome, and hepatocellular carcinoma.

A physical exam reveals muscle wasting, peripheral neuropathy, dementia, pedal edema, as well as the stigmata of chronic liver disease including spider angiomata, palmar erythema, ascites, splenomegaly, asterixis, gynecomastia, testicular atrophy, and Dupuytren's contractures.

Investigations

Laboratory studies reveal macrocytic anemia, thrombocytopenia, elevated PT/INR, hyperbilirubinemia, and hypoalbuminemia. An ultrasound or CT scan suggests the presence of liver cirrhosis. Liver biopsy may show micronodular or micro-macronodular cirrhosis.

Treatment

The only specific treatment is liver transplantation. Most transplant centers require at least 6 months of abstinence. Contrary to perception, patients undergoing transplantation for alcoholic liver disease have excellent post-transplantation survival.

Prognosis

It depends upon whether patient maintains abstinence. Patients with compensated cirrhosis who continue to abstain have a greater than 80% 5-year survival rate. However, patients who continue to drink have a less than 30% 5-year survival rate.

Special Situations

1. *Alcohol and HCV*: There is 10-fold higher prevalence of HCV infection in alcoholic patients as compared to the general population. HCV infection in alcoholics tends to have a more aggressive course and worse prognosis compared to those with HCV infection alone. These patients have a much higher risk for hepatocellular carcinoma. Antiviral therapy for HCV is contraindicated in patients who continue to abuse alcohol.

2. *Acetaminophen toxicity*: Alcoholics are also at increased risk for acetaminophen toxicity, even when used at recommended doses. Acetaminophen toxicity can be distinguished by the fact that transaminase elevations are markedly higher, often exceeding 1,000 IU/L. Patients who abuse alcohol should not use acetaminophen.

PEARLS

○ Nonalcoholic fatty liver disease cannot be differentiated from alcoholic fatty liver disease based on clinical and histologic parameters.

○ Only about 20% of patients with prolonged history of alcohol abuse go on to develop cirrhosis.

○ Females have a lower threshold for developing alcoholic liver disease.

BIBLIOGRAPHY

Stewart SF, Day CP. The management of alcoholic liver disease. *J Hepatol.* 2003;38(Suppl 1):S2-13.

Diehl AM. Liver disease in alcohol abusers: clinical perspective. *Alcohol.* 2002;27(1):7-11.

Arteel G, Marsano L, Mendez C, Bentley F, McClain CJ. Advances in alcoholic liver disease. *Best Pract Res Clin Gastroenterol.* 2003;17(4):625-47.

Chapter

43 *Nonalcoholic Fatty Liver Disease*

NAFLD encompasses hepatic steatosis and nonalcoholic steatohepatitis (NASH). NASH is characterized by hepatic histology consistent with alcoholic liver disease (steatosis and inflammation), but without any history of alcohol abuse. The cut-off value for alcohol intake to distinguish between alcoholic and NAFLD is 20.0 to 30.0 g of alcohol per day. Some experts recommend higher thresholds of alcohol intake. Since the likelihood of NAFLD increases with increasing weight, and there is a high prevalence of obesity in American society, NAFLD is a major health care problem with considerable morbidity and mortality.

EPIDEMIOLOGY

In the absence of direct population based studies, the prevalence estimates of NAFLD vary depending upon the criteria used. NAFLD affects 20 to 30% of the population, and 7 to 11% have histologic evidence of NASH.

Risk factors include diabetes mellitus, obesity, hyperlipidemia, and rapid weight loss. Less common risk factors include acute starvation, parenteral nutrition, extensive small bowel resection, drugs (corticosteroids, amiodarone, tamoxifen, perhexilene, chloroquine, diltiazem, estrogens, methotrexate), Wilson's disease, and jejunal diverticulosis.

It should also be suspected in patients with persistent abnormal liver enzymes in whom no other cause can be identified.

PATHOGENESIS

The initiating factor is insulin resistance leading to steatosis and possibly steatohepatitis. An oxidative injury due to other factors like hepatic iron, leptin, antioxidant deficiency, and intestinal bacteria may be involved in transformation of steatosis to steatohepatitis.

EVALUATION

Patients at risk for NAFLD should have serum ALT checked on a regular basis. If it is normal, observation should be continued. If the ALT is elevated, liver disease should be suspected and further evaluation undertaken. In some cases, NAFLD, including NASH, may be present despite normal ALT levels.

Nonalcoholic Fatty Liver Disease vs Alcoholic Liver Disease

The clues that suggest alcoholic liver disease, especially amongst the hospitalized patients, include the fact that alcoholic patients are sicker, have elevated serum bilirubin, and have a AST/ALT ratio is greater than 2.0. An AST to ALT ratio less than 1.0 can be seen in alcoholic patients in ambulatory settings.

Exclusion of Alternate Diagnosis

Alternate etiologies for chronic liver disease should be excluded including the possibility of alcohol abuse. Abstinence should be recommended to patients who abuse alcohol. In the absence of history of alcohol abuse and any other alternate diagnosis, an imaging study is performed. Liver ultrasound cannot distinguish between fatty liver, steatohepatitis, or fibrosis. A CT scan cannot distinguish between steatosis and steatohepatitis, and can not assess the severity of fibrosis. MRI is expensive and has similar limitations.

In the presence of fatty liver on an imaging study, and after exclusion of other etiologies (viral hepatitis, hemochromatosis, Wilson's disease, AIH, alpha$_1$ antitrypsin deficiency, and primary biliary cirrhosis), a liver biopsy should be considered after assessment of risk vs benefits.

A liver biopsy shows macrovesicular or microvesicular steatosis and/or steatohepatitis. It remains the standard for diagnosis.

To Biopsy or Not?

Whether or not a liver biopsy should be preformed in all cases is controversial. A liver biopsy is the only way of establishing the diagnosis of NAFLD and differentiating steatosis from NASH. Opponents argue that NAFLD is generally a benign disease with a good outcome. In addition, there is no effective therapy for it, while there are risks associated with the liver biopsy.

Proponents argue that liver biopsy has the potential to change the diagnosis and alter the frequency of monitoring the labs and treatment recommendations in significant number of patients.

Potential for a low threshold for liver biopsy should be considered for patients with stigmata of chronic liver disease, splenomegaly, cytopenia, abnormal iron studies, diabetes, and/or significant obesity in an individual over the age of 45.

PROGNOSIS

NAFLD is usually a chronic disorder, and liver insufficiency does not occur in the absence of cirrhosis or rapid weight loss. Prognosis can be determined based on hepatic histology that can be classified into four groups:

1. Fatty liver or steatosis alone.
2. Fatty liver and scattered inflammation.
3. Fatty liver and ballooning degeneration.
4. Fatty liver, ballooning degeneration, plus Mallory bodies or pericellular fibrosis.

There is a greater risk for development of cirrhosis in groups 3 and 4. Fatty liver alone can occasionally progress to steatohepatitis especially following rapid weight loss.

MANAGEMENT

Patients who are overweight with a body mass index (BMI) greater than 25 kg/m^2 should receive weight loss counseling with a target of 10% weight loss at a rate of 1.0 to 2.0 lbs/week. Weight loss greater than 2.0/week can worsen NAFLD and even cause subacute liver failure.

Both a reduction of caloric intake and saturated fat, as well as reducing total fats to less than 30%, is recommended. A regular exercise program may be helpful. Patients with a BMI greater than 35.0 kg/m^2 and NAFLD should be considered for aggressive weight reduction including bariatric surgery. Tight glucose control should be maintained in diabetic patients.

Medical therapy for weight loss may include diet drugs including phentermine, sibutramine, and orlistat. While weight loss in obese subjects is overall beneficial, its usefulness in NAFLD has not been established. Other drugs commonly used (but of unproven value) include vitamin E and ursodeoxycholic acid.

The use of drugs to lower insulin resistance, including metformin and thiazolidendiones, should be considered investigational. Probiotics may help minimize exposure to endogenous intestinal factors that promote hepatic inflammation.

PEARLS

- ○ Nonalcoholic fatty liver disease is not always a benign disease and can progress to cirrhosis and liver failure.
- ○ Patients who are overweight or diabetic should be assessed for the possibility of nonalcoholic fatty liver disease.
- ○ Alternate diagnosis should be excluded before attributing the clinical or diagnostic abnormalities to nonalcoholic fatty liver disease.
- ○ Liver biopsy establishes the diagnosis of nonalcoholic fatty liver disease and provides prognosis.

BIBLIOGRAPHY

Sanyal AJ. AGA technical review on nonalcoholic fatty liver disease. *Gastroenterology*. 2002;123:1705.

Chapter

44 *Drug-Induced Liver Disease*

EPIDEMIOLOGY

Over 600 medications are known to cause liver injury. Drugs are the cause for less than 5% of hospital admissions for jaundice and about 15% of cases of fulminant hepatic failure.

PATHOGENESIS

The spectrum of drug-induced liver injury varies widely and may mimic any type of liver disease. The risk usually increases with age, and women tend to be more susceptible. The injury pattern may be classified as hepatocellular, cholestatic, or mixed hepatocellular/cholestatic.

PATHOLOGY

Acute microvesicular steatosis is caused by aspirin, ketoprofen, valproate, tetracycline, didanosine, zidovudine, and L-asparaginase.

Macrovesicular steatosis manifests from injury due to tamoxifen, alcoholic hepatitis, methotrexate, corticosteroids, and amiodarone.

Acute hepatitis occurs due to acitretin, acetaminophen, acetohexamide, amphetamines (especially ecstasy), celecoxib, piroxicam, cocaine, INH, dantrolene, nitrofurantoin, anesthetics (halothane, enflurane, methoxyflurane, isoflurane), glyburide, M-Dopa, diclofenac, sulfonamides, phenytoin, disulfiram, histamine-2 receptor antagonists, niacin, omeprazole, beta-blockers (acebutolol, labetalol), calcium channel blockers (nifedipine, verapamil, diltiazem), fluconazole, and ketoconazole.

Chronic drug-induced hepatitis is uncommon. It usually starts as acute hepatitis and continued exposure leads to chronic changes and even fibrosis and cirrhosis. Common offenders include M-Dopa, nitrofurantoin, methotrexate, hypervitaminosis A, amiodarone, oxyphenisatin, perhexiline, trazodone, diclofenac, INH, dantrolene, etretinate, acetaminophen, sulfonamides, salicylates, and cimetidine.

Granulomatous hepatitis occurs as a result of M-Dopa, allopurinol, carbamazepine, phenylbutazone, hydralazine, quinidine, procainamide, sulfonamides, nitrofurantoin, diltiazem, gold, chlorpromazine, phenytoin, and quinine. Liver enzymes reflect acute hepatitis with or without cholestasis.

Cholestatic picture may be seen with M-Dopa, niacin, androgens, chlorpropamide, tolbutamide, glipizide, tolazamide, sulindac, oral contraceptives, chlorpromazine, piroxicam, flucloxacillin, cyclosporine, propylthiouracil, methimazole, erythromycin, and tetracycline.

A mixed cholestatic-hepatitis-type picture may be seen with tricyclic antidepressants, amoxicillin, ampicillin, carbamazepine, H_2RAs, nitrofurantoin, quinidine, sulfa drugs, sulindac, naproxen, acetohexamide, glyburide, allopurinol, azathioprine, carbamazepine, chlorpromazine, terbinafine, erythromycin, clavulanic acid, griseofulvin, ketoconazole, tamoxifen, warfarin, ibuprofen, and ACE-inhibitors.

Bile duct injury superimposed on cholestasis occurs due to carbamazepine, dextroproxyphene, chlorpromazine, and flucloxacillin. Patients present as cholangitis. An ERCP will help exclude biliary obstruction.

Chronic cholestasis with biliary strictures is a side effect of intralesional therapy using formalin for hydatid cysts and floxuridine used for metastatic colorectal cancer. Flucloxacillin also causes cholestasis with vanishing bile duct syndrome, which mimics sclerosing cholangitis.

DRUG-INDUCED VASCULAR INJURY

It may manifest as veno-occlusive disease, peliosis hepatis, noncirrhotic portal hypertension, and nodular regenerative hyperplasia. One type may evolve into other.

Veno-occlusive disease affects terminal hepatic venules and veins. It occurs 2 to 10 weeks after starting cytotoxic therapy with vincristine, 6-thioguanine, busulfan, dactinomycin, azathioprine, doxorubicin, pyrrolizidine, and mitomycin. Patients with bone marrow transplants are particularly vulnerable. Patients present with right upper quadrant pain, hepatomegaly, jaundice, and edema. Serum transaminases may be normal or elevated. Imaging studies show large vessels as patent. Biopsy is frequently required for diagnosis. Patients may rapidly progress to liver failure.

Peliosis hepatitis is characterized by small venular lakes in the liver due to sinusoidal injury caused by treatment with oral contraceptives and anabolic steroids. Patients may be asymptomatic or may develop bleeding and liver failure.

Budd-Chiari syndrome occurs with oral contraceptives.

DRUG-INDUCED NEOPLASIA

Nodular regenerative hyperplasia occurs due to anticancer agents like azathioprine. Patients present with manifestations of portal hypertension. Wedge liver biopsy is required for diagnosis. It shows regenerative nodules without fibrosis. Prognosis varies from complete recovery to progression to veno-occlusive disease.

Hepatic adenomas can occur due to exposure to oral contraceptives and anabolic steroids. The risk for adenoma increases over 100-fold after 5 years of therapy with oral contraceptives. Although usually asymptomatic, they may cause abdominal discomfort due to hepatomegaly. Large adenomas may bleed or rupture and surgery may be needed. Adenomas usually regress after stopping therapy but tend to recur during pregnancy.

Angiosarcoma is caused by vinyl chloride, arsenic, anabolic steroids, and thorostat dye.

EXAMPLES OF HEPATOTOXIC DRUGS

1. *Acetaminophen*: It is a common cause of adult poisoning, both intentional and iatrogenic. Liver injury occurs due to a toxic metabolite, N-acetyl-p-benzoquinone. Patients with a history of alcohol abuse and liver cirrhosis are particularly vulnerable. Nonalcoholics without liver disease can easily tolerate up to 7.5 g/day of acetaminophen. Although some patients may be able to tolerate 20.0 to 25.0 g, death can occur at doses as low as 10.0 g/day. Rumack-Matthew nomogram is used to direct management. N-acetylcysteine is a specific antidote and may be of help even after liver injury has occurred.

2. *Amiodarone*: Abnormal liver tests occur in 80% patients. The drug accumulates in lysosomes and inhibits lysosomal phospholipases. Clinically significant toxicity is related to duration of treatment and not the dose. Iodine in amiodarone makes liver appear opaque on CT and is not significant. Cirrhosis occurs in 15 to 50% cases. Liver biopsy is needed for diagnosis. In mild cases, lab abnormalities may resolve in a few weeks after cessation while severe cases have bad outcome. Routine liver test monitoring is recommended but is of unproven benefit.

3. *Chlorpromazine*: It causes cholestatic hepatitis 1 to 6 weeks after starting treatment. Insignificant liver enzyme abnormalities occur in up to half of the patients. Toxicity is not dose-related. Most patients recover completely after drug cessation.

4. *Dantrolene*: It causes acute hepatocellular injury. Check liver enzyme levels every 2 weeks. If tests are normal, and the patient is responding, continue treatment. Discontinue treatment if liver enzymes become abnormal.

5. *Diclofenac*: Acute or chronic hepatitis occurs with or without cholestasis. Warn patients about possible toxicity. Recovery occurs usually after stopping therapy, although fulminant hepatitis and even death may occur.

6. *Didanosine*: Fulminant liver failure with severe lactic acidosis may occur after 10 to 15 weeks of therapy. Biopsy shows microvesicular fatty changes with cholestasis. Monitor symptoms, AST/ALT, PT/INR, and serum bicarbonate during first 4 months of therapy.

7. *Etretinate*: Liver enzymes become abnormal in 25% cases and may resolve on dose reduction. Acute or chronic hepatitis may

occur. Monitor ALT. If levels exceed twice the normal limit, do a liver biopsy or discontinue the drug.

8. *Halothane hepatitis*: It occurs rarely, although the risk increases with repeated exposure. Patients present within 2 weeks after exposure with fever, nausea, vomiting, abdominal pain, arthralgias, malaise, jaundice, and even altered mental status. Liver chemistries reflect hepatocellular injury (AST/ALT 500 to 1000 IU/L). There is no role for corticosteroids or exchange transfusions in management. Patients with fulminant hepatitis usually die without liver transplantation.

9. *INH or isoniazid*: Potential for injury increases with age and is not dose-related. Risk is increased among slow acetylators, alcoholics, as well as those taking rifampin, and pyrazinamide. The risk of INH hepatitis is 0.3% for those younger than 35, and as high as 2.3% above the age of 50. INH hepatitis preceded by prodromal symptoms may develop 1 week to 6 months after starting treatment. Death may occur especially if INH is continued after onset of symptoms. Only a 1-month supply of INH should be provided at any one time. Watch for clinical signs and symptoms of toxicity. Check liver enzymes every month, although it may not prevent toxicity in all cases. Mild liver enzyme elevations occur in one-third of the cases within first 10 weeks but resolve spontaneously. Reevaluate the risk and benefits of continuation of treatment if ALT persists above 100 IU/L. The drug should be withdrawn if the transaminases are greater than 3-fold in patients with symptoms. INH should also be withdrawn in patients with elevations greater than 5-fold irrespective of symptoms.

10. *L-asparaginase*: It causes microvesicular steatosis but liver failure may ensue.

11. *Methotrexate (MTX)*: Carries low risk of hepatic injury (more in patients with psoriasis than rheumatoid arthritis). Baseline laboratory tests including CBC, AST/ALT, serum albumin, bilirubin, and viral hepatitis profile should be obtained prior to therapy. Pretreatment liver biopsy is done in patients with abnormal liver tests, history of alcohol abuse and presence of HBV or HCV. Some experts recommend an index biopsy in all psoriatic patients at 2 to 4 months after starting treatment. Check serum AST/ALT and albumin at 4 to 6 week intervals.

In patients with RA, a liver biopsy is done if over half of the tests performed over a 1 year period are abnormal. Re-evaluate the risk versus the benefits of therapy and biopsy if AST/ALT exceed 3-fold. A repeat biopsy in RA is done as indicated by liver test abnormalities. Many experts perform liver biopsy at every 2 to 3 years or every 1.5 g of cumulative dose.

In psoriasis patients without risk factors, a liver biopsy is usually done after cumulative 1.0 to 1.5 g of MTX. It is repeated at 3.0 and 4.0 g of the cumulative dose. In patients with risk factors, first biopsy is done after 2 to 4 months of therapy, then at 1.0 to1.5 g, 3.0 g, and 4.0 g.

Patients with Grade I and II liver injury on histology can continue the drug. For Grade III-A, biopsy is repeated at 6 months. MTX should be stopped for liver injury Grades III-B and IV with close follow-up, including a consideration for a follow-up biopsy for monitoring.

12. *M-Dopa*: Liver injury occurs more amongst women and usually manifests within 2 to 8 weeks after starting therapy. Liver enzymes should be monitored every month for first 4 months.

13. *Niacin*: It causes a mixed pattern of liver injury and the toxicity is dose dependent. Toxicity is most common with the use of slow release preparations of niacin. Liver enzymes should be monitored and the drug discontinued if the enzymes are persistently elevated.

14. *Nitrofurantoin*: The toxicity is dose dependent. Patients usually present with mildly abnormal liver enzymes. Cholestatic pattern is more common than hepatocellular injury. Onset is within a few days to few weeks after starting therapy and manifests as fever, rash and eosinophilia. Chronic active hepatitis, usually in women, may develop in patients treated for greater than 6 months. There is a marked increase in ALT/AST, gamma globulins, along with a positive ANA in 20% of cases. Significant liver dysfunction and liver failure may occur and is associated with a high mortality of up to 20%. There is no specific treatment. Corticosteroids are not beneficial even when there is autoimmune pattern of hepatitis. Routine liver enzyme monitoring is not helpful.

15. *Phenytoin*: It may cause allergic hepatitis, granulomatous liver disease, and even fulminant liver failure. Initial mild elevations of liver enzymes occur in majority of patients as an adaptive response. After a lag period of 2 to 8 weeks, a pseudomononucleosis-like syndrome develops and patients present with fever, rash, pharyngitis, lymphadenopathy, and eosinophilia. Death occurs in 10 to 40% of patients with severe injury.

16. *Pyrazinamide*: Liver injury is increased among those taking INH or rifampin. Monitor ALT throughout pyrazinamide treatment.

17. *Sulindac*: It usually presents with fever, rash, and constitutional symptoms. Steven-Johnson syndrome may occur. Labs show a cholestatic pattern of liver injury.

18. *Tacrine*: Injury is mild in most cases. Monitor ALT every week for 3 months and discontinue the drug if ALT levels exceed three times the normal limits.

19. *Valproate*: Toxicity occurs more commonly in children. Symptoms occur after lag period of 4 to 12 weeks. Clinical presentation mimics Reye's syndrome. Neurologic features may predominate over hepatic problems. Liver enzyme abnormalities occur in 40% patients and do not predict toxicity. A CT scan may show small liver. Treatment is supportive. Do not use valproate in combination with other antiseizure agents in children less than 3 years of age. Key is to watch for signs and symptoms of possible toxicity during first 6 months of treatment.

20. *Vitamin A*: Toxicity usually occurs due to excessive intake over months to years. Manifestations range from asymptomatic lab abnormalities to fatal liver failure. There is yellow discoloration of skin, neurological and psychological disturbances, hypercalcemia, along with hepatomegaly. The plasma vitamin A level may be normal. Resolution usually occurs after withdrawal of vitamin A. Injury may continue to worsen in some cases.

PEARLS

○ Mild liver enzyme elevation may represent an adaptive response to therapy and not necessarily drug toxicity.

○ Drug-induced liver injury may mimic any and all types of liver diseases and more than one pattern may be seen due to any drug.

BIBLIOGRAPHY

Lee WM. Drug-induced hepatotoxicity. *N Engl J Med*. 2003;349(5):474-85.

Chapter
45 *Autoimmune Hepatitis* ▬▬▬

AIH is a chronic hepatitis of uncertain etiology characterized by considerable heterogeneity in immunological markers, histological findings, and clinical features.

EPIDEMIOLOGY

It may occur at any age, including during infancy and older individuals, but is usually diagnosed before the age of 40. Over 70% of the cases occur in females.

CLASSIFICATION

It is classified into Type I and Type II, based on the type of antibodies present.

Type I AIH

It is the classic form of AIH in which patients are positive for ANA and/or anti-SMA. Antibodies to soluble liver antigens (SLA) occur in about 10% of the patients. Antineutrophilic cytosplasmic antibody may also be seen. On rare occasions antimitochondrial antibodies may also be positive.

Type II AIH

This type of AIH is characterized by antibodies to liver, kidney microsomes (LKM-I), and is generally seen in children and young adults.

Type IA AIH

Ten percent of patients with Type I AIH have antibodies to soluble liver antigens/liver pancreas (anti-SLA/LP). Some experts categorize this as Type III AIH.

Variants of AIH

Various variants of AIH have been described including overlap syndrome with PBC, PSC, viral hepatitis, and autoimmune cholangitis.

SIGNIFICANCE OF SEROLOGIES

The antibodies ANA, SMA, and anti-LKM-I are useful only for diagnostic purposes. They do not have any pathogenic properties and do not correlate with disease activity or response to treatment.

PATHOGENESIS

There is a host predisposition to high immune-reactivity which is genetically determined and triggered by an unknown agent like infection or medication. Further pathogenic mechanisms are unclear. Defective T cell and/or B-cell function may be involved. Another theory proposes a cellular form of cytotoxicity in association with HLA Class II antigens. AIH is probably a polygenic disorder and no single susceptibility gene has been identified.

CLINICAL MANIFESTATIONS

The spectrum varies from asymptomatic patients to fulminant hepatic failure. Some patients may have constitutional symptoms like easy fatigability, lethargy, malaise, anorexia, abdominal discomfort, and pruritus.

Similarly, physical examination may be normal or patients may exhibit hepatosplenomegaly, jaundice, and stigmata of chronic liver disease. Patients with acute presentation are frequently found to have cirrhosis upon biopsy suggesting a preceding subclinical phase prior to presentation.

COMPLICATIONS

The complications of AIH are similar to that of any other chronic liver disease including portal hypertension, hepatic encephalopathy, and increased risk for hepatocellular carcinoma.

LABORATORY TESTS

Liver enzymes usually reflect a hepatocellular pattern with serum aminotransferases (ALT/AST) levels disproportionately greater than the elevation in bilirubin and alkaline phosphatase. However, in some cases, a cholestatic picture with high bilirubin levels may be seen; extra-hepatic obstruction, viral hepatitis, and primary biliary cirrhosis, as well as overlap syndromes, must be excluded in such cases. Elevation of serum globulins especially gamma globulins associated with appropriate circulating autoantibodies help establish the diagnosis in most cases.

HISTOLOGY

Liver biopsy shows portal and lobular inflammatory infiltrate, piecemeal necrosis, fibrosis, and even cirrhosis. Although not diagnostic, histologic features are useful in establishing the diagnosis and grading severity of disease.

Bile duct changes such as cholangitis and ductopenia are rare, and when prominent raise the possibility of an alternate diagnosis. Portal plasma cell infiltrate is typically seen. Fibrosis is evident in most cases, and if left untreated, cirrhosis invariably develops.

DIAGNOSIS

No single test is pathognomic and requires exclusion of other chronic liver diseases like chronic viral hepatitis, drug-induced liver disease, hemochromatosis, Wilson's disease, etc. Since the histologic findings are nonspecific, the ultimate diagnosis is made by the total picture of clinical features, presence of circulating antibodies, hyper-gammaglobulinemia, liver histology, as well as the response to immune-suppressive agents. Presence of other autoimmune diseases like hemolytic anemia, idiopathic thrombocytopenic purpura, Type I diabetes mellitus, thyroiditis, and IBD favor the possibility for AIH.

International diagnostic scoring system for the diagnosis of AIH has a sensitivity of 97 to 100%. While the scoring system may not be necessary in typical cases, it may be useful in atypical cases and low threshold should be used to utilize it for an accurate diagnosis.

Features favoring AIH (the relative score in parenthesis) are female sex (+2); alkaline phosphatase to AST ratio <1.5 (+2); elevated serum gammaglobulins (+1 to +3); serum ANA, SMA or LKMI (+1 to +3); negative viral hepatitis markers (+3); negative medication history (+1); average alcohol intake less than 25.0 g/day (+2); supportive histologic findings (+1 to +5); concurrent immune disease (+2); novel antibodies (+2); HLA DR3 or DR4 (+1); response to steroids (+2); and relapse after withdrawal (+3). Features arguing against AIH include alkaline phosphatase to AST ratio >3.0 (-2), positive AMA (-4), positive drug history (-4), alcohol intake >60.0 g/day (-2), and a lack of supportive or contradictory histologic findings (-3 to −11). An aggregate score greater than 15 prior to treatment establishes the diagnosis of AIH, whereas score of 10 to 15 implies probable diagnosis. An aggregate score after treatment greater than 17 establishes the diagnosis, whereas 12 to 17 makes it probable.

DIFFERENTIAL DIAGNOSIS

AIH in its acute stage needs to be differentiated from various forms of viral hepatitis. Measurement of HCV RNA level in the blood is required for excluding HCV because false positive HCV antibodies are seen in AIH. In addition, patients with chronic HCV may show autoantibodies to rheumatoid factor and cryoglobulins. Rarely both HCV and AIH may be seen in the same individual. About 5% of patients with chronic HCV may have moderate elevations of ANA or SMA titers greater than 1:100. The two may be distinguished by further studies on anti-LKM I antibodies since the anti-LKM I antibodies in HCV are targeted at different epitopes of cytochrome P450 than those seen in AIH.

Differentiating AIH from a patient with nonalcoholic steatohepatitis when ANA is positive may be difficult. Typically gamma-globulin level is elevated in AIH, while it is normal in nonalcoholic steatohepatitis; the biopsy plays an important role, as steatosis is not typically seen in AIH. Serum ferritin can be raised in AIH; as such, hemochromatosis should be excluded by hepatic iron concentration and index.

Drugs can produce a clinical picture similar to autoimmune hepatitis. Possible offenders include minocycline, nitrofurantion, isoniazid, hydralazine, carbamazepine, propylthiouracil, and procainamide. Discontinuation of the drug may result in resolution of the injury, progression to chronic liver disease, or even fulminant liver failure can occur despite cessation of the drug.

OVERLAP SYNDROMES

The prevalence of AMA is 5 to 10% in the general population, thus biopsy is the key to diagnosis. About 25% of AIH patients have a bile duct lesion but not like PBC or PSC. Patients with AIH compatible histology and a positive AMA should be treated as AIH.

Patients with histology compatible with PBC without AMA or other autoimmune markers may be called AMA-negative PBC. In such cases, it should be treated as PBC. In patients with a mixed biochemical picture, the treatment may be a combination of immune-suppressive drugs plus ursodeoxycholic acid.

TREATMENT

Criteria for Treatment

Treatment results in improvement of clinical and histological features as well as survival in patients with severe AIH. However, indications for treatment in mild cases remain a matter of debate.

Absolute indications for treatment include symptomatic disease, serum AST/ALT equal or greater than 10-fold of upper normal limit, serum AST/ALT equal or greater than 5-fold of upper normal limit with a total globulin level equal or greater than twice of normal, or bridging necrosis or multiacinar necrosis on histological examination. In addition, most children with a diagnosis of AIH should undergo treatment.

Relative Indications

In the absence of biochemical and histologic indications outlined above, the role of treatment is controversial. Relative indications include constitutional symptoms like severe malaise and fatigue, arthralgias, with serum AST/ALT and/or gammaglobulin levels less than those in the absolute criteria, or presence of interface hepatitis on a liver biopsy. Patients with nonspecific symptoms without a firm laboratory diagnosis may be followed clinically.

When is Treatment Not Required?

Effect of therapy on asymptomatic individuals with mild (<5 times times normal) elevation of transaminases is unknown even if biochemical and histologic diagnosis is firm. Treatment is not indicated in patients with inactive cirrhosis, pre-existing co-morbid conditions, or drug intolerance.

Treatment Regimens

The preferred treatment is a combination therapy of a prednisone starting at 30.0 mg/day with azathioprine starting with 50.0 to 100.0 mg/day. The prednisone is gradually tapered to 15.0 mg/day by week 4 followed by a maintenance of 5.0 to 10.0 mg/day until end point. Azathioprine is continued at 50.0/150.0 mg/day. Patients should be monitored for drug related side effects.

Initial single drug treatment may be undertaken using prednisone alone starting with 60.0 mg/day of week 1, taper to 40.0 mg/day of week 2, 30.0 mg/day on week 3 and 4, and then continue with 20.0 mg/day maintenance dose until end point. This regimen may be preferable in patients with cytopenia, pregnancy, and malignancy. Some experts recommend starting monotherapy with prednisone starting at 40.0 mg/day. Doses of prednisone greater than 40.0 mg/day are associated with side effects of osteoporosis and uncontrolled diabetes.

Treatment Endpoints

Endpoints of initial treatment include a remission, treatment failure, incomplete response, and drug toxicity.

Remission

Remission is characterized by disappearance of symptoms with normalization of serum bilirubin and gammaglobulins plus serum ALT levels at less than twice the normal level with minimal or no inflammation on biopsy. A liver biopsy must always be done before withdrawing medications to establish remission, since inflammation may be present in over half the patients who satisfy biochemical criteria. Histologic resolution lags behind biochemical improvement, thus a liver biopsy should be done at least 6 months or more after the liver enzymes and gammaglobulin levels have normalized.

Withdrawing Treatment

The preferred option is to reduce prednisone while maintaining azathioprine if ALT levels fall to less than a 2-fold elevation; continue to taper further by 2.5 to 5.0 mg every 1 to 3 months if ALT remains less than 1.5-fold. Continue the lowest dose of prednisone plus azathioprine required to keep ALT less than 1.5-fold. Discontinue prednisone and azathioprine if ALT levels remain normal for 1 to 2 years. Another strategy is to withdraw prednisone over a 6-week period and discontinue azathioprine with regular monitoring for relapse.

Relapse

Relapse occurs in 83% after initial treatment and 47% after repeat treatment. As such, a liver biopsy should be done approximately 6 months after resolution of clinical and laboratory abnormalities and prior to drug withdrawal. Liver biopsy should be done any time a patient deteriorates despite compliance with treatment.

Incomplete Responders

In patients exhibiting incomplete response by some parameter, no improvement in clinical or histological features, or no remission after 3 years of therapy, the medication dose should be reduced to the lowest possible level to prevent worsening since some patients may require indefinite treatment. In patients exhibiting drug toxicity, a reduction in dose or discontinuation of the drug may be needed depending on the severity of the toxicity.

Treatment Failures

In patients exhibiting treatment failure by worsening clinical, laboratory, and histological features despite drug compliance, options include starting high dose prednisone 60.0 mg/day or prednisone 30.0 to 60.0 mg/day plus high dose azathioprine 150.0 mg/day for at least 1 month. Then gradually reduce the doses until a standard maintenance dose is achieved. Low threshold should be maintained for referral to a transplant center.

Drug Precautions

Warn patients about potential for weight gain and to maintain (and not increase) caloric intake. Calcium and vitamin D supplementation reduces the risk for osteoporosis. Monitor CBC every 3 months during azathioprine treatment. Screen stools for parasites especially Strongyloides prior to prednisone therapy, particularly if peripheral eosinophilia is present. Screen annually for diabetes, cataract, bone density, and systemic blood pressure.

Fulminant Hepatic Failure

This may occur rarely as the presenting manifestation and patients needs to be transferred to transplant center. Autoimmune markers are usually not available immediately and diagnosis is frequently made on clinical grounds.

Recurrent AIH Post-Transplantation

As many as 40 to 70% of patients have recurrence of AIH within 5 years after transplantation. Recurrence is treated with standard immune-suppressive regimen. Rarely will retransplantation be required.

Young Patients

Chances of complete remission are less and, as such, the need for eventual liver transplantation is greater. There is a higher likelihood of overlap with PSC. Biliary imaging using MRCP should be done to exclude PSC, which may require ursodeoxycholic acid in addition to standard AIH therapy.

Pregnancy

Although pregnancy is rare in untreated AIH females, fertility is restored with effective therapy. Prednisone and azathioprine appear not to have fetotoxity although reduced doses may be required during pregnancy. Flare-up during pregnancy and after delivery may occur rarely. EGD should be performed during second trimester to look for varices and treat with nonselective beta-blocker if present. A short second stage of labor is the goal in the presence of portal hypertension, otherwise a Caesarian section should be performed.

PROGNOSIS

There are no clinical features at presentation that predict a response to treatment. Most people will show improvement in at least one parameter within 2 weeks of therapy. Patients in whom there is no improvement in hyperbilirubinemia within 2 weeks of therapy should be assessed for liver transplantation.

Patients have a normal life expectancy over a period of 20 years if effectively treated. Over one-third of the patients develop cirrhosis despite treatment. Fifty percent of the patients who achieve remission, relapse within 6 months after stopping treatment and 70% relapse within 3 years.

The 5-year survival rate after liver transplantation is over 85%.

PEARLS

○ International scoring system should be used for accurate diagnosis.

○ Not every patient with the diagnosis of AIH requires treatment.

○ Patients with overlap syndromes are managed based on the predominant features.

BIBLIOGRAPHY

Medina J, Garcia-Buey L, Moreno-Otero R. Review article: immunopathogenetic and therapeutic aspects of autoimmune hepatitis. *Aliment Pharmacol Ther.* 2003;17(1):1-16.

Czaja AJ. Treatment of autoimmune hepatitis. *Semin Liver Dis.* 2002;22(4): 365-78.

Durazzo M, Premoli A, Fagoonee S, Pellicano R. Overlap syndromes of autoimmune hepatitis: what is known so far. *Dig Dis Sci.* 2003; 48(3):423-30.

Chapter
46 *Hemochromatosis*

Hereditary hemochromatosis (HH) is characterized by excessive absorption of iron resulting in its deposition in the liver, heart, pancreas, skin, joints, and pituitary. This leads to long-term sequelae including liver cirrhosis, hepatocellular carcinoma, diabetes, congestive heart failure, bronze pigmentation of the skin, arthritis, and hypogonadism.

EPIDEMIOLOGY

HH is the most common genetic disease with a prevalence of one in 200 to one in 500 persons in population of Northern European descent. The prevalence of homozygous C282Y mutation is between 1:200 to 1:300, whereas about 10% of the people of Northern European descent may be heterozygous carriers. Approximately 5 to 7% of the patients are compound heterozygous. The inheritance follows an autosomal recessive pattern.

PATHOGENESIS

The pathogenesis involves mutation of the hemochromatosis gene called HFE. The two common forms of mutations are C282Y and H63D. There is increased iron absorption because of increase in expression or activity of iron transport mechanisms similar to that seen in iron deficiency anemia.

Phenotypic expression is seen in subjects who are homozygous to C282Y mutation or compound heterozygous for C282Y/H63D mutations. Clinical significance of homozygous H63D is unknown. About 3 to 10% of patients with hemochromatosis are heterozygous for either C282Y or H63D mutations suggesting that these patients are compound heterozygous with these already identified mutations and some additional as yet unidentified mutations. A small percentage of HH patients lack either of the identified mutations. While a single heterozygous mutation often causes elevated transferrin saturation, it is usually not associated with end-organ damage In contrast, some patients with compound heterozygous mutation may develop end-organ damage. Up to 15% of African Americans may have iron overload without any of the typical HFE mutations.

CLINICAL FEATURES

Patients are usually asymptomatic if HH is detected early or they may have nonspecific symptoms like mild weakness, easy fatigue, abdominal pain, arthralgias, and myalgias. Patients with advanced disease may present with manifestations of diabetes mellitus, liver cirrhosis, CHF, impotence and arthritis. It takes about 30 to 60 years for the development of advanced end organ damage. The risk for hepatocellular carcinoma in HH is increased 200-fold.

DIAGNOSIS

Screening Tests

These include serum iron, total iron binding capacity or transferrin saturation, and ferritin. Transferrin saturation greater than 45% in a fasting state should prompt confirmatory tests including genetic testing and biopsy. Serum ferritin greater than 200.0 ng/mL is sensitive but nonspecific. The negative predictive value of combined transferrin saturation less than 45% and serum ferritin less than 200 is greater than 97%.

Genetic Tests

Genetic testing involves testing for both mutations of HFE gene. Only C282Y homozygotes and compound heterozygotes C282Y/H63D are considered diagnostic.

Role of Liver Biopsy

Liver biopsy is not essential in young patients (<40 years) who are found to have normal liver enzymes and are diagnosed as HH by elevated transferrin saturation plus genetic testing (C282Y homozygous or compound heterozygous). Patients with serum ferritin less than 1000.0 ng/mL and without any history of alcohol abuse, chronic hepatitis, or NASH need not undergo liver biopsy because the risk for cirrhosis is low.

Liver biopsy should be done in all homozygotes greater than 40 years of age or those with serum ferritin greater than 1000.0 ng/mL, those with evidence of chronic liver disease, chronic hepatitis, or alcoholism. Biopsy should also be considered in patients who are compound heterozygotes or C282Y heterozygotes with elevated transferrin saturation and ferritin level >1000.0 ng/mL.

Hepatic Iron Overload

Histology shows predominant iron deposition in hepatocytes and bile ducts as compared to Kupffer cells. Hepatic iron concentration may be measured in selected cases. Normal values are <36.0 μmol/g, while values >71.0 μmol/g are seen in homozygous HH. Similarly hepatic iron index is usually greater than 1.9 in most cases of HH.

DIFFERENTIAL DIAGNOSIS

Iron overload may be primary or secondary. Primary overload is usually related to hereditary hemochromatosis although it may be due to non-HFE associated HH, juvenile hemochromatosis, and African iron overload.

African overload or *Bantu hemosiderosis* was initially thought to be due to beer drinking but is now believed to have a non-HFE genetic basis.

Secondary iron overload occurs as a result of ineffective erythropoiesis, iatrogenic iron administration, multiple blood transfusions, or in patients with alcoholism, chronic viral hepatitis, or liver cirrhosis.

Neonatal iron overload occurs as a result of an intrauterine infection. Survival in such cases without liver transplantation is poor.

TREATMENT

Phlebotomy is the cornerstone of therapy and should be undertaken even if the patient is asymptomatic. A weekly phlebotomy of a unit of blood removes approximately 250.0 mg of iron. Induction therapy should include phlebotomy once every week until the goal of a serum ferritin less than 50.0 ng/mL and transferrin saturation less than 50% is achieved. Thereafter maintenance therapy is undertaken including one units of phlebotomy every 2 to 4 months. Each unit of blood removed results in a decline of serum ferritin by 30.0 ng/mL. Patients usually require 3 to 6 phlebotomies per year during the maintenance phase. Presence of cirrhosis is not a contraindication to phlebotomy.

Patients should avoid vitamin C, which increases iron absorption. Phlebotomy results in improvement of fatigue, liver enzymes abnormalities, hepatomegaly and cardiac functions especially if undertaken prior to development of dilated cardiomyopathy. However, there is no impact on arthropathy.

Orthotopic liver transplantation may be undertaken; however the outcome is disappointing with a 1-year survival rate of 50 to 60%.

COMPLICATIONS

Complications of HH include liver cirrhosis, hepatocellular carcinoma, skin pigmentation, diabetes mellitus, arthropathy, cardiomyopathy, secondary hypogonadism, hypothyroidism, and increased risk for infections with Listeria, Yersinia enterocolitica, and Vibrio vulnificus.

PROGNOSIS

Most cases have mild disease, less degrees of iron overload, and as such, mild to minimal phenotypic expression. Patients who undergo treatment prior to development of cirrhosis have normal life expectancy. Those diagnosed after the development of cirrhosis have reduced survival rate and an increased risk for hepatocellular carcinoma despite effective phlebotomy.

SCREENING

Screening is recommended for siblings and children of patients with hemochromatosis. Mass screening of population is controversial and is not recommended.

PEARLS

○ Most cases of hemochromatosis remain undiagnosed.

○ Not all cases of suspected hemochromatosis require a liver biopsy for diagnosis.

○ Liver cirrhosis is not a contraindication to phlebotomy.

○ Screening for hemochromatosis should be part of the evaluation of all patients with elevated liver enzymes.

BIBLIOGRAPHY

Pietrangelo A. Hemochromatosis. *Gut*. 2003;52 Suppl 2:ii23-30.

Chapter
47 *Wilson's Disease* ▬▬▬

Wilson's disease is an autosomal recessive disorder characterized by excessive copper deposition in the liver, red blood cells, central nervous system (CNS), and other tissues.

EPIDEMIOLOGY

It occurs in about 1 in 30 000 persons with a heterozygous carrier rate of 1 in 90 persons. It affects both sexes and occurs in all races.

GENETICS

A Wilson's disease protein named ATP7B is involved in copper transport. The genetic defect has been localized to chromosome 13. Marked diversity in clinical presentation and course suggests that environmental and other genetic factors affect the phenotypic expression.

PATHOGENESIS

Biliary secretion of cooper is important in maintaining copper homeostasis. Impaired biliary secretion of copper in Wilson's disease results in excess deposition in tissues. This causes damage through generation of free radicals leading to hemolysis, chronic hepatitis, fibrosis, and cirrhosis. Copper levels in CSF are elevated in patients with neuropsychiatric manifestations; the levels decline with treatment.

CLINICAL FEATURES

Even though it is a genetic disorder, patients usually present as teenagers or young adults depending on the predominant presentation. Patients with predominant hepatic manifestations present as teenagers, whereas neuropsychiatric symptoms usually present from 19 to 24 years. Symptoms are rare before 6 or after the age of 40.

Kayser-Fleischer (K-F) Rings are classically seen by slit lamp, but may also be visible to the naked eye. Patients may present as chronic hepatitis syndrome, asymptomatic abnormal liver enzymes, advanced portal hypertension including splenomegaly, thrombocytopenia, bleeding varices, or fulminant hepatic failure. The presence of hemolysis in a young person with chronic liver disease suggests Wilson's disease.

Neurological symptoms include tremors, rigidity, slurring of speech, depression, mood disorders, personality changes, or choreoathetosis. Patients with neurological presentation usually have concomitant liver disease. Other findings may include renal tubular acidosis, polyarthritis, cardiac dysrhythmias, CHF, diabetes mellitus, and menstrual abnormalities.

DIAGNOSIS

There is no single test diagnostic for Wilson's disease; a combination of clinical, biochemical, and histologic findings is used. Liver enzymes are abnormal with AST greater than ALT and alkaline phosphatase below normal levels.

The K-F Ring is seen in about 50 to 60% of the cases but may also be seen in primary biliary cirrhosis and biliary atresia.

Most patients have low serum ceruloplasmin less than 20.0 mg/dl. A 24-hour urinary copper excretion is greater than 100.0 μg, but may be normal in patients who are asymptomatic. Serum total copper concentration is reduced due to low ceruloplasmin levels, although free copper concentration (nonceruloplasmin bound) is actually increased.

Some experts advocate the use of pencillamine provocation test of urinary excretion.

Liver biopsy with hepatic copper concentration helps make the diagnosis and is the gold standard. More than 250.0 μg of copper per gram of dry weight is seen in most cases of Wilson's disease (normal <50.0 μg/g of dry weight). The role of genetic testing in diagnosis is limited.

DIFFERENTIAL DIAGNOSIS

Elevated liver copper may be seen in cholestatic liver disorders like primary biliary cirrhosis and primary sclerosing cholangitis.

TREATMENT

Treatment includes two phases. The first phase involves removing tissue copper followed by maintenance phase of prevention of reaccumulation. D-penicillamine (1.0 to 2.0 g/day in four divided doses given 30 minutes before meals and at bedtime) along with pyridoxine (25.0 mg/day) is the therapy of choice in patients with predominant hepatic manifestations.

In patients with neurological problems, trientine is preferred because D-pencillamine may worsen neurological symptoms. However, trientine is less potent than D-pencillamine.

Once de-coppering has been accomplished (urine copper excretion is 250.0 to 500.0 mcg/day), prevention of reaccumulation is accomplished by administration of a lower dose of penicillamine daily to maintain a 24-hour urine copper excretion of 200.0 to 500.0 μg /day. Another option is zinc acetate 50.0 mg PO tid.

LIVER TRANSPLANTATION

Liver transplantation is the treatment of choice for those who are nonresponsive to treatment or who exhibit fulminant hepatic failure. Outcome after transplantation is excellent. Liver transplantation is curative since the primary defect resides in the liver.

GENETIC SCREENING

Because of numerous mutations resulting in genetic heterogeneity, routine testing is not recommended. However, it may be helpful in screening the first-degree relatives once the genetic defect in the index case has been identified.

PEARLS

- ○ Wilson's disease may present as asymptomatic elevation of liver enzymes, chronic hepatitis, or fulminant hepatic failure.
- ○ Patients may present with predominant hepatic or neurological symptoms.
- ○ The inherited defect in Wilson's disease is in the liver, in contrast to hereditary hemochromatosis where the inherited defect lies in the increased iron absorption from the small intestine.

BIBLIOGRAPHY

Schilsky ML. Diagnosis and treatment of Wilson's disease. *Pediatr Transplant.* 2002;6(1):15-9.

Chapter 48 *Alpha₁ Antitrypsin Deficiency*

EPIDEMIOLOGY

Alpha₁ antitrypsin (AAT) deficiency is the most common genetic liver disease in infants and children. It affects one in 2000 to 3000 live births in the United States. Even severe deficiency may remain unrecognized in many cases.

PATHOGENESIS

The abnormal gene is located on chromosome 14. Alleles leading to the reduction of AAT are called deficiency alleles, of which, PiZZ is the most common. PiMM is associated with normal levels of AAT.

Patients homozygous for PiZZ have less than 20% of normal circulating AAT levels. Even though the serum level of AAT is low, hepatic concentration of AAT is high because the abnormal molecule is unable to exit the liver cells and enter the circulation.

PiMZ heterozygotes may present with liver disease if they have concomitant liver disease such as viral or AIH. It is unknown why only some and not everyone with low AAT levels develops hepatic or pulmonary disease.

CLINICAL FEATURES

Clinical presentation varies from persistent jaundice in the newborn to asymptomatic subjects during childhood and early adulthood. Most common presentation is with complications of chronic liver disease (eg, variceal hemorrhage and ascites). Risk for hepatocellular cancer in the presence of cirrhosis is high. Adults with pulmonary involvement present with premature emphysema.

DIAGNOSIS

Diagnosis is established by AAT levels and phenotype. Most patients are homozygous for PiZZ or compound heterozygous for PiSZ. Serum AAT levels are less than 15 to 20% usually. However, the levels can be normal in the presence of high stress states since it is an acute phase reactant, thus it is important to also check for the phenotype. Liver biopsy shows PAS-positive, diastase-resistant globules within liver cells. However, since the globules are distributed unevenly in the liver, their absence does not exclude the disease.

TREATMENT

In addition to alcohol abstinence, patients should abstain from tobacco to prevent emphysema. Liver transplantation is the only effective cure since the recipient assumes the Pi phenotype of the donor. Orthotopic liver transplant has a 5-year survival rate of 83% in children and 60% in adult recipients.

PEARLS

○ Alpha$_1$ antitrypsin levels do not correlate with severity of liver disease.
○ Liver transplantation is curative.

BIBLIOGRAPHY

Carrell RW, Lomas DA. Alpha$_1$-antitrypsin deficiency—a model for conformational diseases. *N Engl J Med.* 2002;346(1):45-53.

de Serres FJ. Worldwide racial and ethnic distribution of alpha1-antitrypsin deficiency: summary of an analysis of published genetic epidemiologic surveys. *Chest.* 2002;122(5):1818-29.

Chapter
49 *Liver Cirrhosis*

Liver cirrhosis is usually a pathological diagnosis and is characterized by extensive fibrosis, a distorted hepatic architecture, and formation of nodules. It is usually irreversible, especially in advanced stages.

EPIDEMIOLOGY

It accounts for more than 25 000 deaths per year.

CLINICAL FEATURES

Cirrhosis may be suspected based on routine physical examination and laboratory studies performed for some unrelated reason. Patients may present with nonspecific complaints like weakness, fatigue, anorexia, weight loss, and low-grade fever. Others may present for the first time with serious complications such as variceal hemorrhage, ascites, spontaneous bacterial peritonitis, hepatic encephalopathy, or hepatocellular carcinoma.

The stigmata of chronic liver disease include spider angiomata, palmar erythema affecting the thenar and hypothenar prominences while sparing the central portion, clubbing, Dupuytren's contractures, gynecomastia, testicular atrophy, hepatomegaly, splenomegaly, ascites, caput medusa, fetor hepaticus, jaundice, and asterixis. Thrombocytopenia is commonly seen in portal hypertension.

Patients may present for the first time with extrahepatic manifestations of liver diseases. These include porphyria cutanea tarda and mixed cryoglobulinemia in patients with HCV or diabetes mellitus and arthropathy in case of hemochromatosis. Parotid gland enlargement may be seen due to chronic alcoholism.

LABORATORY TESTS

The commonly-used term liver function tests (LFTs) is a misnomer since the most commonly ordered tests are the liver enzyme tests including serum aminotransferases (AST and ALT) and alkaline phosphatase which are not tests of liver function. True liver function tests include serum albumin, prothrombin time as well as serum bilirubin. Abnormalities of synthetic function may be seen in acute severe hepatitis as well as cirrhosis.

CBC may show anemia of multifactorial origin, thrombocytopenia, and leukopenia. Use of biochemical markers of hepatic fibrosis is in its infancy. Imaging studies like ultrasound, CT, and MRI scan may show findings suggestive of cirrhosis, but are not diagnostic. Radionuclide liver-spleen scan shows colloid shift with increased uptake in the spleen and bone marrow, but only detects advanced disease.

DIAGNOSIS

Confirmation of the diagnosis requires liver biopsy. However, in cases of stable disease, where all the clinical laboratory and radiological data point to cirrhosis, liver biopsy may not be essential. For example, a patient with ascites, severe coagulopathy, and imaging studies suggestive of a nodular liver does not need a liver biopsy to establish the presence of cirrhosis. The morphological classification of cirrhosis into micronodular, macronodular, and mixed has largely been abandoned.

ETIOLOGIC DIAGNOSIS

1. The most common causes of cirrhosis are alcohol and chronic viral hepatitis.

2. Patients with alcoholic liver disease show serum AST greater than ALT. Both are less than 400 IU/L with a AST/ALT ratio greater than 2.0 although a ratio of less than 1.0 may be seen in alcoholic patients in ambulatory settings (see Chapter 42).

3. Chronic HCV is diagnosed by antibody to HCV and further confirmation by presence of HCV RNA (see Chapter 38).

4. Primary biliary cirrhosis usually occurs in females and patients have markedly elevated alkaline phosphatase of hepatic origin in addition to elevated serum cholesterol and serum IgM. Antimitochondrial antibodies are seen in over 90% of the cases. Persistently elevated serum bilirubin suggests a poor prognosis (see Chapter 40).

5. Primary sclerosing cholangitis is usually associated with inflammatory bowel disease. Patients may present with pruritus and steatorrhea. ERCP shows biliary strictures and there may be evidence of cholelithiasis and cholangiocarcinoma. Over 70% of the patients with PSC have IBD, especially UC. However, less than 5% of patients with IBD develop PSC.

6. An accurate diagnosis of AIH is important since patients with advanced cirrhosis respond to immunosuppressive treatment. Patients have elevated serum globulins, especially gamma-globulins, along with circulating autoantibodies. Serum ANA,

serum anti-SMA, and ANCA are seen in Type I AIH, while anti-liver/kidney microsomal antibody (anti-LKM-1) is characteristic of Type II AIH. Liver biopsy findings are not diagnostic and as such sometime a trial of therapy may be initiated. Anti-HCV antibody may be false positive. International scoring system is helpful in making accurate diagnosis (see Chapter 45).

7. The diagnosis of HBV infection is made by presence of HB surface antigen for greater than 6 months after initial infection plus abnormal liver tests. Additional tests obtained include HB core-antibody, HBeAg, serum HBV DNA, imaging studies, and liver biopsy (see Chapter 37).

8. Hereditary hemochromatosis may manifest with skin hyperpigmentation, diabetes mellitus, pseudogout, and cardiomyopathy. Serum iron, transferrin saturation, and ferritin levels are elevated. Genetic testing (HFE gene mutations) with or without liver biopsy is needed to confirm the diagnosis (see Chapter 46).

9. Wilson's disease should be suspected in patients who present with liver cirrhosis or fulminant hepatic failure under the age of 45. Results show low serum ceruloplasmin concentration in as many as 95% of the patients. Liver biopsy shows increased copper content (see Chapter 47).

10. AAT deficiency also presents with cirrhosis at an early age. Phenotyping should be done for patients with low AAT levels (see Chapter 48).

11. NAFLD is usually diagnosed by liver biopsy which shows findings of alcoholic liver disease in patients without a history of significant alcohol use. Risk factors include obesity and diabetes mellitus (see Chapter 43).

COMPLICATIONS OF CIRRHOSIS

Complications of liver cirrhosis include ascites, spontaneous bacterial peritonitis, hepatorenal syndrome, variceal hemorrhage, hepatopulmonary syndrome, hepatic encephalopathy, and hepatocellular carcinoma.

PROGNOSIS

A variety of models have been used to predict the prognosis. Child's classification is the most commonly used. The Child-Turcotte model uses five variables including serum albumin, bilirubin, ascites, encephalopathy, and nutritional status. A modified Child-Pugh clas-

Table 49-1 Child-Pugh Criteria			
Parameter	#1	#2	#3
Grade of encephalopathy	None	Mild	Moderate
Ascites	None	Mild	Moderate
Albumin (g/dl)	≥3.5	2.8 to 3.5	≤2.7
Bilirubin (mg/dl)	1 to 2	2.1 to 3	≥3.1
PT (seconds >control)	0 to 4	4.1 to 6	≥6.1

Child class A = 5 to 6; class B = 7 to 9; class C = 10 to 15.

sification is useful for assessing surgical risk and overall survival. The Child-Pugh classification incorporates ascites, serum bilirubin, serum albumin, prothrombin time or INR, and encephalopathy.

PREDICTING SEVERITY

Liver biopsy only establishes the diagnosis of cirrhosis and can not detect the severity. The severity of cirrhosis is determined by clinical parameters like Child-Pugh classification.

CHILD-PUGH CRITERIA

This is elaborated in Table 49-1.

In patients undergoing abdominal surgery, the mortality for Class A is 10%, whereas it is 30% for Class B, and 80% for patients with Class C. One year survival for the three categories is 100%, 80%, and 45%, respectively.

More recently Mayo End-stage Liver Disease (MELD) Score has become very popular for predicting 3 month mortality and as such a need for liver transplantation. MELD score takes into account INR, bilirubin, and creatinine using a complex formula. The scoring system gives special consideration to certain conditions like hepatocellular carcinoma. A MELD score of less than 20 predicts a less than 10% chance of mortality over 3 months; a score of greater than 30 predicts more than 50% of mortality in the ensuing 3 months.

MANAGEMENT

It includes slowing or reversing of the disease's progress. Specific treatments are available for certain conditions like using immunosuppressive agents in the treatment of AIH, abstinence in alcoholic cirrhosis, interferon plus ribavirin therapy in chronic HCV infection, and interferon or lamivudine or adefovir therapy in chronic HBV. In most cases, management focuses on treatment of complications. In patients with end-stage liver disease, liver transplantation is the only option.

PEARLS

○ Cirrhosis can be slowed or even reversed in conditions like autoimmune hepatitis.

○ Patients may be diagnosed on routine history and physical exam. Patients may present for the first time with nonspecific symptoms, extrahepatic manifestations, or complications like variceal bleed.

○ Liver biopsy is not essential for diagnosis in all cases.

○ Severe acute hepatitis cannot be distinguished from cirrhosis based on clinical and biochemical parameters alone.

BIBLIOGRAPHY

Kamath PS, Wiesner RH, Malinchoc M, et al. A model to predict survival in patients with end-stage liver disease. *Hepatology*. 2001;33(2):464-70.

Chapter 50 *Medical Care of the Cirrhotic Patient*

Knowledge of the general medical care of cirrhotic patients is important because patients with compensated cirrhosis may remain stable over the next 10 to 20 years. For example, over 75% of patients with compensated cirrhosis due to HCV may survive beyond 10 years.

PRESUMPTIVE DIAGNOSIS OF CIRRHOSIS

Patients may be presumed to have liver cirrhosis if there is evidence of abnormal liver enzymes, synthetic liver dysfunction, portal hypertension, known etiology for liver disease, plus an absence of any other explanation. Cirrhosis is not an etiologic diagnosis, but a manifestation of an etiology. As such, search for etiology is paramount. Twenty percent of the cases of cirrhosis remain cryptogenic; most of these are probably the result of longstanding fatty liver disease (steatohepatitis).

For stable patients with cirrhosis, the management involves education, prevention, general medical management, and determination for referral to liver transplant center.

EDUCATION

Alcohol, Smoking, and Acetaminophen

It involves guidance on strict abstinence from alcohol. Similarly, smokers should quit smoking. In addition to other disadvantages, poor pulmonary function could be a contraindication for transplantation.

Acetaminophen is poorly-tolerated by patients who continue to drink. In patients with advanced liver cirrhosis, no more than 2.0 g of acetaminophen per day (in divided doses) may be given. Patients with compensated cirrhosis can tolerate up to 3.0 to 4.0 g/day in divided doses. Doses greater than 2.0 g/day are avoided in most cases. Acetaminophen is preferred over NSAIDs in patients with ascites.

Nutritional Supplements

Patients should be educated about multivitamins and herbal supplements. Vitamin E supplementation may be helpful. There is potential for toxicity with vitamin A that accumulates in the liver. Vitamin A may worsen portal hypertension. No more than 5000 units/day of vitamin A may be taken. However, beta-carotene is not hepatotoxic, although its ingestion may simulate jaundice. Iron supplements should be avoided unless a patient has iron deficiency.

Infections

Patients with advanced liver disease are relatively immune-compromised and are at a greater risk for infections in general include Traveler's diarrhea, small bowel bacterial overgrowth, etc.

Vibrio vulnificus infection can be lethal in cirrhosis. Risk factors include the ingestion of raw or undercooked seafood and exposure to salt water when a patient has open sores on the body. Presentation includes high fever, hypotension, and renal failure, which can rapidly progress to septic shock.

PREVENTATIVE STRATEGIES

Immunizations

Patients with liver cirrhosis, who do not have immunity to HAV or HBV, should be vaccinated. Similarly, they should get pneumococcal vaccine every 5 years and an influenza vaccine every year.

Dental Care

Patients should undergo a dental examination every 6 to 12 months. Poor dentition creates a high risk for spontaneous bacterial peritonitis in patients with ascites. Presence of gingivitis or a dental abscess when the liver becomes available for transplantation would create a contraindication for liver transplantation.

Variceal Bleeding

In patients who do not have any varices at diagnosis, varices will develop in about 15 to 50%. Initial hemorrhage occurs in 25 to 35% of patients with large varices within a period of 1 year. Each episode of variceal bleeding carries a mortality rate of 20 to 50%.

Patients with cirrhosis should undergo routine base line endoscopy to detect varices. In patients with no found varices, a repeat endoscopy may be undertaken in 2 years. In patients with medium or large varices, prophylaxis with nonselective beta-blockers (propranolol, nadolol) should be undertaken. Prophylactic banding may be considered in patients with large varices if beta-blockers are contraindicated. The need to perform surveillance after initiating beta-blocker therapy is controversial.

SBP Prophylaxis

Prolonged outpatient secondary prophylaxis with norfloxacin 400.0 mg/day PO or trimethoprim/sulfamethoxazale DS 1 tablet every day is effective in patients with prior history of SBP. Prophylaxis should also be undertaken in hospitalized patients who have ascitic fluid protein less than 1.0 g/dl at the time of admission (norfloxacin 400.0 mg/day PO). Antibiotics may be discontinued upon discharge from hospital except in patients with prior history of SBP or patients awaiting liver transplantation. Patients admitted with GI bleeding should have cultures drawn and antibiotic prophylaxis initiated. Long-term antibiotic prophylaxis of SBP in other situations is controversial. General measures for prophylaxis include aggressive attempts at reducing the amount of ascitic fluid by diuresis and early recognition/treatment of any infections elsewhere in the body.

Hepatocellular Carcinoma

Liver cirrhosis, regardless of the etiology, predisposes to development of HCC. HCV is the most common cause of HCC in the United States. Screening for HCC provides the theoretical advantage of early diagnosis, leading to possible early diagnosis and treatment. The benefit and cost-effectiveness of screening has not been established.

An alpha-fetoprotein (AFP) level and liver ultrasound every 6 months has been recommended. Some experts perform a CT scan every 6 months, whereas others undertake an ultrasound every 12 months. These strategies are based not on any scientific studies but on "expert opinion."

AFP levels may be normal in 35% of patients with HCC. Elevated AFP levels of less than 100.0 ng/mL are common in patients with cirrhosis. Significant elevations of AFP as high as 400.0 ng/mL may sometimes be seen in acute necroinflammatory states. In case of an elevated AFP level of less than 100.0 ng/mL after a normal ultrasound, a repeat AFP level should be undertaken in 1 to 3 months. Patients with an AFP level greater than 100.0 ng/mL after a normal ultrasound should undergo a complementary imaging study such as a triple-phase CT scan or MRI with contrast to detect HCC.

Miscellaneous Health Care Issues

Patients should undergo screening for gynecological, breast, colon, and prostate cancer. The medication list should be reviewed, especially antihypertensive medications that may no longer be needed. Medications with hepatotoxic or nephrotoxic potential should be avoided. Patients with well-compensated liver cirrhosis can tolerate standard doses of most medications. In patients with advanced liver cirrhosis, reduce the dose of medications by 50% if the medication is metabolized in the liver. Patients should be screened for osteoporosis and treated appropriately.

Nutrition

Protein-calorie malnutrition is rampant among patients with advanced liver disease. Protein restriction should be undertaken only in cases of severe encephalopathy or persistent encephalopathy despite medical management. Depending upon the nutritional status, diet should contain at 27.0 to 30.0 K_{cal}/kg ideal body weight and 1.0 to 1.5 g/kg/day of protein. About 30% of calories should be in the form of a fat, whereas the rest are administered as carbohydrates. Use of specialized diets, such as branched-chain amino-acids, is controversial, probably not cost-effective, and not favored by most experts.

Referral to Gastroenterologist

A patient should be referred when cirrhosis is first suspected or the diagnosis is established. For routine follow-up, a patient may be seen by a gastroenterologist every 6 to 12 months in cases of stable cirrhosis, and every 3 to 6 months (or more often) in cases of advanced disease. Patients should also be referred if the complications like ascites, encephalopathy, and variceal bleeding occur.

Referral to Transplant Center

Referral to a liver transplantation center should be based on the personal and social history as well as severity of liver disease. Patients with continued substance abuse, severe comorbid conditions, and lack of social and/or financial support are unlikely to be accepted for transplantation.

Initial referral to the transplant center should be considered in patients with a Child-Pugh score equal to or greater than 8, refractory ascites, or renal insufficiency. Most patients undergo transplantation when renal insufficiency and coagulopathy develop. Patients with a MELD score of 15 to 20 are usually listed; patients undergoing transplantation usually have a MELD score greater than 25.

PEARLS

- ○ Many patients with asymptomatic cirrhosis live greater than 15 years. The presence of liver disease should not overshadow the need to address preventative and educational medical strategies.
- ○ Acetaminophen in cirrhosis-adjusted doses may be a better choice as analgesic than the use of NSAIDs for cirrhosis complicated by ascites.

BIBLIOGRAPHY

Plauth M, Schutz ET. Cachexia in liver cirrhosis. *Int J Cardiol.* 2002;85(1):83-7.

Chapter
51 *Ascites*

Ascites is a pathological accumulation of fluid in the peritoneal cavity.

ETIOLOGY

It is caused by liver cirrhosis in as many as 85% of the cases. Less common causes include malignancy (peritoneal carcinomatosis), CHF, tuberculosis, dialysis, and pancreatitis. Unusual causes include abdominal trauma, intraoperative lymphatic tear, injury to intraabdominal blood vessels, lupus, myxedema, *Chlamydia*, AIDS-related opportunistic infections, and *C. difficile* colitis. Adults with ascites and nephrotic syndrome frequently have concomitant liver cirrhosis as cause of the ascites. More than one cause may be found in about 5% of the patients.

PATHOGENESIS

An elevated portal pressure greater than 12.0 mmHg is required for formation of ascites. The increased portal pressure leads to an increase in hydrostatic pressure and exudation of fluid into the peritoneum.

Recently, peripheral arterial vasodilatation theory has been proposed. Patients have arterial vasodilatation and hyperdynamic circulation leading to a decrease in effective intravascular volume, activation of the rennin-angiotensin system, and increased sodium and water retention. Nitric oxide is a primary mediator of vasodilatation.

DIAGNOSIS

Diagnosis is based on history and physical examination and confirmed on imaging studies. The sensitivity and specificity of physical examination varies from 30 to 95%. History should focus on the multiple etiologies and risk factors for chronic liver disease, as well as to the possibility of other causes. Stigmata of chronic liver disease on physical exam point to a hepatic etiology.

Findings of ascites include distended abdomen, flank dullness, fluid wave, and shifting dullness. In contrast to cardiac ascites, jugular venous pressure is low or normal. This is especially important in patients who are alcoholics and who may have alcoholic cardiomyopathy. An umbilical nodule with ascites is seen in gastric or colon cancer, lymphoma, or hepatocellular carcinoma.

Imaging Studies

Ultrasound is the initial test of choice and is the most cost-effective. Splenomegaly (greater than 12.0 cm) or a recanalization of umbilical vein points to portal hypertension.

A chest x-ray and echocardiogram may be helpful in distinguishing between ascites due to cardiac from a noncardiac cause.

Paracentesis

Abdominal paracentesis confirms the presence of ascites, determines the etiology, and evaluates for infection. The risk for serious infections due to paracentesis is less than 1%. Routine prophylactic use of fresh frozen plasma or platelets should be discouraged. Paracentesis should be avoided in patients with clinically evident fibrinolysis or DIC.

The fluid is clear if bilirubin is normal, but is usually translucent yellow in cirrhosis patients. Fluid may be brown in patients with deep jaundice. While infected fluid is turbid or cloudy, opalescent fluid is seen in hypertriglyceridemia and may be misinterpreted as pus. Milky fluid is seen in chylous ascites. Chylous ascites is more likely to be caused by liver cirrhosis than malignancy. Hemorrhagic fluid may occur due to trauma to a collateral vessel or malignancy. RBC greater than $10\,000/mm^3$ leads to pink color of the fluid.

Tests on Ascitic Fluid

The primary focus of testing ascitic fluid is whether portal hypertension is present and whether the fluid is infected. Routine tests include total cell count and differential, albumin concentration, total protein concentration, and bacterial cultures. Blood culture bottles should be inoculated at bedside and 10 mL of fluid should be sent in blood culture bottles for cultures.

Optional tests include glucose concentration, LDH, Gram stain, and amylase. Gram stain of ascitic fluid is only helpful if secondary peritonitis due to gut perforation is suspected. Test for acid-fast bacilli (AFB) smear and culture, cytology, triglycerides, and bilirubin levels are occasionally needed. Testing for pH and lactate is not useful.

Serum albumin should be measured at the same time as fluid albumin. A serum to ascites albumin gradient (SAAG) of 1.1 or greater suggests portal hypertension. The SAAG needs to be done only on the first specimen and does not need to be repeated.

In patients with portal hypertension, fluid protein less than 2.5 g/dl is seen in patients with uncomplicated cirrhosis; a fluid protein greater than 2.5 g/dl points to cardiac ascites. The diagnostic accuracy of fluid protein in diagnosing the cause of ascites is 55%, whereas SAAG is accurate in 97%. Patients with fluid protein less than 1.0 g/dl have high risk of SBP. The concept of exudate/transudate is outdated.

Cell count and differential should be performed on every specimen. It helps determine presence of infection (see also Chapter 52). Subtract one WBC for every 750 RBCs and one neutrophil for every 250 RBCs present in the fluid. A PMN count of greater than 250/mm^3 or WBC count of 500/mm^3 suggests SBP.

SBP is unlikely if patient has positive cultures with polymicrobial flora. Suspect secondary peritonitis if neutrophil count greater than 250/mm^3 is present along with any two of the following:

1. A total fluid protein greater than 1.0 g/dl.
2. Glucose less than 50.0 mg/dl.
3. LDH greater than upper limit of normal for serum. In such cases, intestinal perforation or malignancy should be considered.

In patients with cell count suggestive of SBP but SAAG less than 1.1, polymicrobial infection and pancreatic ascites should be considered.

Normal ascitic fluid to serum amylase ratio is 0.4 in liver cirrhosis. Markedly elevated fluid amylase, with ascitic fluid to serum ratio of approximately 5.0 or greater is seen in patients with pancreatitis or gut perforation.

Abnormal cell counts with predominance of mononuclear cells in patients with routine culture negative ascitic fluid points to tuberculosis. In patients with an elevated fluid WBC with less than 50% PMNs, peritoneal carcinomatosis, and tuberculous peritonitis should be considered. A direct AFB smear is not helpful, whereas peritoneoscopy is 100% sensitive for detecting tuberculous peritonitis.

An ascitic fluid bilirubin greater than the serum bilirubin suggests bile leak. The sensitivity of cytology for malignant ascites is 60 to 75%.

TREATMENT

Treatment includes treatment of the underlying cause as well as a reduction of the amount of ascitic fluid. Although management of ascitic fluid does not improve outcome, patients feel better and it also reduces the risk for spontaneous bacterial peritonitis, hydrothorax, hernia, and cellulitis.

Traditionally a sodium diet of 2.0 g/day has been recommended. Many experts now recommend a moderate restriction of 5.2 g/day.

Fluid restriction should only be undertaken if serum sodium is less than 120.0 meq/L. Bed rest is not helpful.

Spironolactone is the diuretic of choice and is more effective than furosemide alone. Patients may develop painful gynecomastia due to spironolactone. Amiloride (Midamor 5.0 to 20.0 mg/day) is an alternate option but less effective as compared to spironolactone.

Initial starting dose is spironolactone 100.0 mg alone or in addition to furosemide 40.0 mg taken as a single dose in the morning. The dose may be doubled, slowly titrating up to four times the dose. Both the drugs may be given in a single dose. Weight loss should not exceed 1.0 kg/day in patients with edema and 500.0 g/day in patients without edema. Spironolactone should be decreased or stopped in patients who develop hyperkalemia.

Refractory Ascites

Less than 10% of ascites is refractory to conventional therapy. Refractory ascites is defined as a lack of response in patients on intensive diuretic regimen for at least 1 week with salt-restricted diet, an early reappearance of ascites within 4 weeks after mobilization, or presence of diuretic-induced complications.

Noncompliance with dietary restriction is a common cause of diuretic resistance. A 24-hour urinary sodium excretion provides an objective measure of dietary compliance, but is rarely used in clinical practice. A sodium excretion of greater than 90.0 mmol per 24 hours without weight loss points to dietary noncompliance. A spot sodium to potassium ratio of greater than 1.0 in ascitic fluid is seen in patients with a 24-hour sodium excretion of greater than 78.0 meq/day.

Large Volume Paracentesis

Large volume therapeutic paracentesis is the initial treatment of choice in patients with refractory ascites. Removal of less than 5 L at any one time does not have significant impact on hemodynamic parameters. Albumin infusion (6.0 to 8.0 g albumin per L of fluid removed) should be administered in case of patients having greater than 5 L fluid removal at a time.

Transjugular Intrahepatic Portosystemic Shunts

Patients requiring frequent therapeutic taps every 2 weeks or more may benefit from transjugular intrahepatic portosystemic shunts (TIPS). Although TIPS is superior to large volume paracentesis for refractory ascites, it is associated with high costs as well as 30% incidence of hepatic encephalopathy.

SURGERY

Surgically placed peritoneovenous or portosystemic shunts have limited utility. Repair of abdominal hernias in the presence of ascites has a high complication and recurrence rate and should be avoided until liver transplantation.

PROGNOSIS

Ascites is a marker for advanced liver disease and patients should be referred for liver transplantation. Hospitalized patients with ascites have a 40% mortality by 2 years. Prognosis is worse in patients with refractory ascites and SBP.

PEARLS

○ Liver disease is the cause of ascites in 85% of cases.

○ All patients with new onset ascites or a change in their clinical status should undergo prompt paracentesis to characterize the ascites and exclude infection.

○ The use of ascitic fluid protein and the concept of exudate/ transudate for assessing the etiology of ascites is outdated.

○ Presence of ascites is a marker for advanced liver disease and patients should be considered for referral for evaluation to a liver transplant center.

BIBLIOGRAPHY

Moore KP, Wong F, Gines P, et al. The management of ascites in cirrhosis: report on the consensus conference of the International Ascites Club. *Hepatology*. 2003;38(1):258-66.

Chapter 52 *Spontaneous Bacterial Peritonitis* ▬▬▬▬▬

Spontaneous bacterial peritonitis (SBP) is defined as an infection of the ascitic fluid in the absence of a surgically correctable intra-abdominal source of infection. It usually occurs in patients with advanced liver cirrhosis.

PATHOGENESIS

Intestinal hypomotility and localized intestinal immune-deficiency in the presence of portal hypertension promotes bacterial translocation to the mesenteric lymph nodes as well as to the blood stream. This results in bacterial seeding and SBP. Increased risk in patients with advanced liver disease develops due to impaired host defenses such as low complement and cytokine levels, defective PMN, and macrophage function, and decreased complement activation system. A low ascitic fluid total protein concentration (<1.0 g/dl), prior history of SBP, an episode of acute GI bleeding, serum bilirubin above 2.5 mg/dl, and malnutrition increase the risk for SBP. Malignant and cardiac ascites do not usually get infected.

CLINICAL FEATURES

Clinical features may be subtle or absent. About 25% of hospitalized patients with ascites have SBP. Low-grade temperature is the most common manifestation and should be taken seriously because patients are normally hypothermic. Other manifestations include diffuse, mild, and continuous abdominal pain; altered mental status; and abdominal tenderness with or without peritoneal signs. Diarrhea, paralytic ileus, hypothermia, and hypotension occur in severe cases.

DIAGNOSIS

Laboratory tests may reveal leukocytosis, metabolic acidosis, and azotemia. Abdominal paracentesis should be carried out every time a patient with ascites is admitted to the hospital regardless of features of peritonitis. Ascitic fluid should be cultured at bedside in blood culture bottles with at least 10 mL of fluid.

It is important that patients undergo paracentesis before antibiotic administration since as many as 80 to 90% of culture positive ascitic fluid becomes culture-negative within 6 hours of a single dose of antibiotic. Blood, urine, and sputum should also be cultured in patients with suspected of bacteremia.

Ascitic fluid PMN count of greater than $250/mm^3$ suggests the diagnosis and empiric treatment should be started while awaiting the results of cultures.

Culture Negative Neutrocytic Ascites

Culture negative neutrocytic ascites (CNNA) is defined as ascitic fluid with >250 PMN/mm^3, but with negative cultures. It carries the same prognosis and clinical significance as SBP and should be treated with antibiotics. CNNA in the presence of high ascitic fluid total protein (>2.0 g/dl) is seen in peritoneal carcinomatosis and secondary bacterial peritonitis. The PMN count may be falsely elevated in patients with traumatic tap. Subtract 1 PMN for every 250 RBCs.

Differential diagnosis of culture-negative neutrocytic ascites include:

1. Antibiotic treatment prior to paracentesis.
2. Suboptimal culture technique.
3. Inadequate volume of fluid used for culture (<10 mL).
4. Hemorrhagic tap.
5. Pancreatitis.
6. Spontaneous resolution of SBP when the tap is performed or delayed until a time when the bacterial count has declined significantly.

Non-Neutrocytic Bacterial Ascites

Monomicrobial non-neutrocytic bacterial ascites may be seen during the colonization phase of the ascitic fluid. It resolves spontaneously in majority of the cases without going to SBP. A repeat paracentesis in 48 to 72 hours is recommended to exclude progression to SBP.

Polymicrobial bacterial ascites may occur when the paracentesis needle inadvertently enters the bowel. In such cases, the PMN count stays below $250/mm^3$ even though Gram stain and culture shows presence of multiple bacteria. A surgical source of infection should be considered in patients who develop infected ascites while undergoing a course of broad spectrum antibiotic.

TREATMENT

Treatment should be started with cefotaxime 2.0 g every 8 to 12 hours intravenously. Amoxicillin/clavulanic acid is safe, effective, and cheaper. Ampicillin/sulbactam is also effective while aminoglycosides should be avoided.

Other options include ceftriaxone (2.0 g IV q 24 hours) or cefoncid (2.0 g IV q 12 hours). Aztreonam is not a adequate for empiric treatment. Treatment of SBP is usually undertaken for 5 to 10 days and discontinued if there is evidence of clinical response.

Administration of intravenous albumin 1.5 g/kg at time of diagnosis and then 1.0 g/kg on day 3 prevents renal insufficiency and reduces mortality in patients with SBP.

Asymptomatic patients without any other significant problem like bleeding or encephalopathy may be treated with oral ofloxacin 400.0 mg bid or ciprofloxacin 500.0 mg PO bid for 5 to 7 days. Patients with secondary bacterial peritonitis also need appropriate antibiotic coverage in addition to surgical consultation.

COMPLICATIONS

SBP may be complicated by renal failure and hepatorenal syndrome. While there is no consensus on standard of care, we treat such cases with a combination of octreotide 200.0 mcg SQ tid plus midodrine (ProAmatine).

Follow-Up Paracentesis

Repeat paracentesis should be undertaken if warranted clinically by lack of or for an atypical response to antibiotics. In patients with persistent fever or pain, repeat paracentesis should be undertaken. If the PMN count is less than $250/mm^3$, a 5-day course of antibiotics should be completed. If the PMN count is greater than $250/mm^3$ but less than the initial baseline value, treatment should be continued for another 48 to 72 hours before repeat paracentesis.

On the other hand, if evidence of infection persists especially if the PMN count is greater than the initial baseline value, a surgical source of infection should be considered.

PROGNOSIS

Since SBP occurs usually in advanced liver disease, it carries a poor prognosis overall with 70% mortality at 1 year. Consider referral to a liver transplantation center.

SBP PROPHYLAXIS

1. Prolonged outpatient secondary prophylaxis with norfloxacin 400.0 mg/day PO or trimethoprim/sulfamethoxazale DS 1 tablet every day is effective in patients with prior history of SBP.

2. Prophylaxis should also be undertaken in hospitalized patients who have ascitic fluid protein less than 1.0 g/dl at the time of admission (norfloxacin 400.0 mg/day PO). Antibiotics may be discontinued upon discharge from hospital except in patients with prior history of SBP or patients awaiting liver transplantation.

3. Patients admitted with GI bleeding should have cultures drawn and antibiotic prophylaxis initiated. Third generation cephalosporin (cefotaxime 2.0 g IV q 8 hours) is usually used. If cultures are negative at 48 hours, IV antibiotic is switched to a PO formulation (norfloxacin 400.0 mg PO bid for 7 days).

4. Long-term antibiotic prophylaxis of SBP in other situations is controversial. General measures for prophylaxis include aggressive attempts at reducing the amount of ascitic fluid by diuresis, and early recognition and treatment of any infections elsewhere in the body.

PEARLS

○ About 25% of patients admitted to the hospital with ascites have SBP at the time of admission.

○ Culture of ascitic fluid should be done in blood culture bottles at bedside using at least 10.0 mL of fluid.

○ Routine long-term use of SBP prophylaxis in outpatients without a prior history of SBP is controversial.

BIBLIOGRAPHY

Mowat C, Stanley AJ. Review article: spontaneous bacterial peritonitis—diagnosis, treatment, and prevention. *Aliment Pharmacol Ther*. 2001; 15(12):1851-9.

Chapter
53 *Hepatic Encephalopathy*

Hepatic encephalopathy (HE) or portosystemic encephalopathy (PSE) is a reversible state of cerebral dysfunction and altered mental status in patients with liver insufficiency due to acute liver failure or chronic liver disease. A wide spectrum of neuropsychiatric abnormalities with or without major portosystemic shunting may be seen. Although frequently a complication of liver cirrhosis, it may be seen in acute conditions like acute alcoholic hepatitis.

PATHOGENESIS

It is multifactorial involving metabolic and biochemical derangements, brain atrophy and edema, impaired cerebral perfusion, and hyperpermeability of blood-brain barrier. Evidence for the role of elevated ammonia and inhibitory neurotransmission through GABA receptors in CNS is strong. Endogenous benzodiazepines have been identified in the brain of animal models of HE. Alterations in concentrations of neurotransmitters like norepinephrine, serotonin, histamine, and melatonin have been seen. The role of Hp in ammonia production through its urease activity has not been established.

PRECIPITATING FACTORS

HE may be precipitated by sedatives, narcotics, alcohol, excessive dietary intake of protein, GI bleed, infection, electrolyte derangements, constipation, dehydration, large volume paracentesis, portosystemic shunt procedures, and vascular occlusion of the portal or hepatic vein.

CLINICAL FEATURES

In addition to subtle or worsening signs of altered mental status, patients may show stigmata of chronic liver disease such as cachexia, jaundice, ascites, palmar erythema, spider angiomata, or fetor hepaticus. These stigmata are likely to be absent in previously healthy patients presenting with fulminant hepatic failure. Altered sleep pattern such as insomnia or hypersomnia may be the only complaint in early stages. Patients with advance HE show asterixis and hyperactive deep tendon reflexes. Focal neurological deficits like hemiplegia are rare.

LABORATORY DIAGNOSIS

Diagnosis is based on clinical and laboratory testing with an exclusion of organic etiologies using a CT and/or MRI scan. Ammonia levels are elevated and arterial ammonia concentration correlates better with the amount of ammonia at the blood-brain barrier than the venous concentration. Arterial ammonia level may not be elevated in 10% of patients with HE.

Measurement of venous ammonia blood levels may be helpful in the initial evaluation when there is doubt about the presence of significant liver disease or of other causes for an alteration in mental status. Follow-up with repeated ammonia levels is unnecessary and does not replace the evaluation of the patient's mental state.

HE may be classified into mild, moderate, and severe HE and coma. A Glasgow coma scale has also been used. Psychometric tests are more sensitive, but are cumbersome and time consuming. The Number Connection Test (NCT or Reitan Test) is most commonly used. Assessment of reaction time to auditory and visual stimulus may be helpful.

EEG, auditory, or visual evoked potentials are used in research protocols.

TREATMENT

Specific treatment along with removal of precipitating cause results in prompt improvement in most cases.

General Measures

Correct dehydration or electrolyte imbalance. Check for SBP and treat if present. Patients with GI bleeding should receive nasogastric lavage and a rapid GI purge. Unless otherwise contraindicated, a bottle of magnesium citrate (300 mL) accomplishes the latter goal. Any sedatives or tranquilizers should be discontinued. Flumazenil should be administered to patients who have been on benzodiazepines.

Synthetic Disaccharides

Lactulose and lactitol are converted to short change fatty acids in the colon that lowers the colonic pH. The low pH <5.0 favors the formation of nonabsorbable ammonium ion from ammonia resulting in reduction of ammonia available for absorption into the body. The cathartic effect also improves GI transit resulting in elimination of any toxins in the gut lumen.

Lactulose is effective in 70 to 80% of patients. Start at 40 mL/hour until bowel movement occurs, and then use 40 to 90 mL/day titrated to achieve two to three soft stools per day. In patients with ileus, 300 mL of lactulose in 1 L solution may be administered as an enema to be retained for an hour, preferably in trendelenburg position. Lactitol is as effective as lactulose but more palatable.

Colonic Cleansing

Colonic cleansing upon presentation can rapidly remove ammoniagenic substances from the colon and is especially helpful in constipated patients. The use of 1 to 3 L of 20% lactulose or lactitol enema is superior to tap water enema and achieves a favorable response in about 80% of the patients. Although enemas are likely to be superior to oral therapy on theoretical grounds, oral use of lactulose is more convenient and preferred. Colonic lavage using mannitol 1.0 g/kg in a 5 L solution has been shown to be helpful in patients with GI bleed.

Protein Restriction

Protein may be withdrawn initially in cases of severe HE. Protein restricted diet of 40.0 to 60.0 g/day should be administered with gradual increase of protein to 1.0 to 1.5 g/kg/day. Vegetable proteins are preferred. Patients with history of prior HE may not tolerate greater than 70.0 g/day of protein. Oral dietary supplementation with the branched-chain amino acids may be helpful in severely protein-intolerant patients; however, their use is controversial.

Antibiotics

Antibiotics are effective and should be used in patients who cannot tolerate (or who do not respond to) disaccharide therapy within 48 hours. Options include neomycin 2.0 to 8.0 g/day in four divided doses per day, but carries the risk of ototoxicity and nephrotoxicity. We prefer metronidazole (250.0 mg PO tid). Patients not responding to treatment should be monitored in the intensive care unit and treated with intravenous antibiotics.

Miscellaneous

The use of parenteral branched-chain amino acid infusion for treatment of hepatic encephalopathy is controversial and is not cost-effective.

Flumazenil although useful, is not recommended for routine use because of the short lasting effect; however, it may be used to distinguish between drug-induced coma and hepatic encephalopathy.

Treatment of Recurrent Encephalopathy

Patients with recurrent or chronic encephalopathy require chronic use of lactulose with protein restriction of up to 70.0 g/day. Vegetable proteins are superior to animal proteins. Patients who are intolerant to protein may benefit from branched amino acid supplementation. Treatment of constipation is also very important in such cases.

The role of probiotics is evolving. The probiotic Enterococcus faecium SF 68 has been shown to be as effective as lactulose for long-term treatment without any side effects.

Use of zinc supplementation and melatonin is controversial. Zinc acetate (220.0 mg bid) can be administered especially to those who have low zinc levels. Hp should be eradicated if present. Select cases may benefit from neomycin 1.0 to 2.0 g/day PO with monitoring for toxicity. Metronidazole 250.0 to 500.0 mg/day is an alternate option to neomycin.

PEARLS

○ Removal of the precipitating cause along with specific treatment is effective in most cases.

○ Routine use of branched-chain amino acids for nutrition is not recommended.

BIBLIOGRAPHY

Andres T. Blei, Juan Córdoba, and The Practice Parameters Committee of the American College of Gastroenterology. Hepatic encephalopathy. *Am J Gastroenterol.* 2001;96:1968-1976.

Chapter 54 *Hepatorenal Syndrome*

Hepatorenal syndrome is the presence of progressive renal failure occurring in a patient with advanced liver disease and portal hypertension in the absence of specific causes of renal failure.

PATHOGENESIS

A decline in glomerular filtration rate (GFR) and sodium excretion is seen. This occurs due to poor renal perfusion as a result of increased renal vasoconstriction caused by activation of endogenous vasoactive systems in the presence of intense splanchnic vasodilatation. Because of decreased liver function and muscle mass, the serum creatinine may be within normal range despite significant declines in GFR.

PRECIPITATING FACTORS

Although insidious in onset, it may be precipitated by NSAID use, GI bleed, infection, aggressive diuresis, or spontaneous bacterial peritonitis.

CLINICAL FEATURES

There is oliguria with low urinary sodium excretion in the absence of volume contraction. Stigmata of chronic liver disease are seen.

DIAGNOSIS

Serum creatinine rises slowly and progressively worsens in the presence of severe liver disease but in the absence of any apparent renal disease. Urine sodium excretion is less than 10 meq/L. Blood urea nitrogen (BUN) levels are variable. Renal function does not improve in response to volume challenge. Renal ultrasound is performed to exclude obstruction.

Differential diagnosis includes acute tubular necrosis and other causes of prerenal disease like severe bleeding or aggressive diuretic therapy.

TREATMENT

The only proven effective treatment for hepatorenal syndrome is a liver transplantation. Albumin infusion plus terlipressin (an ADH analog not available in the United States) significantly improves renal function. Although there is no consensus on standard of care, we use a combination of midodrine, a selective alpha-1 adrenergic agonist plus octreotide in addition to albumin. Midodrine (ProAmatine 7.5 to 12.5 mg tid) and octreotide (100.0 to 200.0 mcg SQ tid) are titrated to increase the mean arterial pressure by at least 15 mmHg.

Renal failure can be effectively treated with dialysis. However, survival depends upon the severity of liver disease. Hemodialysis may be difficult to perform because of hemodynamic instability. TIPS provides short-term benefit and should be used as a last resort.

PREVENTION

The main focus should be to prevent and eliminate precipitating factors such as GI bleed, electrolyte abnormalities, or infection. A successful liver transplantation is the only hope for a cure.

PEARLS

- ○ Serum creatinine may initially be normal in cases of hepatorenal syndrome.
- ○ Hypovolumia and urinary obstruction should always be excluded by a fluid challenge and imaging studies.
- ○ NSAID use, including the newer selective COX-2 inhibitors, is a frequent cause of renal insufficiency in patients with cirrhosis.

BIBLIOGRAPHY

Kramer L, Horl WH. Hepatorenal syndrome. *Semin Nephrol.* 2002;22(4): 290-301.

Chapter

55 *Hepatocellular Carcinoma* ▬

While the most common malignancy affecting the liver is metastatic carcinoma, the most common primary malignancy is HCC.

EPIDEMIOLOGY

HCC represents about 5% of all cancers and the incidence is rising. The annual incidence in the United States is 2 to 3 per 100 000 persons. Eastern Africa and Eastern Asia have the highest age-adjusted incidence rates. Males outnumber females by 4:1. HCC is the leading cause of death in patients with compensated cirrhosis. About one-third of patients who die of liver cirrhosis have HCC on autopsy.

ETIOLOGY

Most patients have underlying cirrhosis. HCV is the most common underlying etiology for cirrhosis followed by chronic HBV, hemochromatosis, AAT deficiency, and alcoholic liver cirrhosis. Fibrolamellar form of HCC is a slow growing variant of HCC and is not associated with liver cirrhosis.

Other risk factors for HCC include aflatoxin, Budd-Chiari syndrome, and thorostat dye. Role of oral contraceptives and tobacco use is controversial. The risk of HCC is lower among those consuming high intake of vegetable and fruits.

CLINICAL FEATURES

Patients present with abdominal pain, weight loss, fever, and hepatomegaly along with features of liver cirrhosis. Hepatic bruit may be heard. Less common features include blood-tinged ascitic fluid and acute hemoperitoneum. Asymptomatic cases may be detected on screening imaging studies.

DIAGNOSIS

Chemistries show elevated serum alkaline phosphatase, as well as serum AST/ALT. Persistent leukocytosis, polycythemia, hypoglycemia, hypercalcemia, and hypercholestrolemia may be seen. Serum alpha-fetoprotein levels are elevated. The tumor usually appears as multiple nodules on CT scan of the liver. A large solitary mass is less common, and usually occurs in the right lobe. A fine needle biopsy should be performed for suspicious lesions; however many experts feel that biopsy should not be considered absolutely essential for diagnosis. Patients with findings of HCC on two imaging techniques (eg, 3-phase CT and angiography) or with typical findings of HCC on one imaging study plus an elevated AFP greater than 400.0 ng/mL may also be presumed to have HCC. Forty percent of the tumors less than 2.0 cm in size have microscopic evidence of vascular invasion.

TREATMENT

Patients with a normal liver and well-preserved liver function should undergo hepatic resection. Patients with liver cirrhosis and early liver cancer (one single lesion less than 5.0 cm or up to three lesions less than 3.0 cm each) are candidates for liver transplantation. In case orthotopic liver transplant (OLT) is not available for patients with single lesion, segmentectomy or subsegmentectomy may be undertaken; however, these are less desirable options. Resection is contraindicated in cases of decompensated cirrhosis or severe portal hypertension.

Patients with inoperable tumors are candidates for ultrasound guided intralesional therapy (absolute alcohol, 50% acetic acid, or hot saline solution), radiofrequency thermoablation, or laser therapy. Response to systemic chemotherapy is poor.

PROGNOSIS

The 5-year survival for HCC patients undergoing OLT is 60 to 70%. The 5-year survival of patients undergoing resection for a single lesion is similar in some studies.

SCREENING

Screening for patients at risk for HCC is recommended and is described in Chapter 50.

PEARLS

○ Incidence of hepatocellular carcinoma is rising rapidly worldwide.

○ The screening strategies for preventing hepatocellular carcinoma are not evidence-based, but are founded on expert opinion.

BIBLIOGRAPHY

Wudel LJ Jr, Chapman WC. Indications and limitations of liver transplantation for hepatocellular carcinoma. *Surg Oncol Clin N Am*. 2003;
12(1):77-90.

Chapter 56 *Hepatobiliary Disease During Pregnancy*

Hepatobiliary diseases occurring during pregnancy can be divided
into the following groups:

1. Pregnancy occurring in patients with pre-existing liver disease.
2. Liver diseases exacerbated by pregnancy.
3. Liver diseases unique to pregnancy.
4. Diseases of the biliary system.
5. Vascular diseases.

PHYSIOLOGICAL CHANGES

Normal physiologic changes during pregnancy include spider
angiomas and palmar erythema. Since the liver is forced into the chest,
a palpable liver below the costal margin suggests hepatomegaly. No
histologic changes occur in the liver during pregnancy.

Whereas serum hemoglobin and albumin decrease during pregnancy, serum total cholesterol and triglyceride increase. Serum alkaline phosphatase concentrations may be elevated to up to four times
the normal during the third trimester.

PREGNANCY DURING CHRONIC LIVER DISEASE

Pregnancy may occur in patients with chronic HBV, HCV, AIH,
hemochromatosis, and Wilson's disease. There is no increase in risk of
maternal or fetal toxicity in patients with chronic HBV, although all
infants born to the mother should receive active and passive prophylaxis. The transmission of HCV from mother to newborn is less than
10%, and is more likely if the patient is coinfected with HIV. HCV is
not transmitted by breast-feeding.

Immune-suppressive therapy should be continued during pregnancy in patients with AIH. Similarly chelation therapy should be
continued in patients with Wilson's disease during the pregnancy.

After a successful liver transplant, patients may become pregnant; however, there is increased risk for maternal hypertension as well as prematurity.

LIVER DISEASE EXACERBATED BY PREGNANCY

Some hepatobiliary disorders may be detected during pregnancy. Although the course of HAV during pregnancy is similar to other patients, there may be increased risk for premature labor. Perinatal transmission of the virus does not occur.

Acute HBV does not cause increased maternal or fetal toxicity. Perinatal transmission can occur. Women with potential for exposure to HBV during pregnancy may receive the vaccination without causing any fetal problems.

HEV occurs in developing countries and may cause severe liver failure during third trimester. HEV may also be transmitted to the fetus in-utero resulting in acute hepatitis in the newborn.

Herpes simplex hepatitis causes hepatic failure in about half the cases. Despite markedly elevated AST/ALT and PT/INR, patients may be anicteric. Vesicular eruption suggests the diagnosis and can be confirmed by culture of the vesicular fluid, serology, and liver biopsy. Delivery is not needed and treatment with acyclovir is successful.

Hepatitis due to *CMV*, *Epstein-Barr virus*, and *Adenovirus* can occur during the pregnancy, but the illness is usually self-limited and requires only supportive care.

Liver diseases exacerbated by pregnancy include HEV, *Herpes simplex*, and *Herpes zoster*; these may even lead to fulminant hepatic failure. Serious problems usually occur during the third trimester. Patients with *Herpes simplex*-induced severe hepatic failure may be anicteric. Patients are at increased risk for cholestasis during pregnancy.

LIVER DISEASES UNIQUE TO PREGNANCY

These include hyperemesis gravidarum, cholestasis of pregnancy, disorders associated with pre-eclampsia and HELLP syndrome, hepatic infarction, hepatic rupture, and acute fatty liver of pregnancy.

Hyperemesis Gravidarum

Intractable nausea and vomiting occurs in 0.5 to 2.0% of pregnancies and usually occurs in the first trimester. Risk factors include primagravida, young age, low education, and obesity. Pathogenesis is unknown and appears to be multifactorial including genetic, hormonal, and environmental factors. Patients have nausea, vomiting, weight loss, dehydration, and fluid and electrolyte disturbances. Liver enzyme abnormalities may occur in as many as 50% of the cases. Elevations of serum ALT/AST between 500 to 1000 IU/L may be seen.

Antiemetics and pyridoxine (vitamin B_6 25.0 mg tid) are frequently used as first line agents. PPIs are usually added to relieve the increased heartburn. Ginger (250.0 mg qid) has been shown to be of benefit in clinical trials. Prokinetic agents like metoclopramide and domperidone help in patients with bradygastria. Low dose tricyclic antidepressants (imipramine 50.0 mg qhs) are effective. Corticosteroids result in improved sense of well-being, increased appetite, and weight gain, without improvement in nausea or vomiting. Acupuncture, acupressure, and medical hypnosis are adjunctive therapies.

HELLP Syndrome

The syndrome of hemolysis (H), elevated liver tests (EL), and low platelets (LP)—HELLP syndrome—is seen in about 0.2 to 0.6% of all pregnancies. It usually occurs during the second and third trimester but may occur postpartum. The risk is higher with pre-eclampsia (2 to 12%), multiparity, and older moms.

Patients may be asymptomatic or have upper abdominal discomfort, nausea, vomiting, malaise, and headache. Jaundice occurs in less than 10%. In the absence of hepatic infarction, the serum AST/ALT is less than 500 IU/L (usually less than 300 IU/L), along with an elevation of LDH (>600 IU/L), indirect hyperbilirubinemia (<5.0 mg/dl), and thrombocytopenia (<100 K/mm^3). Occasionally DIC may be present.

A CT with limited views is helpful to exclude hepatic rupture, hemorrhage or infarction. Liver biopsy shows periportal hemorrhage and fibrin deposition but is rarely needed.

General care of patient includes treatment of hypertension and DIC (if present) plus seizure prophylaxis. Intravenous fluid support along with blood and blood products are required in half the cases. Delivery is the only specific treatment. In cases of full-term or near maturity, immediate delivery is undertaken. Some experts recommend C-section. In mild cases at less than 34 weeks of gestation, high-dose corticosteroids are administered to extend the pregnancy and improve fetal maturity.

Conservative management is undertaken for hepatic hemorrhage without rupture. In case of rupture, treatment is aggressive hemodynamic support and surgery.

HELLP resolves in most patients after delivery over the next few days. Plasmapheresis is undertaken in case of lack of improvement or deterioration with life threatening complications over 72 hours. Maternal mortality rates vary from 1 to 20%.

Recurrence of HELLP in subsequent pregnancies varies from 3 to 25%.

Acute Fatty Liver of Pregnancy

Acute fatty liver of pregnancy is seen in about 1 in 10 000 deliveries and is associated with pre-eclampsia in about 50% of the cases. It occurs during the second half of the pregnancy and may be diagnosed after delivery. The majority of mothers are nulliparous, and the risk is greater in teen pregnancies. Long-chain 3-hydroxyacyl CoA dehydrogenase deficiency (LCHAD) has been implicated in the pathogenesis.

Clinical manifestations include anorexia, nausea, vomiting, lethargy, abdominal pain, jaundice, bleeding, and altered mental status. Hypertension, edema, and ascites may be seen. Some patients may be asymptomatic and may be detected on routine liver tests. Extra-hepatic complications include infection, intra-abdominal bleeding, polyurea, and polydypsia.

Liver enzyme elevations may range from normal to 1000 IU/L. Bilirubin elevation is mild (<5.0 mg/dl) except in severe cases. Anemia, leukocytosis, coagulopathy, metabolic acidosis, renal dysfunction and hyperamylasemia are seen. In the absence of DIC, platelet count is normal. Severe cases may have hyperammonemia and hypoglycemia. Two-thirds of the cases may be complicated by acute renal failure.

A CT scan is superior to ultrasound for the diagnosis. Differential diagnosis includes HELLP, preeclampsia, thrombocytopenic purpura, hemolytic-uremic syndrome, and severe viral hepatitis.

Diagnosis is made upon clinical grounds and results of laboratory and imaging studies. Imaging studies are helpful to exclude alternate diagnosis such as hepatic infarction or hematoma. A liver biopsy is diagnostic, but is usually not needed except in atypical cases.

Treatment includes maternal stabilization with correction of hypoglycemia, reversal of coagulopathy, lactulose in cases of hepatic encephalopathy, blood and platelet transfusions as needed, followed by immediate delivery. Some experts recommend C-section in all cases, although rapid controlled vaginal delivery with fetal monitoring may be safe in some incidences. Most patients recover without any sequelae; however, liver may take a few days to months to recover and supportive care needs to be continued. Some complications may develop after delivery.

Plasmapharesis has been used. Corticosteroids have no role. Some patients continue to deteriorate despite delivery. Bleeding and infection are the most common life-threatening complications. Occasionally, a patient may require liver transplantation.

Hepatic Infarction and Rupture

Patients present with right upper quadrant pain and fever. Serum AST/ALT are elevated (usually 1000 to 2000 IU/L or higher). Diagnosis is confirmed by hepatic imaging. Aspiration of the lesions if performed shows sterile necrotic debris. Prognosis is good and follow-up imaging after delivery demonstrates resolution of the infarcts.

Patients with hepatic rupture present with shock. It manifests as transaminases markedly elevated by several thousands, along with elevated temperature. A CT scan is diagnostic; it shows evidence of hepatic rupture as well as ascites. Ultrasound can miss the lesion. Treatment options include embolization or surgery. Management is usually conservative and illness is resolved in most patients within 6 months.

Intrahepatic Cholestasis of Pregnancy

Cholestasis of pregnancy is the most common liver disorder associated with pregnancy. It is seen in 0.1% of pregnancies and occurs during the second half of the pregnancy. Genetic, humoral, and exogenous factors appear to be involved. Enhanced sensitivity to estrogens has been implicated

Although pruritus is the hallmark and predominating symptom, mild jaundice may be present. Abdominal pain is rare. Jaundice usually does not occur in the absence of pruritus. Serum ALT/AST concentrations are variable from mild to exceeding 1000 IU/L. Total bile acid concentrations may be elevated by 10- to 100-fold and correlate with fetal risk. Serum alkaline phosphatase may be elevated up to 4-fold. Bilirubin concentration does not exceed 6.0 mg/dl. Serum GGTP may be normal or only mildly elevated despite significant elevations of alkaline phosphatase. Presence of elevated PT/INR suggests vitamin K deficiency. Ultrasound shows normal biliary tree. Liver biopsy is usually not needed.

The most commonly used drug is ursodeoxycholic acid (1.0 to 2.0 g/day). It should be avoided in the first trimester since its safety in pregnancy has not been well established. Other options include hydroxyzine (25.0 to 50.0 mg/day) and cholestyramine (8.0 to 16.0 g/day). Use of glutathione precursor, S-adenosyl methionine (SAMe) is controversial.

Dexamethasone (12.0 mg/day for 7 days) has been shown to improve symptoms, liver tests, and fetal maturity. Activated charcoal and phenobarbital are usually not recommended.

Complications include vitamin K deficiency, which should be prevented by vitamin K supplementation.

Maternal prognosis is excellent with resolution of pruritus within a few days following delivery. The disease recurs in subsequent pregnancies in over half the cases. Patients are more prone to gallstone disease. Progression to cirrhosis may occur rarely. Fetal complications include prematurity and intrauterine death. Thus, delivery should be considered at 36 weeks in patients with severe problems.

BILIARY DISEASE DURING PREGNANCY

Gallbladder Disease

There is increased incidence of cholelithiasis during pregnancy that may be complicated by cholecystitis, choledocholithiasis, and pancreatitis. The best time to perform surgery is the second trimester or early postpartum. An alternate option is an ERCP with sphincterotomy. However, an ERCP should be performed by a highly skilled endoscopist.

Choledochal Cyst

A choledochal cyst may present for the first time during pregnancy with abdominal pain, right upper quadrant mass, and jaundice. Rupture may occur.

VASCULAR DISEASE DURING PREGNANCY

Budd-Chiari Syndrome

Budd-Chiari syndrome may occur due to the hypercoagulable state during pregnancy or due to exacerbation of pre-existing hypercoagulable state. Prognosis is poor. Conservative treatment includes delivery and anticoagulation. Liver transplantation may be needed. There is a recurrence of Budd-Chiari syndrome in subsequent pregnancies.

DRUG-INDUCED LIVER DISEASE

Pregnancy does not confer increased susceptibility to drug toxicity. However, drug toxicity during pregnancy can occur even though pregnant women take very few medications.

PEARLS

- ○ Pregnancy is associated with elevated levels of alkaline phosphatase.
- ○ Viral hepatitis is the most common cause of jaundice during pregnancy.

O Hyperemesis gravidarum may lead to markedly abnormal liver enzymes.

BIBLIOGRAPHY

Sandhu BS, Sanyal AJ. Pregnancy and liver disease. *Gastroenterol Clin North Am.* 2003;32(1):407-36.

Chapter

57 *Fulminant Hepatic Failure* ▬

Definitions of fulminant hepatic failure (FHF) vary. It may be defined as a rapid onset of encephalopathy within 8 weeks of onset of symptoms in a previously healthy subject or within 2 weeks of development of jaundice in a previously healthy individual. Acute liver failure developing outside of these time ranges may be described as subfulminant hepatic failure.

EPIDEMIOLOGY

It is estimated to account for 3.5 deaths per 1 million people.

ETIOLOGY

Etiology varies with the geography. The predominant causes include drugs like acetaminophen; viral HAV, HBV, and HDV; AIH; Wilson's disease; Budd-Chiari syndrome; acute fatty liver of pregnancy; and Reye's syndrome. HBV is the most common viral cause.

Uncommon causes of FHF include heat stroke, sepsis, and hepatic malignancy. The cause may not be identified in as many as 20 to 40% of cases. FHF due to HAV or HBV and acetaminophen carries better prognosis than that caused by idiosyncratic drug reactions and Wilson's disease.

CLINICAL MANIFESTATIONS

The hallmarks of FHF include altered mental status (hepatic encephalopathy) and coagulopathy. Often, there is multisystem failure characterized by cerebral edema, renal failure, acidosis, sepsis, and shock. A CT scan is not reliable for diagnosing cerebral edema and intracranial hypertension, but helps exclude other causes for altered mental status. Liver biopsy is not helpful and is not routinely recommended.

LIVER TRANSPLANTATION

The only proven and effective treatment is liver transplantation that has a 1-year survival rate of 80%. Thus patients with FHF should be immediately transferred to a transplant center for consideration for liver transplantation. Predictive factors for the outcome of hepatic failure include degree of encephalopathy, patient's age, cause of FHF, prothrombin time, serum bilirubin, and arterial pH. Various formulas to decide on the timing of transplantation have been developed.

Transplantation for Acetaminophen Poisoning

According to King's College criteria, in cases of FHF induced by acetaminophen, OLT is recommended for 1) patients with pH less than 7.3 regardless of the degree of encephalopathy; or 2) patients with prothrombin time greater than 100 seconds, a serum creatinine greater than 3.4 mg/dl, plus Grade 3 or 4 encephalopathy.

Nonacetaminophen-Induced FHF

OLT is recommended for a prothrombin time greater than 100 seconds regardless of the degree of encephalopathy or if any three of the following parameters are positive:

1. Age less than 10 or greater than 40.
2. Non-A, non-B hepatitis.
3. Halothane hepatitis.
4. Idiosyncratic drug reaction.
5. Duration of jaundice prior to encephalopathy more than 7 days.
6. PT greater than 50 seconds.
7. Serum bilirubin more than 18.0 mg/dl.

OTHER TREATMENTS

A multispecialist team approach at a transplant center is required to prevent and treat multisystem organ failure.

Hepatic Encephalopathy

Hepatic encephalopathy is usually a manifestation of increased intracranial pressure and should be treated with mannitol and, if possible, monitoring of intracranial pressure.

Cerebral Edema

Most patients also develop cerebral edema that manifests as decerebrate posturing, hypertension, and pupillary abnormalities. Absence of the clinical manifestations of cerebral edema does not exclude the diagnosis. Direct intracranial pressure (ICP) monitoring is recommended. The head should be elevated to 20 degrees. Sudden, rapid changes in position and tracheal suction should be avoided. Sedatives should be avoided as much as possible.

Mannitol is the drug of choice for cerebral edema and intracranial hypertension. Patients with no response to mannitol undergo pentobarbital coma. Mannitol should be avoided in case of renal failure and thiopental infusion should be administered instead. The role for hyperventilation to keep ICP low is controversial. Steroids are not effective and should not be administered.

Renal Failure

Renal failure occurs in about 50% of the cases. Hemofilteration is usually preferred over conventional hemodialysis.

Infection

Low threshold should be applied for frequent cultures of body fluids. Broad spectrum antibiotics should be instituted empirically as needed.

Nutritional Support

Patients with mild encephalopathy may receive oral or enteral feeding with a low protein diet, whereas TPN should be used in advanced cases. Branched-chain amino acids are expensive but not helpful.

Bleeding

Stress prophylaxis using H_2-receptor antagonists or intravenous PPIs should be undertaken in all patients. Fresh frozen plasma should be used in patients with bleeding or those undergoing procedures. A combination of recombinant human factor VIIA plus fresh frozen plasma may be beneficial.

Respiratory Support

Respiratory failure due to pulmonary edema and infections occurs in about one-third of the patients and may require mechanical ventilation for respiratory support.

TREATMENT OF UNDERLYING CAUSE

N-acetylcystine is used for acetaminophen poisoning. Nasogastric lavage, forced diuresis, silibinin, and activated charcoal may be helpful in mushroom poisoning. Portal decompression by TIPS or surgical shunt with or without thrombolytic therapy may help in acute Budd-Chiari syndrome. Patients with Herpes simplex virus infection should be treated with acyclovir. Liver dialysis system may be of short-term benefit.

PEARLS

○ Liver transplantation is the only proven, effective treatment of FHF.

○ Patients with FHF should be transferred to a transplant center as soon as possible.

BIBLIOGRAPHY

McGuire BM. The critically ill liver patient: fulminant hepatic failure. *Semin Gastrointest Dis.* 2003;14(1):39-42.

Chapter
58 *Liver Transplantation*

About 5,000 liver transplants are performed each year in the United States. Many more patients who do require liver transplantation die without being able to get the transplant because of shortage of organs. Because of the shortage, living donor liver transplantation is being offered at select centers.

INDICATIONS

The most common underlying causes leading to transplantation include viral hepatitis (especially HCV), alcoholic liver disease, acute fatty liver of pregnancy, and cryptogenic cirrhosis. Transplantation is less commonly performed in patients with hepatic malignancy, metabolic and genetic disorders like AAT deficiency, hemochromatosis, cystic fibrosis, Wilson's disease, galactosemia, glycogen storage disease, Crigler-Najjar syndrome, familial hypercholestrolemia, Byler's syndrome, and vascular disorders like Budd-Chiari syndrome and veno-occlusive disease. Other uncommon causes include adult polycystic liver disease, Caroli's disease, severe graft vs host disease, sarcoidosis, hepatic trauma, and lymphangiomatosis.

CONTRAINDICATIONS

Absolute contraindications to OLT (with few exceptions) include active alcohol or drug abuse, cancer or active infection anywhere in the body (except when OLT is for HCC), and severe cardiopulmonary disease uncontrolled with medical therapy. Relative contraindications include elderly subjects older than 65, suboptimal family or social support, severe hepatopulmonary syndrome with severe hypoxemia (pO_2 less than 50 mmHg), and intrahepatic tumor more than 5.0 cm in size for single lesion.

REFERRAL TO TRANSPLANT CENTER

Patients should be referred to a liver transplant center when there is advanced and irreversible liver disease (Child-Pugh score is 8 or greater or a MELD score of 20 or higher). Other conditions that may prompt referral to a transplant center include ascites refractory to therapy, a prior episode of SBP, hepatic encephalopathy, malnutrition, recurrent bacterial cholangitis, hepatopulmonary syndrome, hepatorenal syndrome, FHF, HCC, prothrombin time greater than 5 sec above control, serum bilirubin greater than 5.0 mg/dl, worsening quality of life by intractable pruritus, fractures due to metabolic bone disease, and recurrent variceal bleeding.

TRIAGE OF PATIENTS FOR OLT

The MELD score has high predictive value for 3-month mortality in any given patient. It is based upon serum bilirubin, serum creatinine, and INR, and involves a complex calculations. Patients with scores greater than 25 should have their score updated every week with new lab values. MELD score is modified for conditions like HCC providing additional weight for increased mortality risk.

FHF patients with worsening encephalopathy and coagulopathy receive the highest priority for liver transplantation Disease specific prognostic models are also available for disorders including PBC, alcoholic liver disease, and acute liver failure.

PREOPERATIVE EVALUATION

Cardiopulmonary evaluation is done to assess if the patient can withstand the surgery and includes EKG, echocardiography, chest x-rays, pulmonary function tests, stress test, and sometimes arterial blood gases. Coronary angiogram should be performed if a stress test is abnormal or in patients with a history of coronary artery disease.

Renal work-up includes a 24-hour urinary protein and creatinine or GFR using nuclear medicine techniques. Renal transplantation is performed in some patients undergoing liver transplantation; however renal transplantation is not a requirement in cases of hepatorenal syndrome of less than 2 to 4 weeks duration.

Liver biopsy is usually done to establish the etiology of liver disease but is not essential. Imaging studies including CT scan or MRI should be done to exclude hepatic malignancy. A comprehensive social services consult is required to assess for chemical, drug, or alcohol abuse; psychosocial and financial situation, as well as adequacy of family support.

SPECIAL ISSUES

Hepatitis C

Patients who are HCV-positive and receive OLT have an almost 100% recurrence of HCV infection, and about a third of those patients progress rapidly to cirrhosis over a period of 3 to 5 years. Another third have evidence of slowly progressive disease and the remaining third have no significant histologic evidence of disease. Patients transplanted for HCV infection have a somewhat reduced survival, and as such, aggressive management should be attempted prior to OLT.

Hepatitis B

Patients positive for chronic HBV have recurrence after transplantation. The recurrence of HBV can be reduced by administration of HBIG in the peritransplant period and for at least 6 months thereafter. Some patients are treated with lamivudine and HBIG.

Hepatocellular Carcinoma

Patients with HCC should only be transplanted if they have a single tumor less than 5.0 cm confined to the liver or if there are multiple lesions in the liver (less than three) with each lesion measuring less than 3.0 cm.

Living Donor Liver Transplantation

Living donor liver transplantation (LDLT) is being increasingly used especially for pediatric population. Benefits include a short waiting period and the possibility of a reduced risk of developing complications related to cirrhosis and progression to cancer. Risks to the donor include surgical complications (hemorrhage, infection, liver failure, death), as well as financial risk of unemployment and noninsurability.

Acceptable criteria for the donor include age between 18 and 55 years, ABO compatibility, absence of serious systemic disease, adequate liver volume for recipient, absence of infections (HIV, HBV, HCV), absence of significant abnormality of biliary tree and hepatic vasculature, and less than 10% steatosis on histology.

PEARLS

○ Hepatitis C is the leading cause of liver transplantation in the United States.

○ There is a shortage of available organs and many patients requiring OLT die before they can get a liver.

BIBLIOGRAPHY

Wiesner RH, Rakela J, Ishitani MB, Mulligan DC, Spivey JR, Steers JL, Krom RA. Recent advances in liver transplantation. *Mayo Clin Proc.* 2003;78(2):197-210.

Broelsch CE, Frilling A, Testa G, Malago M. Living donor liver transplantation in adults. *Eur J Gastroenterol Hepatol.* 2003;15(1):3-6.

GALLBLADDER AND PANCREAS

Chapter

59 *Gallstones*

EPIDEMIOLOGY

Gallstones occur in 10 to 20% of the population. These are rare in Asia, whereas North Europeans have higher prevalence than Southern Europeans. They tend to occur more among females. Native American women are particularly at risk.

PATHOGENESIS

Gallstones may be of three types:
1. Yellow or cholesterol stones (80 to 85%).
2. Black pigment stones.
3. Brown pigment stones.

Mixed patterns may be seen. Fifteen percent of patients with gallstones also have stones in the common bile duct.

Precipitation of cholesterol or bilirubin leads to stone formation. In addition to cholesterol supersaturation, factors implicated in synthesis of cholesterol stone include gallbladder dysmotility, mucin hypersecretion that promotes crystal formation, and slowed intestinal transit causing elevated levels of hydrophobic bile acids.

Black stones are comprised of bilirubin plus some calcium. They are relatively radio-opaque, but rarely cause obstruction.

Brown stones are associated with chronic infections and are seen in intra- or extrahepatic ducts but not in the gallbladder.

RISK FACTORS

Risk factors for cholesterol stones include multiparity, oral contraceptives, obesity, rapid weight loss, low vegetable protein intake, sedentary lifestyle, hypertriglyceridemia, diabetes mellitus, insulin resistance, spinal cord injuries, and chronic intestinal pseudo-obstruction.

Black stone formation is determined by amount of degradation of heme. Risk factors include hemolytic anemia (sickle cell disease, beta thalassemia), chronic liver disease and portal hypertension, Crohn's disease, and total parenteral nutrition.

Biliary sludge is an intermediate step in the process of cholesterol and black pigment stone formation. However, sludge leads to stone formation only in a minority of cases.

Brown stones are usually seen in the common bile duct and occur as a result of transient bacterial colonization of foreign body such as suture or retained stone after cholecystectomy. Parasitic infections (*Clonorchis*) are the cause of brown stones in East Asia and may lead to *Oriental cholangiohepatitis.*

The occurrence of primary intrahepatic stones or the stones in the common bile duct is rare.

DIAGNOSTIC MODALITIES

Because the stones are mostly radiolucent, less than 25% can be visualized on plain x-ray. Oral cholecystography is outdated and is not used except prior to consideration for oral dissolution therapy. Ultrasound is the test of choice for gallstones; however, CT scan is superior for visualization of choledocholithiasis. A CT can also assess for any complications like pancreatitis, abscess, perforation, etc.

Cholescintigraphy (HIDA scan) is accurate for the diagnosis of acute cholecystitis in 95% of cases. It is also used to look for postoperative biliary leak.

An ERCP is the standard for diagnosis of common bile duct stones; the stones can also be removed during the exam. An MRCP is as accurate as ERCP, but does not allow the therapeutic option.

Microscopic examination of bile after administration of cholecystokinin (CCK) is useful for assessing microlithiasis in patients with biliary symptoms but without ultrasonographic evidence of gallstones.

CLINICAL FEATURES

Gallstones remain silent in about 75 to 85% of the cases. They do not cause symptoms like bitter taste in mouth, chronic pain, flatulence, and nonspecific complaints of gas, bloating, and belching. The prevalence of fatty food intolerance is the same as in general population. Most common manifestation is biliary colic, which occurs at the rate of 2% per year. Complications of gallstones occur in less than 0.2% per year. The incidence of cancer is 0.02% per year.

Biliary Colic

It occurs as a result of stone impaction in the cystic duct. Once a patient has an episode of biliary colic, recurrence occurs in 30% per year. The word biliary colic is a misnomer since the pain is not colicky. It is a steady, constant pain radiating to back or right shoulder and subsides in a few hours. Nausea and vomiting may be present. Persistence of the pain beyond 6 hours should raise the suspicion for cholecystitis.

A physical exam is normal, as are the laboratory studies. Elevations of liver and pancreatic enzymes and/or bilirubin suggest concomitant choledocholithiasis. Right upper quadrant ultrasound is the test of choice.

Acute Cholecystitis

Patients present with right upper quadrant and epigastric pain radiating to the scapula. There is tenderness in the right upper quadrant, and Murphy's sign (pain and inspiratory arrest during palpation of right subcostal region) can be elicited. A CBC will show leukocytosis. Presence of fever, chills, and leukocytosis exceeding 16 000/mm^3 suggests gallbladder empyema warranting urgent surgical consultation. Ultrasound is excellent for the diagnosis of gallstones, but not for acute cholecystitis. HIDA scan is the test of choice. Nonvisualization of gallbladder is 95% accurate for the diagnosis. A false positive test may occur in cases of prolonged fasting and in patients on TPN.

The patient should be admitted to hospital and given nothing by mouth. Intravenous fluid and broad-spectrum antibiotics are administered. Options for antibiotics include cefoxitin in mild cases and ampicillin plus gentamicin or a third generation cephalosporin plus gentamicin in severe cases. Nasogastric suction may be undertaken in patients with persistent nausea and vomiting. Treatment is cholecystectomy, usually laparoscopic. Surgery is undertaken during the same hospitalization after 24 to 48 hours of medical support. Ultrasound-guided percutaneous cholecystostomy may be undertaken in poor surgical risk candidates who do not respond to medical treatment. High-risk surgical candidates who respond to medical therapy well enough to permit a discharge from hospital, may be candidates for nonsurgical therapies.

Chronic Cholecystitis

It is more of a pathologic than a clinical entity occurring as a result of acute cholecystitis or recurrent biliary colic. Preceding history of pain is not always available.

Choledocholithiasis

This occurs in 15% of patients with gallbladder stones. Although frequently asymptomatic, these stones are more likely to cause problems than the stones in gallbladder alone. Patients present with cholangitis or pancreatitis. They have elevated serum alkaline phosphatase and bilirubin. Longstanding stones may cause biliary stricture or secondary biliary cirrhosis. Ultrasound usually but not always shows a dilated common bile duct. An impaction of stone in cystic duct with obstruction of common bile duct due to edema is called *Mirizzi syndrome*.

Acute bacterial cholangitis presents with right upper quadrant pain, fever, and jaundice (*Charcot's triad*). Infection occurs due to Gram negative organisms. Bacteremia may occur and carries high mortality.

Biliary pancreatitis occurs due to stone impaction at the ampulla of Vater causing obstruction of the pancreatic duct.

Rare Complications

Stone may erode through gallbladder and cause cholecystoenteric fistula. Cholecystocolonic fistula causes bile salt induced diarrhea. Large gallstones may get impacted at ileocecal valve to cause intestinal obstruction also known as gallstone ileus. Gallstone may migrate to the stomach through a fistula causing pyloric obstruction, also known as *Bouveret's syndrome*.

TREATMENT OPTIONS FOR GALLSTONES

Surgery

Laparoscopic cholecystectomy is the treatment of choice. About 5% of the operations have to be converted to an open operation. The incidence of bile leak is 0.2 to 0.5%. About 5% develop postcholecystectomy diarrhea, which can be controlled by cholestyramine. The risk of colon cancer may be slightly increased after surgery, especially among women.

Endoscopic Option

Patients who have choledocholithiasis and are poor surgical risk may have the bile duct cleared endoscopically and surgery deferred.

Some experts assert that patients with stones exclusively in the common bile duct (CBD), and not in the gallbladder, may not need surgery if the CBD has been adequately cleared with an ERCP and sphincterotomy.

Oral Dissolution Therapy

UDCA can be an option in select patients who have small cholesterol stones (less than 5.0 mm) and a functioning gallbladder. UDCA should be considered only for symptomatic patients with small stones that have not caused complications. Complementary extracorporeal shock wave lithotripsy (EWSL) may be undertaken along with oral dissolution therapy in patients with large single stone up to 2.0 cm in size.

Contact solvent dissolution using Methyl-tert-butyl ether (MTBE) is not popular because of risk for serious complications.

Treatment of Microlithiasis

Persistent microlithiasis in the absence of significant symptoms can be treated with oral dissolution therapy, although surgery is the only definitive treatment in most cases.

Management Strategy for Biliary Symptoms

1. Patients should undergo gallbladder ultrasound. In case of normal gallbladder, consider repeat examination, examination for crystals in bile, or an EUS. The role of biliary manometry is controversial and select cases may benefit from it.
2. Patients with gallstones on ultrasound and good surgical candidates should undergo laparoscopic cholecystectomy. Those at high-risk for concomitant choledocholithiasis may benefit from a preoperative ERCP. An MRCP is another option but does not provide the benefit of therapeutics.
3. Patients who are poor surgical candidates and have <5.0 mm radiolucent stone burden or a single radiolucent stone should be considered for bile acid dissolution therapy with or without EWSL.

Role of Prophylactic Cholecystectomy

Routine cholecystectomy for a finding of incidental cholelithiasis is not recommended. Candidates for prophylactic surgery include:

1. Patients with high risk of gallbladder cancer (ie, gallbladder polyp greater than 1.0 cm, porcelain gallbladder, and native American females).
2. Young sickle cell disease patients.

3. Patients awaiting organ transplantation.
4. Patients travelling to remote areas or space for prolonged periods.

PEARLS

○ Most patients never have any problems related to their gallstones.

○ Routine use of prophylactic cholecystectomy is not recommended.

BIBLIOGRAPHY

Mark DH, Flamm CR, Aronson N. Evidence-based assessment of diagnostic modalities for common bile duct stones. *Gastrointest Endosc.* 2002;56(6 Suppl):S190-4.

Shaffer EA. Gallbladder sludge: what is its clinical significance? *Curr Gastroenterol Rep.* 2001;3(2):166-73.

Cohen S, Bacon BR, Berlin JA, et al. NIH State-of-the-Science Conference Statement: ERCP for diagnosis and therapy, January 14-16, 2002. *Gastrointest Endosc.* 2002;56(6):803-9.

Chapter
60 *Acute Pancreatitis*

EPIDEMIOLOGY

Acute pancreatitis is an inflammatory condition of the pancreas which occurs in about 5 to 25 persons per 100 000 population. While gallstone pancreatitis is more common in women, alcoholic pancreatitis is predominantly seen in men. The incidence of pancreatitis in African Americans is three times greater than in White men. The incidence also increases with age.

ETIOLOGY

Cholelithiasis and chronic alcoholism account for about 75% of the cases.

The role of biliary sludge is controversial. Many experts recommend cholecystectomy in such cases. Most patients with alcohol induced pancreatitis have acute on chronic pancreatitis.

Other etiologies include genetic mutations; metabolic disorders (hypertriglyceridemia with concentrations greater than 1000.0 mg/dl, hypercalcemia, hyperparathyroidism); medications (didanosine, pentamidine, metronidazole, sulfonamides, tetracycline, furosemide, thiazides, sulfasalazine, aminosalicylates, azathioprine, L-asparaginase, valproic acid, sulindac, estrogen, tamoxifen); viral infections (mumps, *Coxsackie virus, hepatitis B, Cytomegalovirus (CMV), Herpes zoster, Herpes simplex,* HIV); bacteria (*Mycoplasma, Legionella, Leptospira, Salmonella*); fungal infections (*Aspergillus*); parasites (*Toxoplasma, Cryptosporidium, Ascaris*); blunt or penetrating trauma to the abdomen; pancreatic ischemia due to vasculitis, thromboembolism, hypotension and shock; pregnancy; and post-ERCP.

Idiopathic pancreatitis occurs in about 30% of the cases. The role of pancreas divisum is controversial.

PATHOGENESIS

While a large number of etiologies have been implicated, only a small fraction of these patients with such underlying disorders like cholelithiasis or alcoholism develop pancreatitis. Mechanisms probably vary according to the etiology. In case of gallstone pancreatitis, the inciting event is an obstruction due to the impaction of stone or due to edema leading to reflux of bile into the pancreatic ducts.

High concentration of free fatty acids released from triglycerides in patients with hypertriglyceridemia causes edema within the pancreatic capillaries precipitating an inflammatory/toxic event. This leads to autodigestive injury to the pancreas.

Premature activation of pancreatic zymogens within the pancreas precipitates an attack of acute pancreatitis in patients with hereditary pancreatitis.

The initial injury may progress to systemic complications including fever, dehydration, renal failure, shock, adult respiratory distress syndrome (ARDS), and multiorgan failure. Bacterial translocation occurs due to breakdown of gut barrier as a result of ischemia, leading to sepsis.

CLINICAL FEATURES

Patients typically present with acute upper abdominal pain that may be localized or diffused. The pain may radiate to the back and may be preceded by a bout of biliary colic. Alcohol-induced pancreatitis typically occurs 24 to 72 hours after last alcohol intake. There may be associated nausea, vomiting, restlessness, and agitation.

Findings on physical exam are variable and may include fever, tachycardia, abdominal distention, epigastric tenderness and guarding, shallow respirations, Grey Turner's sign (hemorrhagic discoloration in the flank), or Cullen's sign (ecchymosis of periumbilical region). These two signs occur in less than 1% of the cases and reflect intra-abdominal hemorrhage.

Jaundice may occur due to the obstruction of the CBD either due to a stone or inflamed pancreas. A pancreatic pseudocyst may be palpable in the epigastrium. In rare cases, subcutaneous nodular fat necrosis, thrombophlebitis, and arthritis may be seen. Xanthoma may be seen in patients with hyperlipidemia.

DIAGNOSIS

Pancreatic Enzymes

Serum amylase concentrations rise within 12 hours and stay elevated for 3 to 5 days. Serum amylase may occasionally be normal in very severe cases. Urinary amylase levels are increased, but are not used in clinical practice.

Serum lipase elevations last longer than serum amylase. Combined assessment of serum amylase and lipase levels is not superior to assessment of serum amylase alone for the diagnosis. The diagnostic role of the measurement of urinary and serum trypsinogen-2, pancreatitis associated protein (PAP), trypsinogen activation peptide (TAP), and C-reactive protein remains to be established.

Plain X-Rays

Plain x-rays of the abdomen should be done to exclude bowel obstruction or perforation. They are usually normal or may show sentinal loop (ie, localized ileus of a part of small intestine) or a colon cut-off sign manifesting as very little air distal to the splenic flexure due to functional spasm of the descending colon. A chest x-ray may show an elevation of hemidiaphragm, pleural effusion, or atelectasis.

Ultrasound and Computerized Tomography Scan

An abdominal ultrasound is important for detection of gallstones, as well as the size of the CBD. The overlying bowel gas frequently precludes assessment of pancreas.

A CT scan is the test of choice for the diagnosis of acute pancreatitis as well as its complications. It should be done in severe cases or when a patient is not responding to conservative treatment or complications are suspected. It should be done with both oral and IV contrast with pancreatic protocol.

The severity of acute pancreatitis can be estimated by a CT scan severity index on the basis of findings on an unenhanced (score 0 to 4) and enhanced CT scan (score 0 to 6). Grade A reflects normal pancreas; Grade B shows focal or diffuse enlargement or irregularity of the pancreas without peripancreatic inflammation; Grade C reflects a peripancreatic inflammation; Grade D shows findings of Grade C plus a single fluid collection; and Grade E manifests as two or more peripancreatic fluid collections or gas in the pancreas or retroperitoneum. An assessment of pancreatic necrosis is made based on the intravenous contrast enhanced CT. The maximum score is 10; patients with a score equal to or greater than 6 are characterized as severe.

Miscellaneous

An ERCP should be done in patients with severe acute biliary pancreatitis with suspected obstruction. A laparoscopic exploration of common bile duct is as safe and effective as postoperative ERCP.

DIFFERENTIAL DIAGNOSIS

Elevated amylase levels can also be seen in patients with acute cholecystitis, abdominal surgery, trauma, radiation therapy, malignancy with ectopic amylase production, metabolic acidosis, renal failure, macroamylasemia, ruptured ectopic pregnancy, alcoholism, liver cirrhosis, and anorexia bulimia.

A serum ALT concentration of greater than 150 IU/L has a positive predictive value of 95% for gallstone induced pancreatitis. A serum lipase to amylase ratio greater than 2.0 favors alcoholic pancreatitis.

ASSESSMENT OF SEVERITY

Although scoring systems such as Ranson's criteria and Apache II score are used by some physicians, their use for assessing the severity is no better than clinical assessment. A hematocrit of 44% or greater suggests the possibility of severe pancreatitis. A contrast-enhanced CT should be undertaken in patients with suspected severe pancreatitis in order to look for necrosis.

TREATMENT

General Measures

Treatment involves supportive care, correction of underlying cause (if possible), and treatment of complications. Patients suspected of severe pancreatitis should be managed in an ICU setting. Any possible offending drugs should be withdrawn as soon as possible.

Supportive care involves nothing orally by mouth, intravenous fluids, and pain control.

Morphine (5.0 to 15.0 mg IM or slow IV q 4 to 6 hours) may be a better choice than meperidine (25.0 to 50.0 mg IM or IV q 4 to 6 hours) for pain control. A combination of an opiate and promethazine (Phenergan 25.0 to 50.0 mg q 4 to 6 hours) is frequently employed. Nasogastric tube placement with intermittent suction is useful for patients with persistent nausea and vomiting.

Elemental feedings through a nasoenteric tube placed distal to Ligament of Treitz or total parenteral nutrition should be undertaken in severe cases.

Treatment of infection

Consider empiric antibiotics in patients with greater than 30% of pancreatic necrosis. Options include imipenem-cilastatin (Primaxin), a third generation cephalosporin, piperacillin, or a fluoroquinolone. Antifungal therapy with fluconazole has also been used as part of empiric regimen. First generation cephalosporins and aminoglycosides should be avoided.

A CT-guided fine needle aspiration of the necrotic pancreas should be performed if there is no improvement on antibiotics for 1 week. Patients with bacterial infections should undergo necrosectomy. Patients with sterile necrosis are continued on conservative therapy for at least 3 weeks.

Role of ERCP

An ERCP should be performed for ascending cholangitis, as well as for severe biliary pancreatitis with suspected biliary obstruction.

Oral Feeding

Oral feedings are started with clear liquids at about 100 to 200 mL every 4 hours for 24 hours. They are gradually advanced to solid foods over the next 4 to 5 days. Patients with postparandial abdominal pain, nausea, and vomiting after oral feedings may be able to tolerate feeding via nasoenteric tube. Oral or enteric feedings are not contraindicated in the presence of fluid collections or elevated pancreatic enzymes.

Cholecystectomy

Cholecystectomy should be undertaken in patients with gallstone pancreatitis prior to discharge from the hospital since there is a 25% risk of recurrent pancreatitis, cholecystitis or cholangitis within the next 6 weeks. In patients with evidence of dilated bile duct or persistent bile duct stone, a cholangiogram should be undertaken via ERCP or intraoperatively in order to prevent further recurrence. An MRCP or endoscopic ultrasound to exclude a bile duct stone may be undertaken in patients with liver enzymes that are slow to normalize.

APPROACH TO PATIENT WITH IDIOPATHIC PANCREATITIS

The management of such patients should be individualized. Different approaches have been favored by different experts.

1. Laparoscopic cholecystectomy.
2. Examination of bile for microlithiasis and, if positive, cholecystectomy.
3. Pursuit of the diagnosis of the sphincter of Oddi dysfunction is controversial. Sphincter of Oddi manometry as well as ERCP carry significant risk for complications. I recommend that such patients be referred to tertiary care center for diagnosis and treatment.

PEARLS

- ○ Most cases of acute pancreatitis are caused by alcoholism or gallstones.
- ○ Cholecystectomy should be performed during the same hospitalization in cases of gallstone pancreatitis.
- ○ Pancreatic enzymes may be normal in pancreatitis.

BIBLIOGRAPHY

Fogel EL, Sherman S. Acute biliary pancreatitis: when should the endoscopist intervene? *Gastroenterology*. 2003;125(1):229-35.

Mitchell RM, Byrne MF, Baillie J. Pancreatitis. *Lancet*. 2003;361(9367):1447-55.

Yousaf M, McCallion K, Diamond T. Management of severe acute pancreatitis. *Br J Surg*. 2003;90(4):407-20.

Chapter

61 *Chronic Pancreatitis* ▬▬▬

Chronic pancreatitis is a progressive inflammatory condition characterized by morphological changes leading to permanent exocrine, as well as endocrine dysfunction.

EPIDEMIOLOGY

It occurs in about 8 to 10 persons per 100 000 population. It is listed as a discharge diagnosis in about 60 000 hospital admissions each year in the United States.

ETIOLOGY

Etiologies include alcohol abuse, hereditary pancreatitis, trauma, tumors, pancreatic duct obstruction, tropical pancreatitis, systemic disorders like SLE, cystic fibrosis, hyperthyroidism, and mutations of the cystic fibrosis gene. Many cases remain idiopathic The majority of the cases are due to alcohol abuse over a period of at least 10 years; however, only about 5 to 10% of the patients with a history of alcohol abuse develop to chronic pancreatitis.

PATHOGENESIS

Chronic pancreatitis is associated with increased secretion of pancreatic proteins resulting in proteinaceous plugs. Calcification of these plugs leads to scarring and obstruction of the pancreatic ducts. Other factors include ischemia, autoimmune derangements, and a decrease in antioxidants like selenium, vitamins C, vitamin E, and methionine.

CLINICAL FEATURES

Patients may be asymptomatic or may have episodic abdominal pain that is usually epigastric and radiates to the back with associated nausea and vomiting. Pain is relieved by leaning forward and made worse by eating. The pain tends to become constant over the long-term. Pancreatic exocrine insufficiency may lead to steatorrhea resulting in loose, greasy, and foul-smelling stools with glucose intolerance and even diabetes mellitus.

COMPLICATIONS

1. Pancreatic pseudocyst.
2. Bile duct or duodenal obstruction.
3. Pancreatic ascites.
4. Splenic vein thrombosis.
5. Pseudoaneurysm.
6. Pancreatic cancer.

DIAGNOSIS

Routine Studies

Pancreatic enzymes may be normal or mildly elevated. CBC, electrolytes, and liver tests are normal. A bile duct obstruction due to edema, fibrosis, or cancer may result in increased alkaline phosphatase. Fecal fat for Sudan III stain is positive in patients with exocrine insufficiency.

Imaging Studies

Pancreatic calcifications are seen in 30% of the patients. Similarly, ductal calcification or dilatation and pancreatic abnormalities, as well as fluid collections like pseudocysts may be seen on CT, MRI, and ultrasound. An ERCP is standard in the absence of precise diagnosis on preceding tests. Pancreatogram shows beading of the main pancreatic duct and its branches. Early cases of chronic pancreatitis may have a normal ERCP. The role of endoscopic ultrasound, as well as MRCP, is evolving.

Pancreatic Function Tests

Secretin stimulation test, bentiromide test and fecal chymotrypsin are rarely used. A modified Schilling's test has been used in the evaluation of unexplained diarrhea.

DIFFERENTIAL DIAGNOSIS

The main issue is usually distinguishing chronic pancreatitis from pancreatic cancer. Other considerations include peptic ulcer, gallstone disease, and functional bowel disorders.

TREATMENT

Treatment of chronic pancreatitis involves pain management and the treatment of complications.

Pancreatic Enzymes

Response to pancreatic enzymes supplements is variable and recommendations are based on tradition, inconsistent data and "expert opinion." High doses of at least 30K lipase and 90K protease units are recommended. We prefer non-enteric preparations (2 to 4 tablets of Viokase 16 with each meal and bedtime) along with acid suppression using H_2RAs or PPIs.

Analgesics

Pain control may be achieved by nonsteroidal anti-inflammatory drugs (NSAIDs), short course of narcotics, and low doses of tricyclic antidepressants. Chronic narcotic analgesia may be employed in select cases using long acting products like MS Contin (10.0 to 30.0 mg PO q 8 to 12 hours) or fentanyl patches. Consultation with a pain specialist should be obtained in such cases.

Drug-Refractory Pain

Celiac nerve block is effective in less than 50% of the patients. The role of pancreatic endotherapy utilizing pancreatic duct decompression is evolving. Octreotide may be helpful in select cases. Patients with a dilated pancreatic duct (>6.0 mm) who fail medical therapy may be candidates for surgical intervention. Total pancreatectomy followed by islet cell transplantation may be helpful in nondiabetic patients.

Management of Steatorrhea

Patients should receive fat restricted diet of 20.0 g/day or less of fat plus supplemental oral pancreatic enzymes (at least 30K lipase units with each meal). Acid suppression should be undertaken along with pancreatic enzymes supplementation for steatorrhea. We prefer enteric-coated preparations. Patients with weight loss and poor response to dietary management may benefit from medium-chain triglycerides supplementation.

TREATMENT OF COMPLICATIONS

Pancreatic Pseudocyst

Most pseudocysts remain asymptomatic and are diagnosed on ultrasound or a CT scan. Drainage of the pseudocyst is recommended in patients with persistent pain, infection, compression of adjacent structures or rapidly enlarging size. The drainage may be undertaken using percutaneous, endoscopic or surgical techniques depending upon the local expertise. About 10% of the patients with chronic pancreatitis develop a bile duct or duodenal obstruction and require surgical drainage procedures. Endoscopic stents have been used for benign bile duct lesions but require frequent changes.

Pancreatic Ascites and Plural Effusion

These occur due to disruption of the pancreatic duct. Fluid amylase concentration is at least five times the serum amylase concentration and is usually greater than 1000 IU/L. Medical management includes repeated aspiration, diuretics, and parenteral nutrition. Octreotide may be helpful in select cases. Pancreatic stents are helpful if pancreatic duct disruption is present. Many patients require surgery.

Splenic Vein Thrombosis

This occurs due to the adjacent inflammation in the pancreas. Splenectomy is the treatment of choice.

Pseudoaneurysm

Chronic pancreatitis can lead to pseudoaneurysm of splenic, hepatic, gastroduodenal, and pancreaticoduodenal arteries. These may be diagnosed by a CT scan or MRI. Blood flow can be documented on doppler ultrasound. Diagnosis is confirmed by mesenteric angiography and therapeutic embolization can be carried out at the same time. Surgical management of bleeding pseudoaneurysms is associated with high morbidity and mortality.

PEARLS

- ❍ Most patients with a history of alcoholism do not develop chronic pancreatitis.
- ❍ High doses of pancreatic enzyme supplementation are used for pain control and treatment of steatorrhea.
- ❍ Majority of the asymptomatic pancreatic pseudocysts can be observed since they may resolve spontaneously.

BIBLIOGRAPHY

Mitchell RM, Byrne MF, Baillie J. Pancreatitis. *Lancet*. 2003;361(9367):1447-55.

Mohan V, Premalatha G, Pitchumoni CS. Tropical chronic pancreatitis: an update. *J Clin Gastroenterol*. 2003;36(4):337-46.

Thuluvath PJ, Imperio D, Nair S, Cameron JL. Chronic pancreatitis. Long-term pain relief with or without surgery, cancer risk, and mortality. *J Clin Gastroenterol*. 2003;36(2):159-65.

Chapter 62 *Pancreatic Cancer*

Pancreatic cancer is the fourth leading cause of cancer-related mortality and the second leading cause of digestive cancer-related mortality in the United States.

EPIDEMIOLOGY

It occurs in 8.8 per 100 000 persons. Approximately 30 000 new cases occur each year. It is more common amongst males than the females and more among Blacks than Whites. It occurs usually after the age of 50.

RISK FACTORS

Heredity plays an important part in as many as 10% of the cases either directly or indirectly through hereditary chronic pancreatitis. The risk for pancreatic cancer is also increased in Peutz-Jeghers syndrome, Von-Hippel-Lindau syndrome, ataxia-telangiectasia, familial adenomatous polyposis, hereditary nonpolyposis colorectal cancer, nonhereditary chronic pancreatitis (tropical and nontropical), diabetes mellitus, tobacco use, obesity, a diet high in fat and meat, and those who have had a partial gastrectomy and cholecystectomy. The roles of *H. pylori* (Hp) infection, NSAIDs, and coffee and alcohol consumption are controversial.

PATHOGENESIS

The pathogenesis involves diverse combinations of multiple genetic events including the activation of oncogenes, inactivation of tumor suppressive genes, and defects in DNA mismatch repair genes.

CLINICAL FEATURES

Patients present with a dull achy upper abdominal pain that radiates to the back. The pain increases after eating. There is associated weight loss, jaundice, pruritus, acholic stools, and dark urine. Painful jaundice may be seen in patients with locally unresectable disease, which is present in about half of the patients.

Clinical findings may include an abdominal mass, ascites, a palpable but nontender gallbladder, left supraclavicular adenopathy (Virchow's node), and subcutaneous areas of nodular fat necrosis.

DIAGNOSIS

Laboratory Studies

Liver panel shows elevated serum bilirubin and alkaline phosphatase along with mild anemia and hypoalbuminemia. Serum CA19-9 has a sensitivity and specificity of 80 to 90%.

Imaging Studies

Abdominal ultrasound shows dilated bile ducts, as well as a mass in the head of the pancreas. A CT scan with pancreatic protocol is superior to ultrasound and shows biliary and pancreatic duct dilatation, pancreatic mass, and may even show evidence of metastasis as well as ascites. A CT angiography is preferred since it can show major vessel involvement.

Endoscopic ultrasound is superior for the diagnosis of tumors less than 2.0 cm in diameter, as well as for detecting the resectability of the tumor by examining lymph nodes and major vascular involvement. However, an EUS is operator dependant, unavailable at most hospitals, and its role is not clearly established.

An ERCP is helpful in patients with atypical mass or when no pancreatic mass is visualized on CT scan. It may show obstruction of the common bile duct and pancreatic duct (double duct sign), pancreatic duct stricture greater than 1.0 cm in length, and/or changes suggestive of chronic pancreatitis. An MRCP is similar to an ERCP in accuracy.

Cytology and Biopsy

Percutaneous fine needle aspiration of the pancreatic mass has sensitivity and specificity of 80 to 100%. The possibility of dissemination of cancer within peritoneal cavity along the needle path has not been evaluated. An EUS-guided FNA biopsy has less likelihood of intraperitoneal spread.

Laparoscopy

The role of laparoscopy, alone or in combination with endoscopic ultrasound or transabdominal ultrasound, is evolving.

DIFFERENTIAL DIAGNOSIS

The focus is usually on distinguishing a suspected pancreatic cancer from chronic pancreatitis.

MANAGEMENT STRATEGY

Investigation vs Surgery

1. In patients with a mass or lesion in the pancreas who are otherwise good candidates for surgical resection, no further investigations are needed. Surgery should be undertaken recognizing that some patients with benign lesions may wind up getting radical resection.

2. If a patient has a mass lesion and is otherwise not a good surgical candidate, a CT or ultrasound-guided fine needle aspiration biopsy may be undertaken.

3. In patients with an atypical mass in the pancreas or no mass is visualized, an ERCP or MRCP is recommended.

Determining Resectability

In patients with a typical pancreatic mass on a CT scan, the resectability is determined by a good quality CT angiography. Endoscopic ultrasound is highly operator dependent and is available only at a few centers. Some surgeons like to follow-up the helical CT angiography with MRI, laparoscopy, and laparoscopic ultrasound.

TREATMENT

Curative Resection

Patients with cancer of the head or uncinate process of pancreas who undergo Whipple's procedure (pancreaticoduodenectomy) have a mortality of less than 4%. A pylorus preserving pancreaticoduodenectomy is being increasingly performed in preference to Whipple's procedure and has a similar outcome.

Patients with tumor in the body or tail of pancreas usually present late with a surgically non-resectable tumor. In patients deemed to be surgically resectable, a laparoscopic exploration is performed because many patients have occult peritoneal metastasis. The surgical resection for cancer in the body or tail of the pancreas involves distal subtotal pancreatectomy usually combined with splenectomy.

Adjuvant Chemotherapy

Patients with curative surgery for pancreatic cancer should be offered adjuvant chemoradiation. Neoadjuvant chemoradiation is an acceptable option compared to postoperative chemoradiation.

Palliation for Nonresectable Disease

Patients with biliary obstruction should undergo endoscopic stent placement. Duodenal obstruction by the tumor can be relieved by a gastric bypass surgery or endoscopically placed stents. Options for pain control include percutaneous celiac block and/or long acting opiates. Exocrine pancreatic insufficiency may be treated with pancreatic enzyme supplementation.

PROGNOSIS

While surgical resection is the only opportunity for cure, the overall five year survival is less than 10%. Whipple's procedure is associated with a 5-year survival of 20 to 30%. The prognosis of cancer in the body and tail of pancreas is poor compared to that of head of pancreas.

SCREENING

Screening strategies for preventing pancreatic cancer have not been established. Patients with history of hereditary pancreatitis and a family history of pancreatic cancer should start screening at 35 years of age or 10 years before the age at which pancreatic cancer was first diagnosed in the family. Spiral CT and endoscopic ultrasound are the preferred modalities.

PEARLS

○ Patients with a typical mass in pancreatic head and who are otherwise deemed surgically resectable should proceed directly to surgery.

○ Pancreatic cancer carries a poor overall prognosis with 5-year survival of less than 10%.

BIBLIOGRAPHY

Tamm EP, Silverman PM, Charnsangavej C, Evans DB. Diagnosis, staging, and surveillance of pancreatic cancer. *Am J Roentgenol.* 2003; 180(5):1311-23.

Clarke DL, Thomson SR, Madiba TE, Sanyika C. Preoperative imaging of pancreatic cancer: a management-oriented approach. *J Am Coll Surg.* 2003;196(1):119-29.

63 Zollinger-Ellison Syndrome

Zollinger-Ellison syndrome (ZES) or gastrinoma is characterized by peptic ulcer disease, gastric hyperacidity and nonbeta-cell tumor of the pancreas Gastrinoma may be sporadic or associated with multiple endocrine neoplasia (MEN) Type I. Most of the patients have a sporadic form.

EPIDEMIOLOGY

The estimated incidence is 0.1 to 0.3 per 1 million. Mean age at diagnosis is 50. It is controversial if there is a male predominance. ZES is associated with up to 2% of patients with peptic ulcer disease.

PATHOGENESIS

In addition to gastrin, gastrinoma cells contain other neuroendocrine peptides like insulin and glucagon. The differentiation between gastrinoma and other islet cell tumors is based on the elevation of serum gastrin concentration. The high gastrin secretion from gastrinoma leads to an increased number of parietal cells, while increased stimulation of parietal cells leads to increased gastric acid secretion.

Diarrhea may occur due to increased gastric acid secretion, leading to a luminal volume load that cannot be fully absorbed in the small and large intestines. Also, the excess gastric acid going into the small intestine inactivates digestive enzymes and damages the intestinal mucosa leading to maldigestion and malabsorption. High serum gastrin concentrations also have an inhibitory effect on sodium and water absorption in the small intestine.

CLINICAL FEATURES

Typically there is a mean delay of about 5 years between the symptom onset and the diagnosis. Peptic ulcer disease is seen in over 90% of patients. The ulcers are solitary in as many as 75% of the cases, and may be less than 1.0 cm in diameter. Most ulcers occur in the first part of the duodenum and in about 10% cases, they are seen in the jejunum. Diarrhea occurs in a majority of patients, while heartburn is the complaint of about half of the patients. As many as 25% of the patients initially present with gastrointestinal (GI) bleeding.

Almost one-third of the patients with gastrinoma present with metastatic disease. The most common site of metastasis is the liver, but spreading to the bones may also occur.

DIAGNOSIS

Gastrinoma should be suspected in patients with multiple ulcers, drug-refractory ulcers, ulcers beyond the duodenal bulb, ulcers associated with diarrhea, severe esophageal symptoms, and those with an extensive history of peptic ulcer disease, as well as a family history for findings of MEN.

Fasting serum gastrin concentration is the initial test of choice. In the presence of a gastric pH of less than 5.0, a gastrin concentration greater than 1000.0 pg/mL is diagnostic. It is important to check gastric pH in order to exclude secondary hypergastrinemia due to hypo- or achlorhydria as seen in patients with pernicious anemia or atrophic gastritis.

Most patients have a serum gastrin levels between 150.0 and 1000.0 pg/mL. Such serum gastrin elevations can also be seen in renal failure, massive small bowel resection, G-cell hyperplasia, gastric outlet obstruction, retained gastric antrum, and patients taking proton pump inhibitors (PPIs).

A secretin stimulation test should be done in patients with a nondiagnostic serum gastrin level. An increase in serum gastrin level by 200 pg/mL within 10 minutes of secretin infusion is 90% sensitive and specific. In contrast, serum gastrin levels do not increase in patients with hypergastrinemia due to other causes.

Gastric acid output studies are no longer performed in most medical centers. In patients who have normal serum gastrin and a negative secretin stimulation test, but with a high index of suspicion, measurement of serum chromogranin A and/or measurement of serum gastrin levels in response to calcium infusion may be undertaken.

Localization of Tumor

Attempts should be made to localize the tumor, except when associated with MEN-1 syndrome or a decision has been taken to treat the patient medically only. Preoperative techniques, including CT scan, MRI, angiography, EUS, and scintigraphy, combined with intraoperative localization techniques, allow the surgeon to identify over 90% of the sporadic gastrinomas.

Somatostatin scintigraphy is the test of choice because of high sensitivity and specificity. If hepatic metastasis are detected, a percutaneous biopsy is performed. If no tumor or metastases is found, endoscopic ultrasound or dual phase helical CT should be undertaken.

Arterial stimulation venous sampling is rarely used. In general, patients are usually taken for exploratory laparotomy for evaluation with intraoperative palpation, transillumination, EUS, and duodenotomy, which help find small gastrinomas that have otherwise not been detected.

TREATMENT

Medical Management

This is undertaken in patients with gastrinoma associated with MEN-1 syndrome. Patients should undergo periodic gastric acid output studies to assess the adequacy of treatment. The goal is gastric acid secretion of less than 10 meq/hour prior to the next dose of the treatment. PPIs like omeprazole, lansoprazole, pantoprazole, rabeprazole, and esomeprazole are usually used. Patients are usually started on three times the usual dose of the drug. Once adequate gastric acid control has been achieved, a reduction of dose may be attempted. However, each reduction should be confirmed with gastric acid output secretion within 2 weeks. Pantoprazole may be intravenously administered in the doses of 80.0 to 120.0 mg twice a day in patients who can not take medications orally. Intravenous lansoprazole is on the horizon.

Surgery

Patients with a sporadic gastrinoma without evidence of metastasis should undergo exploratory laparotomy with curative intent. This approach leads to cure in up to one-third of the patients. Surgery is not routinely recommended for patients with MEN-1.

Postsurgical Management

As many as 40% of the patients require prolonged acid suppression therapy following curative surgery because of the residual excess of gastric parietal cells. As such, many experts recommend parietal cell vagotomy in all patients undergoing exploratory laparotomy for ZES.

Treatment of Metastatic Disease

Options for the treatment of metastatic disease include use of long-acting somatostatin analogs like octreotide, interferon-alpha, palliative surgery by resection of hepatic metastasis, chemotherapy, embolization, and chemo-immobilization of the hepatic artery.

PROGNOSIS

Liver metastasis following curative surgery develops in less than 4% of the patients over a period of 6 years. Reoperation is needed in patients with a recurrent ZES.

Over 80% of the patients without liver metastasis survive 15 years, as compared to a 30% 10-year survival of patients with hepatic metastasis. Patients with MEN-1 usually have a lower rate of metastasis at the time of initial diagnosis, and as such, a higher survival rate. Survival rates can be correlated with initial fasting gastrin levels.

PEARLS

○ Elevations of serum gastrin level up to 700 pg/mL may occur with proton pump inhibitor therapy.

○ Medical treatment is undertaken for gastrinomas related to MEN-1. Surgery is the treatment of choice for patients with sporadic gastrinoma without evidence of hepatic metastasis. However, gastric hyperacidity persists for a long time in majority of patients following curative surgery.

BIBLIOGRAPHY

Tomassetti P, Migliori M, Lalli S, Campana D, Tomassetti V, Corinaldesi R. Epidemiology, clinical features, and diagnosis of gastroenteropancreatic endocrine tumors. *Ann Oncol.* 2001;12 Suppl 2:S95-9.

Azimuddin K, Chamberlain RS. The surgical management of pancreatic neuroendocrine tumors. *Surg Clin North Am.* 2001;81(3):511-25.

SMALL INTESTINE

Chapter

64 *Chronic Intestinal Pseudo-Obstruction*

Chronic intestinal pseudo-obstruction (CIP) is the failure of propagation of gastrointestinal (GI) contents downstream as a result of the breakdown of the GI neuromuscular system. It mimics intestinal obstruction except that no obvious cause of obstruction can be found.

PATHOGENESIS

Familial and sporadic visceral myopathies and neuropathies are uncommon. Most cases are secondary, and many appear to be associated with autoimmune disorders.

Causes include autonomic neuropathies, stroke, diabetes mellitus, multiple sclerosis, spinal cord injury, poliomyelitis, amyloidosis, anorexia nervosa, neurofibromatosis, paraneoplastic syndrome, Parkinsonism, porphyria, scleroderma, and postvagotomy syndrome. GI smooth muscle may be affected by dermatomyoscitis, connective tissue disorders, muscular dystrophy, and SLE.

Medications implicated in CIP include anticholinergics, calcium channel blockers, clonidine, lithium, narcotics, and tricyclic antidepressants. Many cases are idiopathic and, frequently, a preceding history of a viral infection will be elicited.

CLINICAL MANIFESTATIONS

Symptoms may be acute, chronic, or intermittent with small bowel and/or colonic involvement, along with involvement of other segments of the gastrointestinal tract. Most patients complain of nausea, vomiting, abdominal pain, bloating, and abdominal distension. Both diarrhea and/or constipation may occur.

Other symptoms include early satiety, anorexia, weight loss plus urinary symptoms, in addition to manifestations of the underlying disorder. Systemic features may include dizziness, palpitations, orthostasis, dry mucus membranes, impotence and decreased sweating, all of which may be mediated by associated autonomic nervous system (ANS) dysfunction.

Many patients have associated disorders: hypercoagulability, chronic pain, urinary retention, migraine headaches, and sleep disorders, etc.

DIAGNOSIS

In addition to routine blood counts, chemistries, and thyroid function tests, investigations for lead poisoning and porphyria may be undertaken in select cases.

Exclude Intestinal Obstruction

Plain x-rays of the chest and abdomen are undertaken to exclude the possibility of mechanical obstruction. X-rays show distended loops of bowel with air-fluid levels. Small intestinal diverticulosis or pneumatosis intestinalis may be seen. Any focus of mechanical obstruction should be aggressively sought by doing GI endoscopy, an upper GI, a small bowel series, and a barium enema. Small intestinal manometry has been reported to show specific patterns associated with partial obstruction, but it is not routinely used in clinical practice.

Tests for Gastrointestinal Transit

A gastric emptying study, small intestinal transit study, and colonic marker transit study are done as the next step. A 4-hour solid gastric emptying test is the standard for the diagnosis of gastroparesis. A hydrogen breath test may be used for small intestinal transit, but may not be accurate in patients because of possibility of small intestinal bacterial overgrowth. Colonic marker study protocol varies among different institutions. Whole gut scintigraphy can be undertaken and may be cost-effective.

Exclude Bacterial Overgrowth

Patients with suspected small intestinal bacterial overgrowth (especially those with low vitamin B_{12} and high folic acid levels) should preferably undergo testing for small bowel bacterial overgrowth (SBBO) as described in Chapter 66.

Motility Tests

Gastroduodenal manometry may be useful in patients with documented dysmotility on scintigraphy but is not available in most medical centers. It can help distinguish between a myopathy from neuropathic process. Electrogastrography (EGG) can detect abnormalities of gastric rhythm associated with gastroparesis.

Autonomic Function Testing

This is useful in patients with symptoms suggestive of systemic disorder. It can be undertaken by examining the postural changes in blood pressure and changes in RR intervals with deep breathing for cholinergic function. Maneuvers related to blood flow changes in response to postural change or cold stress and thermal response to sweating are undertaken to exclude adrenergic dysfunction.

Role of Computerized Tomography Scan and Magnetic Resonance Imaging Scan

An MRI of the brain and spinal cord should be done if a central nervous system (CNS) lesion is suspected. Similarly, a CT scan of chest is helpful if lung cancer is suspected as the cause of paraneoplastic syndrome.

Biopsy

A full thickness intestinal biopsy is needed for a precise diagnosis but is rarely used in clinical practice. It should be undertaken if a laparotomy is undertaken for any reason.

TREATMENT

Lifestyle measures include eating small frequent meals and limiting fatty foods that delay intestinal motility. Fluid replacement, with the correction of fluid and electrolyte imbalance, is a cornerstone of treatment along with nutritional support.

Nutrition

Patients with nausea, vomiting and malnutrition may benefit from a jejunal placement of nasoenteric tube or jejunostomy tube. TPN may be needed in patients with severe, diffuse dysmotility. Venting gastrostomy is helpful in patients with abdominal pain due to excessive distention and vomiting. Some patients are able to avoid enteral or parenteral nutrition with aggressive use of liquid nutritional supplements.

Control of Nausea and Vomiting

Promethazine (Phenergan 12.5 to 25.0 mg PO or IM every 4 hours or suppository every 12 hours) and prochlorperazine (Compazine 5.0 to 10.0 mg PO or IM every 6 hours or 5.0 to 10.0 mg IV every 3 to 6 hours or 25.0 mg suppository every 12 hours) are helpful.

A continuous intravenous infusion of promethazine at 8.0 mg/hour may be more effective during acute episodes. Select cases may need infusions as high as 16.0 to 24.0 mg/hour. The rate of infusion should be titrated to CNS depression.

Newer antiemetics include ondansetron at 16.0 to 24.0 mg/day PO, granisetron 2.0 mg/day PO, or dolasetron 100.0 mg/day PO.

Severe cases may require a combination of promethazine 8.0 to 24.0 mg/hour infusion plus ondansetron 8.0 to 10.0 mg IV every 6 hours during acute exacerbation.

Pain Control

This is a complex problem since many patients require narcotics for pain control, which of course slows the motility further. There is potential for addiction. Assistance from a pain specialist should be sought.

Prokinetics

Erythromycin is helpful during acute exacerbation (250.0 mg to 500.0 mg IV q 8 hours). Chronic use of erythromycin is not as beneficial due to tachyphylaxis plus significant gastrointestinal side effects. Metoclopramide is a dopamine antagonist and is taken as 10.0 to 20.0 mg PO 30 minutes before each meal and at bedtime. Octreotide 100.0 mcg subcutaneously q HS with or without erythromycin may be used especially during acute exacerbation.

Cisapride is also effective but is not easily available. Domperidone (10.0 to 30.0 mg PO qid) is a peripheral dopamine antagonist that acts like metoclopramide, but with reduced potential for extrapyramidal side effects. It is available in the United States as an orphan drug. Bethanecol can be helpful with gastroparesis but its use is limited by its side effects.

Specific Therapies

Patients with recurrent small bowel bacterial overgrowth may benefit from cyclic use of antibiotics like ciprofloxacin 500.0 mg bid alternating with doxycycline 100.0 mg bid and metronidazole 250.0 mg tid for 1 week each month.

The injection of botulinum toxin into the pyloric sphincter is useful if excessive pyloric sphincter tone is suspected as the cause of functional gastric outlet obstruction.

Emerging Therapies

Tegaserod (Zelnorm 6.0 mg bid), currently approved for constipation-predominant irritable bowel syndrome (IBS), is being increasingly used by some experts for chronic intestinal pseudo-obstruction.

Electro-acupuncture combined with electrical stimulation of certain anatomic sites has been shown to be of benefit in gastroparesis.

Gastric electrical stimulation has been approved by the United States Food and Drug Administration (FDA) for gastroparesis and holds promise for dysfunction of other parts of the GI tract.

Role of Surgery

The role of surgery is limited. In case of involvement of a localized segment of small or large intestine, resection may be appropriate. Bypass of the diseased local segment can be undertaken. Tubes can be placed for venting as well as feeding. Patients with primarily colonic involvement may benefit from subtotal colectomy. Small intestinal transplantation is experimental.

PEARLS

- ○ Most cases of CIP are idiopathic.
- ○ Fluid replacement and nutritional support, in addition to symptomatic relief, are the mainstays of treatment.
- ○ Gastric electrical stimulator is helpful in severe cases and has been shown to maintain or improve nutritional status in patients with drug-refractory gastroparesis.

REFERENCES

Kamm MA. Intestinal pseudo-obstruction. *Gut*. 2000;47 Suppl 4:iv84; discussion iv87.

Lin Z, Chen JD. Advances in gastrointestinal electrical stimulation. *Crit Rev Biomed Eng*. 2002;30(4-6):419-57.

Hirano I, Pandolfino J. Chronic intestinal pseudo-obstruction. *Dig Dis*. 2000;18(2):83-92.

Chapter

65 *Small Bowel Obstruction*

Small bowel obstruction (SBO), as the name implies, is obstruction to the downward flow of intestinal contents.

EPIDEMIOLOGY

While no direct data is available, adhesiolysis alone accounts for 300 000 hospitalizations, 800 000 days of inpatient care, and $1.3 billion in health care costs.

ETIOLOGY

The most common causes are postoperative adhesions and hernias. Intrinsic obstruction is less common and occurs due to tumors and strictures. Other causes include volvulus, congenital malformations, atresia, stenosis, inflammatory or radiation stricture, intussusception, gallstones, and fecal impaction. About 75% of small intestinal obstructions are caused by postoperative adhesions.

NATURAL HISTORY

An interval between laparotomy and SBO due to adhesions varies from 6 months to 65 years. SBO may occur in as many as 15% of laparotomy patients within 2 years after the procedure. The risks for recurrent obstruction over the next 10 years may be as high as 42%. The risk is more likely after lower intestinal surgery and less likely after negative laparotomy for trauma. Mortality in patients with strangulation may be as high as 37%. Over half of the patients admitted for SBO require surgery with an overall mortality of 5%.

PATHOGENESIS

SBO leads to the dilation of the proximal bowel, causing swelling of the intestinal wall and fluid sequestration into the bowel lumen. Increasing intestinal edema leads to third spacing of fluid into the peritoneal cavity.

Strangulation may be seen in 10% of bowel obstructions and leads to necrosis with potential for perforation. Total obstruction usually advances to strangulation. Patients with closed lobe obstruction (ie, obstruction of the lumen at two locations) also rapidly advance to strangulation. Strangulation can occur in partial obstruction as seen in Richter's hernia.

CLINICAL FEATURES

Patients present with abdominal pain, nausea, vomiting, and anorexia. Nausea and vomiting are less severe in patients with distal small bowel obstruction. The abdominal pain is crampy and there is a lack of passage of stool or flatus. A change from crampy to constant localized pain may suggest impending perforation. Bacterial overgrowth leads to feculent vomiting.

Clinical examination shows evidence for dehydration (ie, tachycardia and hypotension). Presence of fever suggests strangulation. Abdomen is distended with high pitched or hypoactive bowel sounds. Presence of rebound, guarding, or rigidity suggests peritonitis.

Abdominal mass on examination may be a clue to the presence of an abscess or tumor. Inguinal, femoral, as well as any sites of previous incisions, must be carefully examined for hernia. The rectal vault is usually empty on digital examination unless there is evidence of a mass. Blood may be seen on the glove finger in patients with neoplasm, ischemia, or intussusception.

DIAGNOSIS

Laboratory Studies

Serum chemistries reflect dehydration with electrolyte abnormalities and an elevation of serum blood urea nitrogen (BUN) and creatinine. Hematocrit may be falsely elevated. Metabolic alkalosis occurs due to persistent vomiting. The presence of metabolic acidosis is an ominous sign and is seen in the presence of ischemic bowel or severe dehydration causing hypoperfusion. Serum lactate is a sensitive sign of strangulation.

Imaging Studies

A chest x-ray and abdominal flat and upright x-rays should be obtained. The presence of free air under the diaphragm suggests perforation. Dilated loops of small bowel with multiple air-fluid levels point to SBO, although they may also be seen in paralytic ileus. A presence of air in the rectum makes the diagnosis of SBO less likely. Abdominal x-rays are nondiagnostic or nonspecific in up to 20% of the cases.

CT scan is preferred over small bowel series to differentiate between SBO and pseudo-obstruction. Abdominal CT with intravenous plus oral water-soluble contrast can define the site of obstruction as well as point towards the etiology of SBO or any other abdominal pathology. Since adhesions are the most common cause, no obvious cause for obstruction is seen in most cases of SBO.

A small bowel series is very sensitive for the diagnosis of SBO and should be carried out if the CT scan is nondiagnostic. An abdominal ultrasound may be used in patients who are pregnant or severely ill.

DIFFERENTIAL DIAGNOSIS

Intestinal pseudo-obstruction presents in a fashion similar to SBO. Paralytic ileus is caused in acute cases by trauma, postoperative state, as well as ischemia and electrolyte disorders. Chronic intestinal pseudo-obstruction presents with intermittent episodes of recurrent abdominal distention and there is relatively greater colonic distention than small bowel distention.

TREATMENT

General Measures

Management includes NPO, nasogastric suction, correction of electrolyte abnormalities, and antibiotics for infection. A Foley catheter for monitoring urine output and a central venous catheter for fluid management are valuable adjuncts. Some patients may require parenteral nutrition

Medical management is likely to be successful in patients with partial obstruction, intra-abdominal malignancy, recurrent obstruction due to adhesions, radiation strictures, or early postoperative obstruction.

Surgery

About 90% of patients with partial obstruction resolve with medical management within 48 hours; nonresponders should be taken to surgery. Some surgeons wait longer than 48 hours in cases where partial obstruction due to adhesions is suspected. Patients with complete obstruction should be observed no more than 12 to 24 hours prior to surgical intervention. Similarly patients with impending strangulation or closed loop bowel obstruction are candidates for prompt surgery. Long decompression tubes are outdated.

The type and extent of surgery depends upon the cause of obstruction and the overall clinical situation. Bowel viability is determined during surgery either clinically or by intravenous injection of fluorescein and visualization under fluorescent light. Fluorescent technique is superior to clinical judgement as well as doppler ultrasound examination. Doppler examination may be helpful if fluorescent technique is nondiagnostic. Laparoscopic surgery may be undertaken in select cases with a success rates of 60 to 80%.

PREVENTION

Focus is on surgical techniques to prevent adhesion formation since adhesions are the most common cause of SBO. Modification of suturing or plicating techniques, placement of intestinal tubes through jejunostomy, as well as chemical agents such as high molecular weight dextran are not helpful. Bioresorbable barrier membranes may be help in preventing adhesions.

PEARLS

- ○ The clinical and radiological presentation of SBO and the paralytic ileus may be similar; a CT of the abdomen is superior to small bowel series for diagnosis.
- ○ Complete bowel obstruction is likely to go to strangulation and should lead to prompt surgical intervention.

BIBLIOGRAPHY

Dijkstra FR, Nieuwenhuijzen M, Reijnen MM, van Goor H. Recent clinical developments in pathophysiology, epidemiology, diagnosis and treatment of intra-abdominal adhesions. *Scand J Gastroenterol.* 2000;(232 Suppl):52-9.

Chapter
66 *Small Bowel Bacterial Overgrowth*

Contrary to popular misconception, the small intestine and the stomach are not entirely sterile. Excessive growth of bacteria is prevented by antegrade peristalsis, bacterial destruction by gastric acidity, bile and proteolytic enzymes, intestinal immune system, and prevention of retrograde translocation of bacteria from colon to small intestine by the ileocecal valve.

BOWEL FLORA

While stomach and duodenum have small numbers of bacteria, jejunum normally contains about 10^4 organisms per mL, which are predominately lactobacilli, enterococci, and Gram-positive aerobes or facultative anaerobes. Terminal ileum has as high as 10^9 organisms per mL.

PREDISPOSING FACTORS

SBBO may occur due to a stasis of intestinal contents (small intestinal diverticulosis), surgically created blind lopes, strictures, impaired intestinal motility due to diabetes mellitus or scleroderma, intestinal pseudo-obstruction, or strictures due to disorders like radiation enteritis and Crohn's disease. Abnormal connections due to gastrocolic or jejunocolic fistula or the removal of ileocecal valve barrier due to surgical resection lead to excessive growth of bacteria. In addition, systemic disorders like immune-deficiency, chronic pancreatitis, liver cirrhosis, alcoholism, and advanced age may predispose to intestinal overgrowth. Hypochlorhydria, including that related to long-term proton pump inhibitor (PPI) therapy, also promotes small bowel bacterial overgrowth—but it is usually not clinically significant.

PATHOGENESIS

Bacterial overgrowth causes problems when jejunal concentrations of bacteria exceed 10^5 organisms per mL. Commonly seen organisms include *Streptococcus, Staphylococcus, Bacteroides, E. coli, Klebsiella, Clostridium, Lactobacillus,* and *Peptostreptococcus.*

Diarrhea and malabsorption occurs due to a variety of mechanisms including epithelial cell injury; bacterial deconjugation of bile acids causing absorption of deconjugated bile salts in the jejunum with a resultant reduced concentrations for fat absorption; toxic effect of deconjugated bile on intestinal mucosa; bacterial degradation of carbohydrates and proteins; a reversible form of protein losing enteropathy; and reduced vitamin B_{12} absorption by competing with the host for absorption.

CLINICAL MANIFESTATIONS

Patients usually present with increased gassiness due to increased intestinal gas production, loose and acidic stools, abdominal distension, and flatulence.

Other features may include anemia, neurological problems related to B_{12} deficiency, steatorrhea, fat-soluble vitamin deficiency due to fat malabsorption, dyspepsia, and weight loss. In severe cases, patients may present with tetany due to hypocalcemia, night blindness due to vitamin A deficiency, arthritis, and dermatitis.

Physical exam may reveal muscle wasting, succussion splash, peripheral neuropathy, and neurological impairment.

PATHOLOGY

Histologic alterations may occur in some cases and include increased cellularity, mild to moderate mucosal inflammation, and subtotal villous atrophy with focal areas of ulcerations.

DIAGNOSIS

A CBC will show anemia that may be microcytic, macrocytic, or mixed. Serum vitamin B_{12} may be low along with normal or high serum folate levels. Diagnostic studies include an upper GI and small bowel series showing hypomotility, stricture, dilated loops, or diverticula. A modified form of Schilling's test in which a course of antibiotic administration normalizes the absorption of B_{12} deficiency is diagnostic; this test is rarely used. Small bowel biopsy is not pathognomic.

Empiric treatment has been used as a diagnostic test. However, some experts recommend establishing a firm diagnosis since treatment may require more than one course of antibiotic or long-term cyclic administrations. In addition, the symptoms may be related to the underlying disease like scleroderma or Crohn's disease, rather than bacterial overgrowth.

Jejunal aspirate is the standard that can be done endoscopically or through jejunal intubation. This is a cumbersome procedure and is not followed at many centers. Concentrations greater than 10^5 organisms per mL suggest the diagnosis.

A radio-labeled [14C]-d-xylose breath test has a sensitivity and specificity of 90%; exposure to a small amount of radioactivity is involved, but the test is not available at most centers. Hydrogen breath test using lactulose is the most commonly used test because it is widely available, safe and easy; however, this test has a 15 to 20% false negative rate.

TREATMENT

Treatment is multifaceted and involves managing the underlying condition, antibiotics, and nutritional support. Structural lesions may be amenable to surgical intervention (eg, stricture). Prokinetic drugs have not been shown to be of benefit.

The goal of antibiotic treatment is not to eliminate the flora in its entirety, but to alter its composition so as to lead to clinical improvement. Traditionally, tetracycline 250.0 mg PO qid has been used but may be ineffective in as many as 40 to 60% of patients due to antibiotic resistance. Alternate options include norfloxacin 800.0 mg/day PO; oral gentamicin 80.0 mg/day plus metronidazole 500.0 mg PO tid; metronidazole 500.0 mg PO tid alone or in combination with a cephalosporin such as cephalexin 250.0 mg PO qid, or a double-strength trimethoprim-sulfamethoxazole bid.

Augmentin (amoxicillin-clavulanate) 875.0 mg bid is highly effective, but may lead to antibiotic-induced diarrhea in about one-third of the patients. The course of therapy is about 7 to 10 days. Rarely a prolonged course of 1 to 2 months may be required before symptomatic relief is seen.

Repeated courses of antibiotics for recurrent SBBO may be required in some patients on a regular basis (eg, course of an antibiotic for first 5 to 10 days each month). Antibiotics should preferably be used in rotation (tetracycline 250.0 mg qid, ciprofloxacin 250.0 mg bid, Augmentin 500.0 mg tid, metronidazole 250.0 to 500.0 mg tid, norfloxacin 800.0 mg/day, and doxycycline 100.0 mg bid) to prevent antibiotic resistance.

Nonantibiotic Treatment

Nutritional support involves correction of micronutrient deficiency. Lactose containing foods should be avoided. Some patients with bacterial overgrowth and unexplained inflammation in the small or large intestine may benefit from a short course of corticosteroids and aminosalicylates.

Adjunctive Treatment

These include intestinal lavage by periodic purgation with polyethylene glycol solution. The role of probiotics is evolving and appears promising. It should be kept in mind that various probiotics vary in their effectiveness and only those species that have been documented to be beneficial should be used. For example, initial studies suggest that Lactobacillus planetarium 299 V may be helpful, whereas Lactobacillus fermentum has not been shown to be of benefit.

PEARLS

- ○ The small intestine is not normally sterile. Bacterial count exceeding 10^5 organisms per mL in jejunal aspirate signifies clinically significant bacterial overgrowth.
- ○ Treatment includes antibiotics plus the treatment of underlying cause.

BIBLIOGRAPHY

Rose S, Young MA, Reynolds JC. Gastrointestinal manifestations of scleroderma. *Gastroenterol Clin North Am.* 1998;27(3):563-94.

67 *Lactose Intolerance* ▬▬▬

Lactase deficiency or lactose intolerance occurs worldwide.

EPIDEMIOLOGY

The prevalence of lactase deficiency varies from about 5% in Northern Europeans to 60 to 95% in Southern Asians, African Americans, and Native Americans.

PATHOGENESIS

Three kinds of syndromes are recognized. The congenital form is rare. Primary lactase deficiency usually presents later in life. Secondary lactase deficiency occurs in conjunction with small intestinal diseases like SBBO, stasis syndrome, Crohn's disease, and giardiasis.

CLINICAL FEATURES

Manifestations are variable. Patients may be asymptomatic or complain of abdominal cramps, bloating, flatulence, diarrhea, and borborygmi. The stools may be bulky and frothy.

However, many patients who complain of lactose intolerance by history are not found to be lactase deficient. Conversely, most patients with lactase deficiency can tolerate at least one glass of milk a day.

DIAGNOSIS

Lactose absorption test involves measurement of blood glucose level after ingestion of 50.0 g of lactose. Lactose hydrogen breath test is the most commonly used test and is very sensitive and specific. Differential diagnosis includes maldigestion of other carbohydrates like fructose and sorbitol.

TREATMENT

It includes a reduction of lactose intake, use of lactose-free products, or administration of commercially available lactase enzymes. Response to various products varies. Yogurt containing live cultures is well-tolerated by most lactose intolerant subjects. Calcium supplementation should be undertaken by patients who avoid milk and diary products.

PEARLS

○ Most patients with lactase deficiency can tolerate at least one glass of milk per day.

○ Most patients who believe that lactose intolerance is the cause of their symptoms do not have lactase deficiency.

BIBLIOGRAPHY

Srinivasan R, Minocha A. When to suspect lactose intolerance. *Postgrad Med*. 1998;104:109-123.

Chapter

68 *Celiac Disease*

EPIDEMIOLOGY

Celiac disease, also known as gluten enteropathy or nontropical sprue occurs primarily amongst Whites of European descent. There is a prevalence rate of one in 200 to 500 persons depending upon the criteria used and the population studied. The majority of these cases are asymptomatic or have nonspecific symptoms.

PATHOGENESIS

Celiac sprue is an inherited immune disorder triggered by an environmental insult in the form of gliadin, which is a component of gluten. In a genetically predisposed individual, this insult triggers the disease. The genetic predisposition is multifactorial and both HLA-linked and other genes are involved.

CLASSIFICATION

Celiac disease may be classified into classic, latent, or potential celiac disease. The classic form is characterized by signs and symptoms of malabsorption along with villous atrophy on histology. The histologic lesion varies from mild alteration with increased intraepithelial lymphocytes to a flat mucosa with a total villous atrophy. Different histologic schemes have been proposed.

Potential celiac disease patients are those with characteristic serologic pattern but with minimal or absent clinical and histologic findings.

CLINICAL FEATURES

Most patients present between the age of 10 and 40 years, but do not have the classical malabsorptive presentation. Manifestations may include diarrhea, including bulky foul smelling and floating stools; increased flatulence; weight loss; growth failure; anemia; and other complications of malabsorption syndrome. Some patients may have only mild and nonspecific symptoms such as fatigue and iron deficiency anemia. Others may be misdiagnosed with IBS.

EXTRAGASTROINTESTINAL ASSOCIATIONS

Celiac disease is associated with infertility and rheumatological disorders, as well as neurological disorders like depression, seizure disorder, migraines, and myopathy, etc. Some patients may initially present with a neuropsychiatric illness like idiopathic ataxia, episodic headaches and osteoporosis. Dermatitis herpetiformis is common and may be seen in about 10 to 20% of patients. Other associations include diabetes mellitus, selective IgA deficiency, Down's syndrome, liver diseases (eg, autoimmune hepatitis (AIH), PSC, PBC), autoimmune thyroid disease, and infertility. Babies born to mothers with untreated celiac disease tend to have low birth weight.

DIAGNOSIS

Diagnosis is suggested by clinical presentation and laboratory studies, and is confirmed with serologic testing and small bowel biopsy.

Serology

The most useful serologic screening test involves antitissue transglutaminase (tTG), but an antigliadin antibodies (AGA) test is also available. For either test, both IgG and IgA antibodies should be tested because of the possible coexisting IgA deficiency. The patient should be on gluten containing diet since the antibody levels decline during gluten-free diet (GFD). The antireticulin antibody test does not offer any advantage over anti-tTG or AGA.

The antiendomysial antibody test is less sensitive, but more specific than an AGA test. The antitissue transglutaminase antibody is as good as an antiendomysial antibody test, but less expensive.

Approach to Diagnosis

The tests ordered depend upon the physician's experience as well as the sensitivity and specificity of the assays at any given laboratory. In a patient with low probability of celiac disease, we recommend checking (both IgG and IgA) antigliadin plus antitissue transglutaminase antibody. Absence of all antibodies excludes the diagnosis, whereas a positive test on either IgA AGA or tTG antibody should prompt a small bowel biopsy. Of note, IgG AGA is very nonspecific.

In patients with high probability of celiac disease, both the serologies as above and small bowel biopsy should be performed. Some experts only do an IgA antitissue transglutaminase antibody or IgA anti-endomysial antibody; still other perform IgA antitissue transglutaminase antibody, plus total IgA levels. About 2 to 6% of celiacs have selective IgA deficiency.

In patients with positive serology but negative histology, biopsy should be reviewed or even repeated. If histology is abnormal but antibodies are negative, other causes of villous atrophy (postgastroenteritis, giardiasis, tropical sprue, SBBO, or Crohn's disease) should be entertained and the biopsy should be reviewed again.

Positive histology and serology establish the diagnosis and treatment should be undertaken.

Gluten Challenge

The role of gluten challenge to document diagnosis is controversial. It may be undertaken in children in whom there is possibility of alternate diagnosis like infectious diarrhea and cow's milk intolerance. Challenge may produce gliadin shock due to severe diarrhea, causing dehydration and acidaosis, requiring treatment with corticosteroids.

TREATMENT

Dietary Restriction

A gluten-free diet forms the cornerstone of treatment. Wheat, rye, and barley are the principle offenders. The issue of oats is a matter of debate. While oats contain gluten, it appears that long-term pure oat ingestion is safe, although a major issue is obtaining pure oats.

Dietary counseling involves providing written information about the variety of foods as well as the resources available to them and perhaps addresses of helpful internet sites.

Soybean, rice, corn, buckwheat, and many other grains are safe. Many additives in food products contain gluten and close attention should be paid to the package label.

Additional Measures

Many patients have lactose intolerance concomitantly, and as such, should avoid dairy products until lactase levels are restored; this may take several weeks.

A gluten-free diet can be low in roughage and may lead to constipation. Gluten-free fiber supplementation may help. Patients have high risk for osteoporosis and sometimes develop osteomalacia. DEXA scan should be done and treatment undertaken accordingly.

Rarely hyposplenism is present. Patients should receive pneumococcal vaccine due to an increased risk for infections.

Treatment of Mild Disease

The benefit of a strict gluten-free diet is questionable in patients with mild symptoms or in whom celiac disease is diagnosed solely on the basis of antibody testing without significant clinical presentation.

There may be theoretic benefits of a strict gluten-free diet even if patient does not have significant symptoms (ie, less potential for micronutrient malabsorption, which may have clinical consequences like a reduction in the risk for malignancy and additional autoimmune disorders when taking gluten in the diet).

Latent Celiac Disease

Patients who are tTG or AGA IgA antibody positive, but negative by histology, are thought to be latent celiacs. A gluten-free diet is not recommended. Patients should be closely monitored with repeat biopsies undertaken as clinically warranted. Micronutrient concentrations for iron, folic acid, calcium, and vitamin B_{12} should be checked and corrected if needed.

MONITORING THERAPY

Symptomatic Relief Without Histologic Improvement

Patients usually have symptomatically relief within 1 to 2 weeks after starting gluten-free diet. Check tTG in 1 to 3 months after starting the diet and sequentially after this if tTG is still elevated. A repeat biopsy should be undertaken in patients who fail to have clinical improvement in spite of antibody responses. A biopsy may also be undertaken to confirm histological healing once antibody elevation normalizes.

If there is no histologic improvement despite symptomatic relief, a repeat biopsy should be undertaken after 6 to 9 months. In patients with lack of symptomatic, serologic, or histologic improvement, an alternate diagnosis, noncompliance, or inadvertent intake of gluten should be considered. A decline in tTG antibodies may be useful for monitoring clinical response as well as compliance.

Lack of Symptomatic and Histologic Response

An absence of improvement of symptoms and histologic response in spite of a truly GFD should raise concern for refractory sprue, ulcerative jejunitis or intestinal lymphoma. However, it should be considered that not all manifestations respond equally fast. For example, dermatitis herpetiformis may take 6 to 12 months to respond. Bone problems and neuropathy may only partially respond despite a rigid gluten-free diet.

Alternate diagnosis in nonresponders include lactose intolerance, IBS, SBBO, Crohn's disease, cow's milk protein intolerance in children, eosinophilic gastroenteritis, giardiasis, tropical sprue, and ZES.

Refractory Sprue

Refractory sprue includes patients who never respond to gluten free diet and those who initially respond but then relapse despite strict adherence to diet. Some of these patients develop collagenous sprue.

Patients with refractory sprue can rapidly deteriorate and death may ensue. Immunosuppression forms the cornerstone of treatment. Corticosteroids are used starting with oral prednisolone 40.0 to 60.0 mg/day with a slow taper after a few weeks in those who respond to the lowest possible dose to keep the patient asymptomatic. Azathioprine and 6-MP may be added as steroid-sparing agents. Cyclosporine has been used as a last resort or as a bridge to azathioprine therapy.

ASSOCIATED CONDITIONS

Ulcerative Jejunitis

Patients have clinical features of malabsorption syndrome. Benign appearing ulcers are seen on endoscopy. Ulcerative jejunitis may be fatal in as many as 30% of the patients. Resection of the ulcerated segment may improve prognosis.

Intestinal Lymphoma

Patients present with fever, hepatosplenomegaly, ascites, intestinal perforation, intestinal obstruction and even hemorrhage. A full thickness biopsy is required for diagnosis. It is rapidly fatal with less than a 10% 5-year survival rate.

Dermatitis Herpetiformis

Dermatitis herpetiformis is the most common dermatological association of celiac sprue. Response to a gluten-free diet may be delayed as long as 6 to 12 months. Therapy frequently includes dapsone in addition to gluten restriction. However, dapsone may not be needed as a gluten-free diet heals both skin and gut lesions, whereas dapsone heals only the skin lesions.

SEROLOGICAL MONITORING

Monitoring of celiac disease may be carried out by serum IgA tTG or antigliadin antibody. However, the test is not useful if the baseline levels were normal. IgA endomysial antibody can also be used for monitoring therapy but costs more.

SCREENING

The benefit of mass screening for asymptomatic celiac disease has not been established.

PEARLS

- ❍ Dietary noncompliance is the most common cause of relapse.
- ❍ Benefit of treating serology-positive and histology-negative celiac disease (latent celiacs) is questionable.

BIBLIOGRAPHY

Ciclitira PJ. AGA technical review on celiac sprue. *Gastroenterology*. 2001; 120:1526-1540.

Crowe SE. Gastrointestinal food allergies: do they exist? *Curr Gastroenterol Rep*. 2001;3(4):351-7.

Chapter
69 *Tropical Sprue*

EPIDEMIOLOGY

Tropical sprue, as the name suggests, occurs in tropical areas and requires at least 1 month of residence in the region.

PATHOGENESIS

It is considered to be an infectious disease, although no particular pathogen has been isolated. Malabsorption occurs due to reduced levels of disaccharidase enzymes, as well as reduced absorptive capacity due to the damaged intestinal mucosa.

PATHOLOGY

The most common site of involvement is the small intestine, although the colon may also be involved. Chronic inflammatory infiltrate with blunting of the villi is seen on histology.

CLINICAL FEATURES

The illness may be acute in onset with rapid progression or it may be chronic, insidious, and follow a slow progression. Symptoms include abdominal cramps, diarrhea, gas, fatigue, and progressive weight loss. Physical exam may show muscle wasting, glossitis, cheilitis, ascites, and pedal edema.

DIAGNOSIS

A stool test for fats is abnormal, as is the serum and urinary D-xylose test. Typically megaloblastic anemia and even pancytopenia may be seen. Small bowel contrast studies show thickened mucosal folds in the small intestine. Other infectious etiologies like *Entamoeba histolytica, Giardia, Strongyloides, Cryptosporidium, Isospora*, etc, need to be excluded.

DIFFERENTIAL DIAGNOSIS

Diseases mimicking tropical sprue include celiac sprue, intestinal lymphoma, giardiasis, and SBBO. Histologic changes on a small bowel biopsy are similar to those seen in untreated celiac sprue.

TREATMENT

Symptoms improve dramatically upon supplementation of folic acid 5.0 mg/day and can be diagnostic of the illness. Folic acid alone can cure acute but not chronic illness. In addition to folic acid 5.0 mg/day for 1 year, tetracycline 250.0 mg qid should be given for at least 6 months or until intestinal function returns to normal. Parenteral vitamin B_{12} supplementation should be undertaken in patients with concomitant vitamin B_{12} deficiency. As many as 10 to 20% of patients living in tropics may suffer from a relapse or reinfection.

PEARLS

O Tropical sprue is a diagnosis of exclusion of other etiologies that may present in a similar fashion.

O Dramatic response to folic acid supplementation can be of diagnostic value.

BIBLIOGRAPHY

Thielman NM, Guerrant RL. Persistent diarrhea in the returned traveler. *Infect Dis Clin North Am.* 1998;12(2):489-501.

Chapter
70 *Intestinal Lymphangiectasia*

EPIDEMIOLOGY

Primary disease (Milroy's disease) usually occurs during childhood.

PATHOGENESIS

There is a malformation of lymphatic system associated with lymphedema, chylothorax, or chylous ascites.

Secondary cases may occur due to congenital hepatic fibrosis, constrictive pericarditis, cancer, tuberculosis, sarcoidosis, retroperitoneal fibrosis, chronic pancreatitis, Crohn's disease, and radiation therapy.

CLINICAL FEATURES

Patients have diarrhea, nausea, vomiting, abdominal pain, and growth retardation.

DIAGNOSIS

There is a reduction in concentrations of serum albumin and globulin. Lymphocyte count is decreased. A small bowel series shows a thickened and nodular mucosa. Scattered white spots are seen on enteroscopy. Biopsy shows dilated lymphatics. Alpha$_1$ antitrypsin (AAT) clearance is useful for diagnosing protein-losing enteropathy.

TREATMENT

A significant component of oral intake should be composed of medium-chain triglycerides. Localized resection may be helpful in some patients. Secondary underlying disorders should be corrected.

PEARLS

- ○ Intestinal lymphangiectasia may be seen secondary to cancer, tuberculosis, and inflammatory bowel disease.
- ○ Treatment involves ingestion of medium chain triglycerides and correction of the underlying cause if possible.

BIBLIOGRAPHY

Guma J, Rubio J, Masip C, Alvaro T, Borras JL. Aggressive bowel lymphoma in a patient with intestinal lymphangiectasia and widespread viral warts. *Ann Oncol.* 1998;9(12):1355-6.

Chapter

71 *Whipple's Disease* ▬▬▬

Whipple's disease is a multisystem infectious disorder involving the gastrointestinal system, lungs, kidneys, eyes, heart, CNS, and joints.

EPIDEMIOLOGY

It usually presents in the fourth and fifth decades of life with a male predominance, and is caused by an acid-fast organism, Tropheryma whippelii. The DNA of the organism can found in small intestine of normal healthy subjects suggesting that host factors play a role in pathogenesis.

CLINICAL FEATURES

Most patients present with weight loss (90%), diarrhea (75%), arthralgias (70%), and occult GI bleeding (80%). Physical findings suggestive of congestive heart failure and valvular heart disease may be present. Pericardial rub may be heard. Other features include lymphadenopathy, dementia, ocular problems, ataxia, clonus, and hyperpigmentation.

DIAGNOSIS

PAS+ macrophages are seen on small bowel biopsy and acid fast organisms can be seen after appropriate staining. Electron microscopy should be performed if the diagnosis is in doubt. PCR techniques are used in investigational setting and are very sensitive for monitoring response to antibiotic therapy.

DIFFERENTIAL DIAGNOSIS

This includes IBD, alcoholism, hyperthyroidism, infections (Mycobacterium avium-intracellulare, histoplasmosis, cryptococcosis), macroglobulinemia, and AIDS. PAS+ macrophages can be present in normal gastric and rectal mucosa.

TREATMENT

Initial therapy includes intravenous Penicillin G (1.2 MU) plus streptomycin (1.0 g) IV every day for 2 weeks, followed by Trimethoprim-sulfamethoxazole DS bid for 1 year. For patients with CNS involvement, ceftriaxone 2.0 g IV should be used instead of Penicillin G. In patients who are allergic to sulfa drugs, cefixime 400.0 mg PO bid or doxycycline 100.0 mg PO bid for 1 year may be used.

Response to therapy may be monitored by hematocrit and weight gain. There is no need to do repeat small intestinal biopsy in order to monitor therapy.

PROGNOSIS

Relapse may occur in 15 to 40% of the patients.

PEARLS

○ Whipple's disease is a multisystem infectious disorder and initial diagnosis is frequently made by neurologists.

○ Relapse is common despite long-term antibiotic therapy.

BIBLIOGRAPHY

Marth T, Raoult D. Whipple's disease. *Lancet*. 2003;361(9353):239-46.

LARGE INTESTINE

Chapter

72 *Acute Appendicitis*

EPIDEMIOLOGY

Acute appendicitis is one of the most common abdominal emergencies and accounts for about 250 000 cases each year in the United States. It is more likely to occur in adolescents and young adults with a slight male predominance. The 15 to 20% rate of negative appendectomy has not declined despite advances in diagnostic modalities over the years.

PATHOGENESIS

An obstruction of the appendiceal lumen due to lymphoid follicular hyperplasia in the young and by fibrosis or fecalith or neoplasia in the elderly subjects leads to increased intralumenal pressure with thrombosis and occlusion of vessels. This results in ischemia, necrosis, and bacterial overgrowth. Necrosis is followed by perforation and localized abscess formation in most cases.

CLINICAL FEATURES

Initially, symptoms are nonspecific including "indigestion" and irregular bowel movements. This is followed by mid-abdominal pain that then localizes to the right lower quadrant. Patients with retrocecal appendix may only have dull nonspecific achy pain.

Physical examination reveals elevated temperature with right lower quadrant tenderness. Specialized maneuvers include Rovsing's sign (pain in the right lower quadrant upon palpation in the left lower quadrant), Obturator sign (pain upon internal rotation of the hip seen with the pelvic appendix), and an Iliopsoas sign (right lower quadrant pain precipitated by extension of the right hip) associated with retrocecal appendix.

LABORATORY

Most patients have leukocytosis, although normal WBC does not exclude acute appendicitis. Urinalysis may show sterile pyuria and helps to exclude a urinary tract infection (UTI) as the cause. Pelvic cultures should be taken in sexually-active menstruating women, and a pregnancy test should be done in young women. Plain x-rays of the abdomen are helpful in excluding any other abdominal catastrophe. Ultrasound has excellent diagnostic accuracy and is used in many medical centers. A CT scan is the imaging modality of choice.

Differential diagnosis includes right-sided diverticulitis, Meckel's diverticulitis, acute infectious ileitis, and pelvic inflammatory disease.

TREATMENT

Surgery is the cornerstone of treatment. Initial steps include intravenous fluids, correction of electrolyte imbalance as well as perioperative antibiotics. Patients who present within 24 to 72 hours of onset of symptoms are usually treated with immediate appendectomy. Colonoscopic drainage of the appendix has been done in patients who are considered poor surgical risks.

Patients With Delayed Presentation

Initial treatment of patients who have had symptoms longer than 5 days is conservative. If an abscess is present, it should be drained subcutaneously. An appendectomy should be performed in 8 to 12 weeks to prevent recurrence, as well as to exclude neoplasm. Patients older than 40 years of age should also undergo a colonoscopy to rule out malignancy. The role of laparoscopic appendectomy is evolving.

Pregnant Patients

Pregnant patients with suspected appendicitis should undergo an ultrasonography, which is safe and accurate. However, because of diagnostic difficulties in pregnant patients, a negative appendectomy rate of up to 35% is acceptable. There is increased risk of fetal mortality if perforation occurs. Pregnancy-related complications are common if surgery is performed in the first or second trimester; however, it is safe in the third trimester.

Chronic Appendicitis

Chronic appendicitis should be considered in patients who have chronic right lower quadrant pain with fever and a mass or abscess on

CT scan. Some experts believe that it is recurrent acute appendicitis and not chronic appendicitis. Appendectomy should be performed in such patients.

PEARLS

○ Despite advances in technology over the last 3 decades, the rate of negative appendectomy has not declined.

○ Appendectomy during the third trimester is safe.

BIBLIOGRAPHY

Minocha A. An endoscopic view of appendicitis. *N Engl J Med.* 1998; 12;339(20):1481.

Junge K, Marx A, Peiper Ch, Klosterhalfen B, Schumpelick V. Cecal-diverticulitis: a rare differential diagnosis for right-sided lower abdominal pain. *Colorectal Dis.* 2003;5(3):241-5.

Chapter
73 *Clostridium Difficile Diarrhea*

Clostridium difficile (or *C. difficile*) causes antibiotic-induced diarrhea after the normal gut flora has been altered by antibiotic therapy. A sporadic form may also occur.

EPIDEMIOLOGY

C. difficile is seen in 1 to 3% of healthy population. As many as 3 million cases of *C. difficile* occur in the United States alone each year. It affects 10% of the patients who have been hospitalized for greater than 2 days but occurs less commonly as a result of outpatient antibiotic use. Risk factors include elderly malnourished patients, exposure to multiple antibiotics, abdominal surgery, ischemic colitis, chemotherapy, enteral tube feedings, and an infected roommate. Role of carriers as an important reservoir of infection in the hospitals is controversial.

PATHOGENESIS

C. difficile spores are ubiquitous in the environment. When intestinal flora is altered, *C. difficile* colonizes the human GI tract and produces two toxins: A (enterotoxin) and B (cytotoxin). This leads to an inflammatory reaction and increased secretions. Both the toxins play a role in pathogenesis of *C. difficile* disease in humans. All strains of *C. difficile* are not toxogenic; no disease occurs in the absence of the toxin. Some strains produce a variant of toxin-A; stool assays in such cases show toxin-B positive but toxin-A as being falsely negative.

Colonization occurs only when microbial barrier is altered (eg, by antibiotic therapy, cancer, chemotherapy, etc). Whether ischemic colitis predisposes to *C. difficile* infection or that the pathologic findings resemble colonic ischemia is controversial.

C. difficile diarrhea may be caused by any or all antibiotics, including metronidazole and vancomycin, that are used to treat it. The risk is the highest with broad spectrum antibiotics like clindamycin, although ampicillin is the most common culprit because of its frequent use.

Of note, most antibiotic-associated diarrhea is not due to *C. difficile*, but occurs due to an alteration of the colonic microflora. The altered flora causes impairment of carbohydrate fermentation leading to increased carbohydrate concentration in the gut lumen. This results in osmotic diarrhea.

CLINICAL FEATURES

C. difficile-associated enteric disease occurs as a spectrum varying from asymptomatic carrier state, to antibiotic-induced diarrhea, to *C. difficile* diarrhea/colitis, to pseudomembranous colitis, and finally to severe and fulminant colitis. Patients usually have lower abdominal pain (especially left-sided), watery diarrhea, and low-grade fever. Rectal bleeding may be present.

Patients may complain of nausea, vomiting, anorexia, malaise, and profuse diarrhea of 10 to 15 bowel movements per day. Symptoms may be more severe in patients with pseudomembranous colitis.

Atypical Presentations

Atypical presentations include a long latent period between discontinuation of antibiotic and onset of diarrhea, which may be as long as 1 to 2 months; *C. difficile* colitis related to cancer chemotherapy; rare *C. difficile* involvement of small intestine; fulminant colitis occurring in 2 to 3% as initial presentation; protein-losing enteropathy; ascites; relapsing infection in about 20 to 30% patients; and toxic megacolon.

DIAGNOSIS

Routine Studies

A CBC shows leukocytosis. Leukemoid reaction may occur. Leukocytes are present in the stool. Serum albumin is usually decreased even early during the course of disease.

Stool Studies

Do not test stool for *C. difficile* if the stool is not diarrheal or to establish a cure after successful treatment.

Diagnosis is established by documenting *C. difficile* toxin usually by immunoassay. Stool culture for *C. difficile* is very sensitive but is positive in case of carriers too.

Cytotoxicity tissue culture assay of the toxin is the standard. The assay looks for the presence of toxin A and toxin B. However, it is expensive and takes 24 to 72 hours.

ELISA test for *C. difficile* toxin provides rapid turnaround (2 to 4 hours) for results. In many labs, the ELISA test is usually done only for toxin A, and as such, it would miss the diagnosis if *C. difficile* produces only toxin B or a mutant of toxin A. Combined ELISA testing for toxins A and B is superior to testing for toxin A alone. False negative tests can occur especially if tested only once.

Latex agglutination assay results can be available within 30 to 60 minutes, but is neither sensitive nor specific. Studies on dot immunobinding assay and PCR appear promising.

Endoscopy

Endoscopy is not required in patients with typical symptoms and positive stool studies. Sigmoidoscopy shows edema, erosions, and ulcerations. Nodular exudates, which appear as pseudomembranes, are yellow or off-white measuring from 0.2 to 2.0 cm in diameter scattered with intervening normal mucosa. Pseudomembranes in rectosigmoid region are pathognomic for *C. difficile* infection. A minority of patients may have only right-sided colonic involvement, and as such, sigmoidoscopy would miss those lesions.

Approach to Management

If the initial stool test is negative and clinical suspicion is high, empiric therapy should be undertaken. Cytotoxicity assay or endoscopy should be done in patients who do not respond to therapy.

Differential Diagnosis

Fasting improves the osmotic diarrhea induced by antibiotics but not the diarrhea due to *C. difficile*. Other considerations include various other etiologies of colitis like Crohn's disease, ischemia, infections, and nonsteroidal anti-inflammatory drugs (NSAIDs).

Treatment

Patients with mild diarrhea usually respond to the cessation of antibiotic therapy and no specific treatment is required. Treatment is not needed for patients with mild symptoms and negative stool studies. Therapy is not recommended for carriers.

Correct fluid and electrolyte balance. Antimotility agents should be avoided. Metronidazole 250.0 to 500.0 mg PO tid for 10 to 14 days is the treatment of choice. It is preferred over vancomycin because of cost as well as to reduce the possibility of vancomycin resistant bacteria. Vancomycin 125.0 mg qid orally is equally effective but more expensive. Intravenous vancomycin is not effective. In patients who are very ill or high risk, we prefer oral vancomycin as the first line drug. Bacitracin (250 000 units qid) is effective but is not readily available. Role of probiotics is evolving (Lactinex 1.0 g PO qid for 10 to 14 days).

Special Situations

Resistance to metronidazole or vancomycin has not been reported. Thus failure to respond to treatment may occur due to misdiagnosis, noncompliance with therapy, or very severe colitis. In case of patients requiring prolonged course of antibiotics for their underlying disorder, the treatment should cover the period of antibiotic use plus an additional week.

Treatment of Severe Cases

Patients with severe infection may benefit from combination of oral vancomycin (125.0 to 500.0 mg PO q 6 hours) and intravenous metronidazole 500.0 mg IV q 8 hours. Vancomycin suspension in 100 mL normal saline administered as enemas is effective and may be used in severe cases with ileus.

Role of Surgery

Up to 3% of patients may require surgery due to impending perforation or refractory septicemia.

Treatment of Relapse

Relapse occurs in about 20% of the patients within 1 to 4 weeks. Another course of the initial antibiotic for 2 weeks should be administered. If relapse recurs, a repeat stool study should be undertaken to confirm diagnosis.

Tapering dose of vancomycin may be administered starting with 125.0 mg qid for 7 days, then 125.0 mg bid for 7 days, 125.0 mg qd for 7 days, 125.0 mg every other day for 7 days, and then 125.0 mg every 3 days for 2 to 3 weeks. Cholestyramine 4.0 g qd may be given in addition to vancomycin. However, vancomycin should be taken at least 2 hours apart from cholestyramine.

Another option is to give vancomycin plus cholestyramine or rifampin alternating with an off-period 1 week at a time. Metronidazole tapering regimens may be used similar to vancomycin.

Probiotic *Saccharomyces boulardii* 500.0 mg bid for 4 weeks reduces the relapse rates in patients with recurrent *C. difficile* diarrhea. Oral administration of *Lactobacillus GG* (1.0 g packet qid or 10^{10}/day PO) after a course of vancomycin or metronidazole may be beneficial. Use of gammaglobulins containing high titer IgG antitoxin A antibodies (400.0 mg/kg q 3 weeks) appears promising. Enemas using fresh feces from healthy subjects (50.0 g in 500 mL of saline), as well as rectal infusion of mixture of various aerobic and anaerobic bacteria, have been used with success.

PEARLS

○ Not all antibiotic-induced diarrhea is related to *C. difficile*.
○ Do not test stool for *C. difficile* if stool is not diarrheal.
○ Initial stool test for nosocomial diarrhea should be to test for *C. difficile* only except among elderly or immune-compromised patients
○ Both metronidazole and vancomycin are equally effective for treatment of *C. difficile* colitis. However, vancomycin is not effective when given intravenously whereas metronidazole is.

REFERENCES

Surawicz CM. Probiotics, antibiotic-associated diarrhea and Clostridium difficile diarrhea in humans. *Best Pract Res Clin Gastroenterol.* 2003;17(5):775-83.

Hurley BW, Nguyen CC. The spectrum of pseudomembranous enterocolitis and antibiotic-associated diarrhea. *Arch Intern Med.* 2002; 162(19):2177-84.

McFarland LV, Elmer GW, Surawicz CM. Breaking the cycle: treatment strategies for 163 cases of recurrent Clostridium difficile disease. *Am J Gastroenterol.* 2002;97(7):1769-75

Chapter 74   *Irritable Bowel Syndrome* ▰▰

Irritable bowel syndrome (IBS) is a functional disorder character-ized by altered gut motility and/or sensation caused by luminal or environmental stimuli, visceral hypersensitivity, and dysregulation of brain-gut axis. It results in abdominal pain associated with altered defecation.

EPIDEMIOLOGY

The estimated prevalence of IBS varies widely depending on the study criteria used and the population studied, but the overall preva-lence of IBS is similar between Western and Eastern cultures. Approximately 10 to 20% of the population suffers from IBS. When the same population is studied at two different time points separated by 1 to 5 years, the prevalence rates remain unchanged. Although as many as 40% of the subjects having symptoms consistent with IBS at one time do not have them when surveyed in follow-up, these are replaced by other symptomatic people such that the prevalence rates remain stable.

The prevalence is greater amongst women than in men in the Western society, but studies from India suggest IBS is more common amongst men. Patients usually present for the first time between the ages of 15 and 50. Prevalence estimates of IBS amongst African Americans and Hispanics are less established; our studies suggest that the prevalence is similar to those in Whites.

USE OF HEALTH CARE

Patients seeking health care attention form the tip of the iceberg. At the same time, as many as 12% of the patients seen in the primary care practice carry the diagnosis of IBS. Physician surveys suggest that as many as 41% of all the outpatient GI diagnosis are accounted for by functional GI disorders of which IBS is the most common.

Patients with IBS seeking medical attention tend to have concur-rent non-GI complaints. There is also a greater likelihood of prior hysterectomy and appendectomy amongst these patients. The cost to the health care system related to IBS is high. IBS accounts for 2.4 to 3.5 million physician visits annually in the United States resulting in 2.2 million prescriptions.

SOCIOECONOMIC IMPACT

The average annual health care cost of a patient with IBS is $4044, compared to $2719 for the patients without this diagnosis. Patients miss three times as many work days as those without IBS. The disorder is associated with $1.6 billion in direct and $19.2 billion in indirect costs annually to the health care system.

CLINICAL FEATURES

The ROME II criteria defines IBS as a group of functional bowel disorders in which the patient complains of at least 12 weeks of abdominal discomfort or pain within the preceding 12 months (which need not be consecutive). The pain must be associated with at least two of the following three features:

1. Improvement of pain with defecation.
2. Onset of pain with change in frequency of stool.
3. Onset of the pain associated with change in appearance of stool.

The diagnosis of IBS also is supported by abnormal stool frequency, abnormal stool form, difficult defecation, urgency or incomplete evacuation, mucus in stools, and a sensation of bloating or abdominal distention. These criteria assume that there is no biochemical or structural explanation for the complaints.

The symptoms of IBS wax and wane over a long period of time. On an average, a patient has about 12 symptom episodes over a period of 12 weeks and each episode lasts about 4 to 6 days.

QUALITY OF LIFE

Patients with IBS have poorer functional status and poorer health-related quality of life as compared to healthy controls, patients with diabetes, or patients with end stage renal disease.

PATHOPHYSIOLOGY

Non-IBS vs IBS Patients

Abdominal pain and altered bowel habit can occur in healthy subjects, as well as IBS patients, in response to abnormal stimuli like infection, dietary indiscretion (eg, alcohol intake), foreign travel, strenuous physical activity, or psychological stress. Thus, the differences between the IBS patients and healthy controls are largely quantitative and not qualitative with respect to pathophysiological mechanisms.

Intestinal Dysmotility

Altered motility patterns in different parts of the gastrointestinal tract are noted in patients with IBS; however, these findings are not consistent. IBS is characterized primarily by increased motor reactivity to psychological and physiological stimuli that normally affect the bowel on an everyday basis.

Visceral Hypersensitivity

Enhanced visceral hypersensitivity is common and leads to a lowering of pain threshold. This may be of primary importance in the pathophysiology of IBS.

Gastrointestinal Immune Function

Alterations in gut immune function have been implicated in some studies. An increased number of mast cells are present in small intestine and colon. Many patients attribute the onset of their symptoms to a bout of gastroenteritis. It appears that psychological distress also may play a role in determining which patients, particularly with postinfectious IBS, have persistent symptoms following intestinal infection.

Nervous System Dysregulation

Autonomic dysfunction is present is noted in about 25% of IBS patients. Bidirectional communication between brain and gut plays an important role in gastrointestinal health and disease. Chronic inflammation increases the perceptual sensitivity as demonstrated by decreased thresholds for sensation and pain. Stress, anxiety, or recall of remote psychological trauma can enhance the perception of painful events.

Role of Stress

Stress may precipitate the symptoms or worsen the symptoms. While not necessarily associated with the disease *per se*, there is a 40 to 80% prevalence of psychiatric diagnosis among patients with IBS. History of sexual or physical abuse, increased stressful life events, chronic social stress or anxiety disorder, or maladaptive coping style are all associated with poor clinical outcome. There are limited differences between the psychological profiles of those who seek health care vs those who do not. Those who seek health care generally report greater levels of psychological distress than those who do not.

DIAGNOSIS

Diagnosis should be a positive one and based on ROME II criteria, as well as the exclusion of any biochemical or structural abnormalities that may present with similar features. This includes exclusion of other functional disorders like functional diarrhea, pelvic floor dysfunction, or slow transit constipation with associated abdominal discomfort.

A more aggressive work-up is required when alarm features such as weight loss, refractory diarrhea, bleeding, abnormal physical examination or laboratory studies, and a family history of colon cancer are present. In the absence of these alarm features, the specificity of diagnostic criteria (ROME I) exceeds 98%.

Depending on the presentation and the possibility of alternative diagnosis, patients should undergo routine studies including CBC, stools for occult blood, ova and parasites, and thyroid function tests. Screen for celiac sprue (antigliadin antibody plus antitissue transglutaminase antibody test) in patients with diarrhea.

Colonoscopy is usually performed in patients above the age of 50, whereas sigmoidoscopy is often considered sufficient in younger subjects. Some experts recommend a colonoscopy in most subjects, regardless of age, since normal colonoscopy removes the fear of cancer—a stressor seen in many patients. In addition, it provides an opportunity to take biopsies for evaluation of microscopic colitis and ileocolonic inflammatory bowel disease (IBD) that might explain the patient's symptoms. The extent and nature of the work-up requires some degree of common sense and is directed by the symptoms and clinical presentation.

MANAGEMENT

A trusting physician/patient relationship with compassionate support is of paramount importance. Patient education and reassurance helps patients cope with the symptoms. Although a generalization regarding food sensitivities cannot be made across all IBS patients, certain foods may exacerbate symptoms in some patients. Diet diaries may help identify if large fatty meals, beans, alcohol, caffeine, or lactose, for example, are offenders. Avoid recommending a diet that is too restrictive. The underlying concept for treatment strategy is to balance two factors, the stool pattern (eg, diarrhea, constipation) or other symptoms (eg, bloating), and the severity of symptoms as determined by the pain.

Step 1

The initial management step involves therapeutic trial based on symptom severity. Fiber is uniformly offered to almost all IBS patients, although its effectiveness in diarrhea-predominant IBS is not clearly established. Patients should be encouraged to use a diary to monitor their symptoms for 2 to 3 weeks. They should document aggravating or relieving factors and stressors encountered during the period. The role of specific diets and stressors in the patients can then be ascertained.

Patients with mild to moderate symptoms usually can be treated symptomatically with medications targeted at the principal GI symptom.

CONSTIPATION

Dietary fiber (25.0 g/day) with plenty of water is recommended for patients with mild to moderate constipation. Tegaserod (Zelnorm 6.0 mg PO bid) has been shown to provide a global relief of symptoms as well as improve constipation. Tegaserod should be discontinued if there is no response by the end of 4 weeks. Osmotic laxatives like Philip's Milk of Magnesia and sorbitol may be used.

DIARRHEA

Patients with diarrhea-predominant IBS of mild to moderate severity should be tried on loperamide (2.0 to 4.0 mg bid to qid) or diphenoxylate (2.5 mg plus 0.025 mg of atropine bid to qid) for symptomatic relief of diarrhea. Alosetron (Lotronex, 1.0 mg/day initially) is available for limited use in severe cases of diarrhea-predominant IBS.

Likewise, in severe cases of diarrhea, cholestyramine (4.0 g tid) may be tried or the diagnostic evaluation may be extended.

ABDOMINAL PAIN

Patients with a predominant symptom of abdominal pain, gaseousness, or bloating should be treated with anticholinergics/antispasmodics or antidepressants. Although antispasmodics like hyoscyamine and dicyclomine are routinely prescribed for these symptoms, their effectiveness has not been easy to demonstrate. As such antispasmodics/anticholinergics should be used on as needed basis for acute attacks. Psychological treatments also may be helpful.

Step 2

If the above mentioned therapeutic trials fail or the patient's symptoms are severe, further investigation should be considered. Colonic transit assessments may be required for patients with constipation. If obstructive defecation is suspected, anorectal manometry with balloon expulsion, defecography, and EMG may be undertaken.

In patients with persistent diarrhea, a 24-hour stool volume, stool for osmolality and fat, as well as laxative screen should be undertaken. Hydrogen breath test for small bowel bacterial overgrowth and a small bowel biopsy for *Giardia* as well as malabsorptive disorders should be considered. We recommend exclusion of microscopic colitis by undertaking colonic biopsies, although this is controversial. Use of hydrogen breath test to exclude lactose intolerance is controversial, although many physicians advise such patients to limit their lactose intake.

An empiric trial of antibiotics may be given for presumed small bowel bacterial overgrowth. Consider a therapeutic trial of cholestyramine, especially if symptoms are temporally related to a history of cholecystectomy. Patients with persistent symptoms of pain-predominant IBS should undergo a plain x-ray of the abdomen during an acute episode to rule out intermittent bowel obstruction, or gastric dilatation from aerophagia.

Further imaging studies including small bowel series, CT scan, and pelvic ultrasound may be considered for patients with persistent symptoms, especially those with vomiting, weight loss, and abnormal chemistries. In general, expensive and invasive studies should not be solely based on patient reports of symptom severity, but also on clinical suspicion as determined by alarm signs.

Step 3

ANTIDEPRESSANTS

Antidepressants, both tricyclic antidepressants (TCA), and more contemporary antidepressants (eg, SSRIs), are frequently prescribed for the treatment of IBS. Their role is synergistic with psychological and the previously-mentioned medical treatments, as they may directly affect the pathophysiological underpinnings of this disorder. The doses of TCAs are typically much lower than those used for depression suggesting that the effects are not related to their antidepressant effects. Drugs like amitriptyline, imipramine, doxepin, desipramine, or nortriptyline (10.0 to 50.0 mg q HS) can help with the abdominal pain as well as improve any sleep disturbance. The effect starts within days.

Side effects of TCAs (eg, sedation, constipation, and xerostomia) limit their use in some patients. SSRIs in usual psychiatric dosages help with the depression, anxiety, and panic that may be present in some of these patients. Side effects include insomnia, agitation, diarrhea, night sweats, weight changes, and possible sexual dysfunction. The SSRIs and other contemporary antidepressants have not been as well studied as the TCAs in this setting.

Many patients refuse to take antidepressants because of their "mind altering" potential and patient education about the rationale for use is helpful. When there is poor response to one antidepressant, a different class of antidepressant may be considered. Some experts prescribe a combination of a tricyclic antidepressant and a SSRI.

BENZODIAZEPINES

There is risk for physical dependence considering the chronic nature of IBS; as such, they should be used for brief periods if required. Buspirone (acts at serotonin 5-HT$_1$A and 5-HT$_2$ receptors as well as dopamine D$_2$ receptors) and SSRIs are better approaches to anxiety if this is the rationale for benzopdiazepine use in the IBS patient.

PSYCHOLOGICAL TREATMENTS

Psychological treatments including psychodynamic therapy, interpersonal therapy, cognitive behavioral therapy, relaxation techniques, and stress management have been shown to improve symptoms. Cognitive-behavioral therapy is superior to education or desipramine for treatment of severe cases. Hypnosis and relaxation decrease perceptual sensitivity. Therapy using IBS classes by a team of physicians, nurses, and dietitians has been shown to be effective.

ALTERNATIVE AND COMPLEMENTARY MEDICINE

Limited data is available, but amongst alternative and complementary therapies, Chinese herbal medicine appears a valid alternative for some patients because of the beneficial effect demonstrated in double blind placebo-controlled trials. Peppermint oil remains under investigation and has had positive outcome in some studies. Certain probiotics have been shown to be of benefit in early studies and their role appears promising.

PEARLS

- ○ Irritable bowel syndrome is a clinical diagnosis based on specific diagnostic criteria and both abdominal pain and bowel problems must be present for diagnosis. Pain, diarrhea, or constipation alone does not qualify for the diagnosis.
- ○ A biopsychosocial model involving multiple exacerbating and perpetuating factors has been implicated in pathogenesis.

BIBLIOGRAPHY

Drossman D, Camilleri M, Mayer EA, Whitehead WE. AGA technical review on irritable bowel syndrome. *Gastroenterology*. 2002;123: 2108.

Clouse RE. Antidepressants for irritable bowel syndrome. *Gut*. 2003; 52(4):598-9.

Bensoussan A, Talley NJ, Hing M, Menzies R, Guo A, Ngu M. Treatment of irritable bowel syndrome with Chinese herbal medicine: a randomized controlled trial. *JAMA*. 1998;280(18):1585-9.

Chapter
75 *Inflammatory Bowel Disease*

IBD is a chronic inflammation of uncertain etiology involving the digestive tract. It is primarily divided into ulcerative colitis (UC) and Crohn's disease. About 10 to 15% of the cases remain indeterminate.

EPIDEMIOLOGY

The incidence of UC varies from 5 to 15 per 100 000 persons, whereas for Crohn's disease it is 3 to 10 per 100 000 population. While the incidence of UC has remained constant, the incidence of Crohn's disease has been progressively rising. IBD is less common in Asia and South America. It is more prevalent in the northern countries than in the southern countries.

Most cases present between the age of 15 to 30 years. There is a second peak incidence manifesting at 50 to 80 years of age especially for Crohn's disease. There is no sex predominance. IBD occurs more among Whites than Blacks, and more among the Jewish than non-Jewish population. It is lower amongst the Hispanic population as compared to Whites.

PATHOGENESIS

There is an increased genetic predisposition although greater than 80% of patients have no family history of IBD. For example, multiple mutations of the NOD2 gene (renamed CARD 15) within chromosome 16 have been implicated in Crohn's disease; NOD2 gene mutations are not involved in UC. However, these mutations may also be present in healthy subjects suggesting that additional gene mutations, as well as environmental factors, are important in phenotypic expression of Crohn's disease.

The role of oral contraceptives in the pathogenesis is controversial. Whereas smoking is protective against UC, it tends to worsen Crohn's disease. Prior appendectomy confers protection against ulcerative colitis and not for Crohn's disease. Nutritional deficiencies do not cause or contribute to the pathogenesis.

The role of infectious agents is controversial and continues to be debated. Studies suggest that "normal" intestinal flora may contribute to the pathogenesis in susceptible individuals. The relationship between breast-feeding and Crohn's disease is controversial. NSAIDs increase the risk for development of IBD or induce flare-up. Stress does not cause IBD but contributes to exacerbation of symptoms.

DISTRIBUTION

Ulcerative Colitis

The inflammation is mucosal, almost always starts in the rectum, and extends proximally in a contiguous fashion. UC may be divided on the basis of location into ulcerative proctitis; distal colitis or proctosigmoiditis, left-sided colitis extending to the splenic flexure; or extensive and pancolitis, extending beyond the splenic flexure and potentially all the way up to the cecum. Backwash ileitis may be present in a few cases.

Crohn's Disease

In contrast to UC, Crohn's disease can involve any part of the GI tract extending from mouth to anus. Rectum is usually spared. About half of the patients have both small and large bowel involvement, 20% have colitis alone and about 35% have ileitis or small bowel involvement alone. A small fraction of patients may have predominant upper gastrointestinal involvement.

The small intestine is involved in overall 80% of Crohn's disease, whereas about one-third of the patients may have perianal disease. The inflammation is transmural and skip lesions are common. The transmural inflammation predisposes to the formation of strictures and fistulae.

HISTORY

Ulcerative Colitis

Patients with proctitis or proctosigmoiditis present with intermittent rectal bleeding with mucus, mild abdominal pain, and tenesmus. Constipation with rectal bleeding may be seen in 25% of such cases. Moderate UC occurs in patients with at least left-sided involvement with frequent loose bloody stools up to ten per day, mild anemia, mild abdominal pain, and low-grade fever. Patients are not malnourished.

Patients with extensive colonic involvement have severe diarrhea (>10 stools per day) with abdominal pain, fever, and bleeding that requires a blood transfusion. Patients are frequently malnourished. Inflammation may extend to submucosal areas all the way to the muscle layers of the colonic wall, increasing the predisposition to toxic megacolon and even perforation.

Crohn's Disease

Crohn's disease, in addition to the classification by anatomic involvement, may also be classified as an *inflammatory, obstructive* (stricturing), or *fistulous* disease.

Clinical presentation depends upon the anatomic location involved and the type of disease. Clinical features include abdominal pain, fever, diarrhea (which may be bloody), weight loss, and low-grade temperature. Patients with predominant gastroduodenal involvement have epigastric pain and early satiety. Dysphagia, odynophagia, oral ulcers, and chest pain may be seen in oral or esophageal Crohn's disease.

Perianal Crohn's disease presents with perianal abscesses, fistulae, and painful external hemorrhoids and fissures. Pneumaturia and recurrent UTIs may be seen in enterovesical fistula. A passage of gas or stool per vagina is seen in rectovaginal fistula.

Most children with Crohn's disease present with weight loss, which may precede intestinal symptoms in about 30% of the patients.

PHYSICAL FINDINGS

Physical exam in UC may be normal or may show mild abdominal tenderness especially in the left lower quadrant. Patients with severe disease may have signs of dehydration, tachycardia, and hypoactive bowel sounds. Diffuse abdominal tenderness with rebound is seen in patients with toxic megacolon or perforation.

Findings in Crohn's disease are variable and include elevated temperature, cachexia, weight loss, muscle wasting, and abdominal tenderness and mass—especially in the right lower quadrant. Perianal exam may reveal evidence of abscess and fistulae. An oral exam may show evidence of aphthous ulcers.

LABORATORY STUDIES

Routine Studies

A routine CBC may be normal or may show evidence of iron deficiency anemia. Additionally, there may be vitamin B_{12} and folate deficiency in Crohn's disease, thus, anemia may be mixed. WBC may be elevated because of the inflammatory process or infection. A metabolic profile may show low serum albumin, abnormal electrolytes and even metabolic acidosis.

Stool studies should always be performed to exclude infections as the cause of inflammation. This includes testing for routine ova and parasites, culture, and sensitivity, including *Yersinia*, *E. coli O157:H7* and *C. difficile* toxin. Up to 25% of cases of relapse may have underlying *C. difficile* diarrhea.

Serology

The perinuclear antineutrophil cytoplasmic antibody (pANCA) is seen in about two-thirds of the patients with UC and about 10 to 20% of the patients with Crohn's disease. In contrast, the anti-Saccharomyces cereviciae antibody (ASCA) is positive in about two-thirds of the patients with Crohn's disease and in about 10% of the patients with UC. Using the two tests in combination may distinguish UC from Crohn's disease in patients with indeterminate colitis.

Endoscopy

Endoscopy is the cornerstone of diagnosis. Findings in UC include edema with loss of normal vascular pattern, mucosal granularity, friability, and ulceration. Patients with left-sided UC may show inflammation in the periappendiceal region, and this does not represent skip lesions of Crohn's disease.

Findings in Crohn's disease include rectal sparing, ulcers (aphthous or deep linear) with edema, erythema and granularity, cobblestoning, pseudopolyps, and skip lesions. Involvement of the upper gastrointestinal tract by Crohn's can be confirmed or excluded by EGD.

The correlation between endoscopic findings and clinical manifestations (ie, signs and symptoms in Crohn's disease) is suboptimal.

Imaging Studies

A plain x-ray series of the abdomen is helpful in acute cases to exclude any perforation or toxic megacolon. Small bowel series can help delineate the small intestinal involvement as well as to document strictures and fistulae. Small bowel enteroclysis or a dedicated small bowel study may be superior. Abdominal ultrasound and CT scans are helpful in excluding intra-abdominal abscesses as well as to document any obstruction or fistula.

Radionuclide WBC scintigraphy is helpful in assessing the extent of inflammation. Transabdominal bowel sonography, which is different from regular abdominal ultrasound (although the device is the same), can help:

1. Define the extent of the disease, location, length, and severity of strictures, as well as fistulae.
2. Exclude intra-abdominal abscess.
3. Define or document postoperative recurrence.
4. Monitor healing of fistula of patients under immunosuppression.

However, it may not be available in many centers.

Histology

Histology is helpful in excluding other diagnosis, although frequently the distinction is not absolute in many cases. Noncaseating granulomas indicate Crohn's disease, but are seen only in about 20 to 40% of the cases. Crypt abscesses are common and nondiagnostic.

DIFFERENTIAL DIAGNOSIS

IBD should be distinguished from other causes of inflammation in the gastrointestinal tract including bacterial infections (*Yersinia, Mycobacterium tuberculosis*), amebiasis, viral infections (*Cytomegalovirus [CMV], Herpes*), microscopic colitis, diverticulitis, medication induced colitis (NSAIDs, gold), ischemic colitis, radiation colitis, appendicitis, Behcet's disease, endometriosis, solitary rectal ulcer syndrome, and even malignancy like carcinoma and lymphoma.

Patients with microscopic colitis usually have diarrhea without any significant endoscopic or radiological findings. Segmental chronic colitis associated with diverticular disease is seen in the region of diverticuli. NSAIDs may induce inflammation and ulceration throughout the GI tract. Radiation enteritis may present with diarrhea, profuse bleeding, or even strictures and fistulae. Solitary rectal ulcer syndrome can be distinguished on the basis of typical histopathological features. Acute diverticulitis may present with intra-abdominal abscess and fistula.

COMPLICATIONS

Complications of UC include massive hemorrhage in up to 3% of patients, fulminant colitis in 10 to 20% of the patients, and rectosigmoid stricture in 5 to 10%. A stricture in patients with UC is considered malignant unless proven otherwise. In addition, Crohn's disease may manifest with intestinal obstruction and abscesses, as well as metastatic Crohn's disease.

EXTRAINTESTINAL MANIFESTATIONS

Patients with IBD have numerous extraintestinal complications that are more likely in patients with colonic involvement. These include involvement of eyes (uveitis, episcleritis), skin (erythema nodosum and pyoderma gangrenosum), joints (spondyloarthropathy, peripheral and axial arthritis, ankylosing spondylitis), liver (autoimmune hepatitis, primary sclerosing cholangitis), secondary amyloidosis, as well as venous and arterial thrombosis.

Patients with Crohn's disease may have complications like bile acid diarrhea, malabsorption syndrome and steatorrhea, malnutrition, coagulopathy, and osteopenia. There is increased incidence of cholelithiasis and renal stones, including oxalate and uric acid stones. Vitamin B_{12} deficiency is common in patients with ileal disease or ileal resection.

COURSE OF INFLAMMATORY BOWEL DISEASE

Most patients with UC have intermittent remissions and relapses although 10 to 20% of patients may have prolonged remission after initial presentation. Patients with ulcerative proctitis or ulcerative proctosigmoiditis have a benign course and 20% of them achieve complete remission. However, extension of the disease may occur in about 10 to 20% of the cases. Recurrence of the disease in patients with severe UC is no more likely than in patients with milder forms once the remission is achieved.

Natural history of Crohn's disease is based on type of Crohn's affecting the patient. Inflammatory Crohn's disease tends to be aggressive with frequent and early recurrences. Obstructive Crohn's disease follows an indolent course and responds well to surgery. The need for repeat surgery is lower in fistulous disease compared to the other forms. Fistulous Crohn's disease responds well to maintenance therapy for preventing recurrences.

TREATMENT OF ULCERATIVE COLITIS

Medical therapy of active UC depends upon disease severity.

Proctitis

Treatment with 5-ASA suppositories (Canasa 500.0 mg bid to tid) with or without steroid foams is effective in most cases of proctitis. Start with one suppository twice a day until patient is in remission. Maintenance therapy may only be undertaken in patients with recurrent proctitis. Patients intolerant to 5-ASA suppositories may benefit from oral 5-ASA agents (mesalamine, balsalazide).

Proctosigmoiditis

Most patients with proctosigmoiditis respond to topical therapy. Treatment is initiated with 5-ASA enema (Rowasa 4.0 g/60 mL) with or without oral 5-ASA preparation. In patients with partial or no response in 3 to 4 weeks, steroid enemas should be added. Patients not responding to topical therapy may benefit from oral corticosteroids. Steroids should be tapered in patients who respond and reinstituted when the flare-up occurs. On the other hand, if there is no response within 4 weeks, options include hospitalization with intravenous corticosteroid therapy or additional immune-suppressants and/or the use of nicotine patch.

Therapeutic failure with 5-ASA products should only be considered when sulfasalazine has been gradually increased up to 6.0 g/day, or mesalamine up to 4.8 g/day given in two to four divided doses. Usual dose for balsalazide (Colazal) is 2.25 g PO tid. Peak effect occurs in 3 to 6 weeks. Maintenance dose should be used once remission is achieved (sulfasalazine 2.0 g/day or mesalamine 1.2 to 2.4 g/day). Some patients require higher doses for maintenance. Folic acid 1.0 mg/day should be given to patients on sulfasalazine. Prednisone when used should be started at 40.0 to 60.0 mg/day with expected response occurring within 2 weeks after which the dose can gradually be tapered by 5.0 mg/week.

Budesonide enemas (not available in the United States) are effective in inducing remission in distal UC.

Left-Sided and Extensive Colitis

Patients are initially treated with a oral 5-ASA compound (mesalamine or balsalazide) plus topical therapy with either 5-ASA or steroid enema. Prednisone at 40.0 to 60.0 mg/day should be undertaken in patients who fail the above therapy or in those with severe symptoms. Additional medical management includes iron supplementation, preferably parenteral iron in patients who can not tolerate oral iron. Antidiarrheal agents should be avoided in acutely sick patients.

Severe Colitis

Severe colitis implies frequent bloody stools with weight loss and signs of volume depletion. Presence of severe toxic symptoms including fever and abdominal pain suggest fulminant colitis. Such a flare-up may occur when a new 5-ASA compound has been started or the dose has just been increased and this is related to 5-ASA compound. 5-ASA drug should be withheld in acute severe flare-ups. Patients are treated with corticosteroids.

Patients with severe colitis or those not responding to oral steroids require hospitalization. Intravenous corticosteroids are used including hydrocortisone 100.0 mg IV q 8 hours or methylprednisolone 20.0 to 40.0 mg IV q 8 hours. In patients not on any corticosteroids previously, ACTH 120 units per 24 hours IV infusion may be superior to parenteral steroids. Hydrocortisone or 5-ASA enema once or twice a day may be added in patients not responding to intravenous therapy within 2 to 3 days.

Broad spectrum antibiotics may be considered in patients with a severe colitis not responding to above therapy, as well as for all the patients with fulminant colitis. A typical regimen may include a third generation cephalosporin plus metronidazole.

Baseline and follow-up abdominal x-rays should be obtained and gastrointestinal decompression may be undertaken using a nasogastric tube with or without a rectal tube as needed. Hyperbaric oxygen has been used with benefit.

Colectomy should be considered in patients with toxic megacolon with a transverse colon diameter greater than 6.0 cm who do not respond to treatment within 72 hours. Cyclosporine should be considered in patients with less severe disease not responding to intravenous corticosteroids within 7 to 10 days. Cyclosporine is administered as 4.0 mg/kg/day continuous IV infusion. A lower dose of 2.0 mg/kg/day infusion appears to be equally effective with reduced potential for toxicity. In patients who respond to IV cyclosporine, oral cyclosporine should be continued at 8.0 mg/kg and azathioprine (1.5 to 2.5 mg/kg/day) or 6-MP should be started for 4 months while following cyclosporine levels.

Adjunctive Measures in Ulcerative Colitis

Lactose, fresh fruit and vegetables, caffeine, carbonated beverages, or sorbitol-containing products should be avoided during active disease. Multivitamins should be taken along with folic acid 1.0 mg/day. There is no role for elemental or parenteral nutrition in UC. Patients with increased stress may benefit from tranquilizers like lorazepam since evidence suggests that stress can worsen the disease. Antidepressants may be useful in select cases.

Patients with refractory UC regardless of extent of colonic involvement may benefit from fish oil, oral antibiotics like ciprofloxacin, nicotine patches, and immunosuppressive agents. Even surgery may be a consideration. Fish oil is used in high doses (up to 15 to 18 capsules per day with each capsule containing 0.18 g EPA per capsule). However, ciprofloxacin and fish oil do not have any role in maintenance therapy. Similarly, transdermal nicotine may be used for inducing, but not for maintenance therapy since it is not effective in maintenance.

Treatment of Medically Refractory Ulcerative Colitis

Refractory patients may benefit from immunomodulator therapy with daily azathioprine (2.0 to 2.5 mg/kg) or 6-MP (1.5 to 2.0 mg/kg). These drugs are slow acting and can take as many as three to eight months for action. Levels of 6-thioguanine, the metabolite of azathioprine/6-MP should be monitored. Some experts recommend checking the thiopurine methyltransferase enzyme (TPMT) activity prior to initiating therapy. Studies with the use of infliximab (Remicade) are on going. The role of probiotics is evolving and looks promising.

MANAGEMENT OF CROHN'S DISEASE

Medical management of Crohn's disease depends on the disease location and severity.

Upper Gastrointestinal Crohn's

Oral lesions are treated with hydrocortisone topically or topical sucralfate. Patients with gastroduodenal disease may benefit from acid suppressive therapy or sucralfate. In nonresponders, mesalamine (Pentasa) may be used. Prednisone is frequently required and is usually effective within 2 weeks. Azathioprine or 6-MP may be used in nonresponders or for maintaining the mission.

Mild to Moderate Crohn's Ilietis

Initial treatment involves the 5-ASA formulation up to 4.8 g/day or budesonide 9.0 mg/day. In nonresponders, antibiotics like ciprofloxacin 500.0 mg bid may be added for 6 weeks. In patients who respond to ciprofloxacin, therapy should be continued for another 6 weeks after which 500.0 mg/day should be given for 6 weeks and then stopped. Clarithromycin 500.0 mg bid has also been used and if effective may be continued for 6 months.

Patients not responding to antibiotics should receive prednisone (40.0 to 60.0 mg/day). Response is seen within 7 to 14 days at which time the dose should be tapered at 5.0 mg/week. Maintenance therapy for ileitis should be undertaken with mesalamine. Sulfasalazine or olsalazine are not effective. Patients with partial response to first line therapy may receive antidiarrheal agents including loperamide or cholestyramine.

Localized Peritonitis

Patients with localized peritonitis are treated with broad spectrum antibiotics including a third generation cephalosporin plus metronidazole. Corticosteroids are usually withheld at this point. However, in case of patients already on corticosteroids, the dose may be increased.

Intra-Abdominal Abscess

In this case, a surgical consult should be obtained. Management includes medical therapy plus percutaneous drainage, which can avoid surgery in about half the cases.

Small Bowel Obstruction

Conservative therapy with IV fluids, nasogastric suction, and parenteral nutrition resolves most cases of small bowel obstruction (SBO). Parenteral steroids may be considered and surgery is needed in nonresponders.

Crohn's Colitis

Patients with ileocolitis or colonic involvement only are initially treated with sulfasalazine or mesalamine. Patients who do not improve within 3 to 4 weeks should receive antibiotics like metronidazole 10.0 mg/day that may be increased to 20.0 mg/day in nonresponders. Other choices include ciprofloxacin or clarithromycin, which may be used in combination with metronidazole. Patients who do not respond or who have severe symptoms on initial presentation should receive prednisone 40.0 to 60.0 mg/day, which may be combined with 5-ASA and antibiotics. Steroids should be tapered once remission is achieved.

Patients with severe or toxic symptoms require hospitalization including parenteral nutrition and corticosteroids. For patients refractory to above therapy, immune-modulator like azathioprine (1.5 to 2.5 mg/kg) or 6-MP (1.0 to 2.0 mg/kg/day) may be used starting at 50.0 to 75.0 mg/day. Monitor 6-thioguanine (6-TG) levels. Consider checking thiopurine methyltransferase (TPMT) enzyme levels prior to initiating therapy. Onset of response takes about 3 to 6 months and occurs in 70% of the cases.

Methotrexate 25.0 mg IM per week or infliximab 5.0 mg/kg IV are alternate options. Folic acid supplementation should be given when methotrexate therapy is used. Patients with continued refractoriness to medical therapy despite aggressive management may benefit from chronic low-dose steroid therapy and TPN. Nutrition using elemental or polymeric diet is an alternate option to TPN.

Perianal Crohn's

Patients benefit from metronidazole, which is initiated at 10.0 mg/kg/day and is increased to 20.0 mg/kg/day if there is no response within 2 to 4 weeks. However, peripheral neuropathy tends to occur at this dose and if it does, the drug should be stopped and may be restarted at the lower dose. Because of high relapse of disease following cessation, long-term therapy may be needed for at least 12 months at the lowest effective dose of metronidazole.

Ciprofloxacin 500.0 mg bid may be used as an alternate to metronidazole or in combination with it. Immune-modulator therapy with azathioprine or 6-MP should be considered with or without surgical management.

Treatment of Fistulae

In case of enteroenteric fistulae, azathioprine or 6-MP should be tried since steroids or sulfasalazine are not effective. Azathioprine should also be considered for treatment for enterovesical fistulae in addition to antibiotics to control UTI. However, most patients will require surgery. Infliximab and 6-MP/azathioprine are effective for perianal fistulizing disease. Injection of fibrin glue in perianal fistulae results in symptomatic relief in many patients.

Prevention of Postoperative Relapse

Relapse is common after surgical resection. Metronidazole and oral 5-ASA agents may help prevent postoperative recurrence after ileal or colonic resection where as sulfasalazine and corticosteroids are not helpful. 5-ASA (3.0 g/day) should be used as initial therapy. In case of patients requiring resection despite 5-ASA, 6-MP may be used.

SURGICAL MANAGEMENT OF INFLAMMATORY BOWEL DISEASE

The most common indication is refractory disease, which includes persistent symptoms despite high dose corticosteroid therapy, steroid-dependence, dysplasia, or cancer. Others indications include uncontrolled hemorrhage, perforation, or toxic megacolon.

Ulcerative Colitis

Options include proctocolectomy with permanent ileostomy or continent ileostomy, abdominal colectomy with ileorectal anastomosis, or colectomy with mucosal proctectomy and ileal pouch-anal canal anastomosis (IPAA). IPAA is the most common surgery used.

Pouchitis occurs in about 10 to 40% of patients with IPAA. Symptoms include abdominal pain, fever, increased stool frequency, urgency, nocturnal defecation, and rectal bleeding. Endoscopy shows erythema, edema, friability, erosions and ulcerations. Etiology is unknown. Recurrence occurs in about 50% of the cases. Acute episodes respond to metronidazole 1.0 to 2.0 g/day PO for 7 to 10 days. An alternate option is ciprofloxacin 500.0 mg bid. Role of probiotics, especially VSL#3 appears promising. Up to 10% of patients develop chronic symptoms and require long-term or continuous therapy. Continued surveillance for cancer is needed. In patients refractory to medical treatment, excision of the pouch and ileostomy may be needed.

Crohn's Disease

Surgery is very common in patients with Crohn's disease. Over a period of 15 years after diagnosis, almost 75% of the patients would have had at least one operation, with over 50% having had multiple operations. The choice of operation depends upon the underlying problem. A stricture may require a resection or stricturoplasty. Patients with perianal abscess and fistula may undergo incision and drainage of abscess, fistulotomy, placement of drains or flap surgery. Drug-resistant inflammatory colitis may require colectomy with ileorectal anastomosis. As a rule, minimalist surgery is the rule.

FERTILITY

Fertility in men or women with IBD is not decreased. Sulfasalazine causes hypospermia in men which is reversible within 2 months of discontinuation. Newer 5-ASA formulations do not affect sperm count. Azathioprine does not reduce the quality of semen. Anatomic defects like tubal occlusions may occur in females. Painful coitus may be a barrier in efforts to conceive.

PREGNANCY AND NURSING

Relapse rate during the pregnancy is similar to the relapse rate in nonpregnant patients provided the conception occurred during remission. However, if conception occurred during active disease, the disease is likely to stay active during pregnancy and may worsen. Remission achieved during pregnancy is likely to be sustained. Pattern of IBD during one pregnancy does not predict the events during subsequent pregnancies.

Complications during pregnancy are similar to those amongst nonpregnant women. Although there may be increased incidence of preterm births and low birth weight babies, there is no increase in congenital abnormalities or stillbirth. Episiotomy is avoided and

Cesarean section undertaken in patients with active perianal Crohn's disease because of concern for fistula formation. However, for patients in remission, the mode of delivery is based on obstetrical issues.

While sigmoidoscopy is safe, colonoscopy should be avoided during pregnancy unless it is absolutely essential. Similarly, x-rays should be avoided.

Sulfasalazine and 5-ASA formulations are safe during pregnancy. Short-term course of metronidazole is safe, whereas the effect of long-term therapy is controversial. Ciprofloxacin is not recommended during pregnancy or for children. Although data is conflicting, risks due to corticosteroids appears to be low and they should not be withheld during pregnancy.

Azathioprine and 6-MP should be continued during pregnancy if patients cannot be managed without these medications. These drugs are secreted in breast milk, and as such, lactation is discouraged.

Methotrexate can induce abortion. Contraception should be initiated at least 3 months prior to starting the methotrexate both in men and women. The use of infliximab appears to be safe.

Antidiarrheal agents like loperamide or diphenoxylate with atropine should be avoided during pregnancy and lactation.

Intra-abdominal surgery may induce premature labor or spontaneous abortion. Female patients with ileoanal pouch have normal pregnancies and deliveries.

RISK FOR MALIGNANCY

Both UC and Crohn's disease have an increased risk for malignancy, although in UC, it is limited to the colon.

There is an increased risk for colon cancer in both UC and Crohn's disease, related to the extent and duration of the disease. Surveillance colonoscopy is probably less effective in Crohn's disease than UC.

Patients with extensive colitis due to UC or Crohn's for greater than 7 to 8 years should undergo an annual colonoscopy with biopsies for surveillance of dysplasia. In patients with left-sided UC, a colonoscopy is initiated at 7 to 8 years; however, further colonoscopies are undertaken every 2 years up to year 15, and then every year. Some experts recommend initiating surveillance at year 12 to 15 in patients with left-sided colitis.

Surveillance for ulcerative proctitis is not recommended and is generally not undertaken for proctosigmoiditis.

Colectomy should be recommended for any patient found to have dysplasia or dysplasia associated with mass lesion during surveillance.

In case of Crohn's disease, in addition to colon, there is increased risk for small intestinal cancer as well as cancer of the anus. The increased risk for lymphoma in Crohn's disease is controversial.

PEARLS

○   Surgery is curative for ulcerative colitis but not Crohn's disease.

○   Corticosteroids are effective for inducing remission but should not be used for maintaining remission.

BIBLIOGRAPHY

Hanauer SB, Sandborn W, and The Practice Parameters Committee of the American College of Gastroenterology. Management of Crohn's disease in adults . *Am J Gastroenterol.* 2001,96:P 635-643.

Lashner BA. Colorectal cancer surveillance for patients with inflammatory bowel disease. *Gastrointest Endosc Clin N Am.* 2002;12(1):135-43, viii. Review.

Sharan R, Schoen RE. Cancer in inflammatory bowel disease. An evidence-based analysis and guide for physicians and patients. *Gastroenterol Clin North Am.* 2002;31(1):237-54.

Chapter
76 *Microscopic Colitis*

Microscopic colitis is an umbrella term used for lymphocytic colitis and collagenous colitis, which manifest with chronic watery diarrhea; however, the findings on contrast studies as well as colonoscopy are normal whereas the histology shows evidence of inflammation.

It is unclear whether lymphocytic colitis and collagenous colitis represent spectrum or part of the same disorder or chronic idiopathic inflammatory bowel disease or whether they are distinct entities. Some experts categorize microscopic colitis into three types:

1.   Lymphocytic colitis.

2.   Collagenous colitis without lymphocytic infiltration of surface epithelium.

3.   A mixed form.

EPIDEMIOLOGY

In North America, it is believed to represent about 10% of cases of watery diarrhea with a female predominance. The female preponderance is seen more for collagenous colitis than lymphocytic colitis. It tends to occur predominantly in the fifth to eighth decade of life.

PATHOGENESIS

Although primarily limited to the colon, ileum may be involved. Pathogenesis is unknown. Theories include abnormal collagen metabolism, diabetes mellitus, bacterial toxins, bile acid malabsorption, infections, autoimmune dysfunction, NSAIDs, and other medications (lansoprazole, simvastatin, ticlopidine, and flutamide).

Microscopic colitis may precede the development of chronic idiopathic IBD. The disease may be associated with arthralgias, celiac sprue, and other autoimmune disorders. Frequently coexisting extraintestinal manifestations like arthritis, thyroiditis lymphocytic gastritis, celiac sprue, and collagenous gastroduodenitis, suggest a systemic pathophysiologic basis.

CLINICAL FEATURES

Patients present with watery diarrhea that may be intermittent or continuous. The diarrhea is voluminous, and may be as high as 1 to 2 L/day. Many patients are misdiagnosed as diarrhea-predominant IBS. Abdominal pain, weight loss, and fatigue may be seen.

DIAGNOSIS

Stools studies are normal. Occasionally, stools may be positive for leukocytes. Stool osmolality suggests secretary diarrhea with the osmotic gap of less than 50 mOsm/L.

A CBC may be normal or show mild anemia. Serum autoantibodies like RA, ANA, AMA, and pANCA are seen in about half the patients. Erythrocyte sedimentation rate (ESR) may be elevated. Colonoscopy is usually normal or may show a mild patchy erythema or edema.

PATHOLOGY

Biopsies obtained only from the left colon during sigmoidoscopy may miss some cases. Histology shows edema and mixed inflammatory infiltrate in lamina propria with an increased number of intraepithelial lymphocytes. Collagenous colitis is distinguished by the presence of a thick subepithelial band of collagen. Crypts are usually well-preserved.

DIFFERENTIAL DIAGNOSIS

Presence of nausea, vomiting, dehydration, hematochezia, hematemesis, and melena should raise suspicion for other etiologies. Differential diagnosis includes IBS, IBD, chronic infectious diarrhea, medications, radiation enteropathy, factitious diarrhea, celiac sprue, chronic IBD, VIPoma, antibiotic-associated diarrhea, and carcinoid syndrome.

TREATMENT

Treatment is conservative and includes reassurance as well as discontinuation of medications implicated in the pathogenesis. A stepwise approach to treatment is usually followed. Most patients respond to symptomatic treatment.

Lifestyles alterations include discontinuation of caffeine, alcohol, and NSAIDs as much as possible.

Patients with celiac disease should be placed on gluten-free diet. Bulking agents and antidiarrheal agents (loperamide, diphenoxylate) are recommended as needed. If there is no response to first line therapy, bismuth subsalicylate (Pepto-Bismol, 262.0-mg tabs, 2 tablets PO tid) is prescribed. In case of nonresponders, anti-inflammatory agents like 5-ASA drugs (Asacol, Pentasa, Colazal) are then recommended. A failure to respond to above treatments may necessitate a need for short-term course for corticosteroids. Budesonide 9.0 mg/day is also effective.

In steroid refractory cases, azathioprine or 6-MP has been used with success. Rarely octreotide and even surgery may be needed. Other regimens that have been tried include metronidazole, verapamil, methotrexate, and other immunosuppressive drugs.

COURSE

Although the course is usually waxing and weaning, spontaneous resolution may occur. Once a particular treatment strategy controls the diarrhea, it should be continued for 8 to 12 weeks and then discontinued in a tapering dose. Relapse of the diarrhea while tapering or upon discontinuation suggests a need for maintenance therapy.

PEARLS

- ○ Microscopic colitis is characterized by diarrhea and histological evidence of inflammation in the presence of normal mucosa upon colonoscopy.
- ○ Asymptomatic cases of microscopic colitis should not be treated.
- ○ Most patients respond to symptomatic measures such as bulking agents and antidiarrheal agents.

BIBLIOGRAPHY

Pardi DS, Smyrk TC, Tremaine WJ, Sandborn WJ. Microscopic colitis: a review. *Am J Gastroenterol*. 2002;97(4):794-802.

Chande N, McDonald JW, MacDonald JK. Interventions for treating collagenous colitis. *Cochrane Database Syst Rev*. 2003;(1):CD003575.

Chapter
77 *Acute Colonic Pseudo-Obstruction (Ogilvie's Syndrome)* ▬▬▬▬▬

Ogilvie's syndrome refers to acute colonic distention, predominantly right-sided, without any evidence of overt obstruction. The entire colon and rectum may be involved.

EPIDEMIOLOGY

Risk factors include the male sex and elderly patients.

PATHOGENESIS

Most cases are related to severe underlying medical or surgical conditions like severe trauma, infection, cardiac disease, electrolyte imbalance, and use of medications that slow down gastrointestinal motility. The exact pathophysiologic mechanism remains to be established. Metabolic disturbances and medications are usually not the underlying cause but exacerbating factors. An underlying autonomic nervous system (ANS) dysfunction is suspected.

CLINICAL FEATURES

Patients complain of abdominal pain, nausea, vomiting, and abdominal distention. Although most patients are constipated, a few may suffer from a paradoxical diarrhea. There may be lack of passage of flatus. Respiratory distress may occur because of distention of the abdomen caused by massive dilation of colon

Physical exam reveals tympanitic abdomen. Contrary to intuition, bowel sounds may be present. Peritoneal signs are absent in most cases; their presence suggests impending perforation.

DIAGNOSIS

A CBC may show leukocytosis; however, this is due to an underlying condition or in patients with impending perforation. A metabolic profile may show electrolyte abnormalities. Abdominal x-ray shows a dilated colon, predominantly right-sided, but the dilatation may occasionally extend all the way to the rectum. Haustral markings are maintained. Diagnosis can be confirmed by a water-soluble contrast enema or a colonoscopy.

DIFFERENTIAL DIAGNOSIS

Acute mechanical obstruction and acute toxic megacolon must be excluded. Lack of left-sided colonic gas, as well as air-fluid levels in the small intestine, can be seen in both mechanical obstruction and Ogilvie's syndrome.

A water-soluble contrast enema can differentiate mechanical obstruction from pseudo-obstruction and may even be therapeutic in some cases like volvulus.

Patients with toxic megacolon appear acutely sick with fever, tachycardia, and have peritoneal signs on physical exam, along with leukocytosis. Thumb-printing may be seen on abdominal x-rays. Endoscopic evaluation shows evidence of acute colitis. Urgent surgical consultation should be obtained.

TREATMENT

General Measures

These include supportive care including maintaining fluid and electrolyte balance and the correction of any underlying of factors that may contribute to pseudo-obstruction (eg, electrolyte abnormalities, medications, possible infection, and congestive heart failure). A nasogastric tube should be inserted and attached to intermittent suction. A rectal tube should be attached with drainage to gravity. Optimum body positioning measures include knee/chest position with hips held high alternating with right and left decubitus position for 15 to 30 minutes each.

Medical Therapy

Neostigmine (1.0 to 2.0 mg IV) produces rapid colonic decompression within a few minutes. A few patients may need a second dose which may be repeated in about 2 hours. Because of the risk for symptomatic bradycardia, patients should stay supine for 60 minutes and monitored preferably on a cardiac bed. Bedside atropine should be available. Neostigmine should be used cautiously in patients who have bradyarrhythmia or those receiving beta-blockers.

Erythromycin 250.0 mg IV q 8 hours for 3 days has been used successfully. However, there are no controlled trials. Cisapride has been used with success but is not available in the United States.

Close clinical and radiological follow-up with abdominal x-rays every 12 to 24 hours should be performed. Medical management should be continued for up to 48 hours in the absence of severe pain or rapid cecal dilation exceeding 12.0 cm.

Colonic Decompression

Although colonic decompression is frequently used, its role in management remains controversial since many cases with a cecal diameter ranging from 9.0 to 18.0 cm have been reported to resolve without decompression within 48 hours. Risks versus benefits should be carefully weighed since colonoscopic decompression for Ogilvie's syndrome carries a mortality rate of 1%. Water enemas may be performed with a rectal tube prior to colonoscopy, although they are rarely effective.

It is not the absolute colonic diameter, but the rate of dilation, that is more important when considering colonoscopic decompression. In acute cases, consider colonoscopic decompression if colonic diameter exceeds 11.0 to 13.0 cm and there is failure of supportive and pharmacological intervention or signs of clinical deterioration.

It is not necessary to examine the entire colon. Advancement of the colonoscope and tube placement in the distal transverse colon may be sufficient. A placement of decompression tube at the time of colonoscopic decompression is frequently recommended although controlled data are lacking. Recurrence following colonoscopic decompression occurs in 40% of the cases.

Surgery

Surgery is indicated in patients who fail medical management or who develop signs of impending perforation or frank perforation. A cecostomy or right hemicolectomy may be performed in patients with no evidence of bowel perforation. Percutaneous cecostomy is also an option. In patients with perforation, a total colectomy with ileostomy and a Hartmann procedure are performed.

PEARLS

O Bowel sounds are present in many of the cases with acute colonic pseudo-obstruction.

O It is not the actual diameter of the colon but the rate at which colonic dilation occurs that is an important consideration for endoscopic decompression.

BIBLIOGRAPHY

De Giorgio R, Barbara G, Stanghellini V, et al. Review article: the pharmacological treatment of acute colonic pseudo-obstruction. *Aliment Pharmacol Thera.* 2001;15(11):1717-27.

Saunders MD, Kimmey MB. Colonic pseudo-obstruction: the dilated colon in the ICU. *Semin Gastrointest Dis.* 2003;14(1):20-7.

Chapter 78
Diverticular Disease of the Colon

Diverticulosis implies presence of diverticuli, while diverticulitis indicates inflammation/infection of the diverticulum due to a micro- or macroperforation. Although diverticula may occur anywhere in GI tract, colonic diverticulosis is the most common.

EPIDEMIOLOGY

Diverticulosis is primarily a disease of the West with prevalence rates as high as 45%, whereas in Africa and Asia the prevalence is less than 2%. In addition, the diverticulosis tends to be predominantly left-sided in the West, while it is right-sided in Asia and Africa. It is uncommon before the age of 40. By the age of 80, as many as 60 to 80% of Americans have it. It effects both sexes equally.

Risk factors include low dietary fiber intake, obesity, and lack of physical exercise. An association with smoking, alcohol, or caffeine has not been clearly established. There may be a correlation with colon cancer; however, a cause and effect relationship has not been established.

PATHOGENESIS

Colonic diverticulum is a false diverticulum because it is comprised of mucosa and submucosa herniating through the muscle layer and covered by serosa. Most patients have left-sided diverticulosis with a predominance in the sigmoid colon, whereas 35% of patients have diverticuli distributed proximal to the sigmoid colon. Less than 5% of patients have diverticulosis exclusively proximal to the sigmoid colon. Most colonic diverticulosis is asymptomatic.

PAINFUL DIVERTICULAR DISEASE

The existence of painful diverticular disease as a pathologic entity is controversial. Patients complain of intermittent abdominal pain, irregular defecation, and passage of pellet-like stools with occasional diarrhea. Such patients may have coexisting IBS. Antibiotics are not helpful. Antispasmodic agents along with a high fiber diet, plenty of fluids, and exercise are recommended. Some of these patients eventually have an episode of acute diverticulitis.

DIVERTICULITIS

Pathogenesis

Diverticulitis is caused by a micro- or macroperforation of the diverticulum with spillage of fecal contents. It is caused by an increased intralumenal pressure and/or inspissated food particles. Most cases are mild because perforation is quickly walled off.

Clinical Features

Patients complain of left lower quadrant pain since right-sided diverticulitis is extremely rare, except amongst Asians and Africans. In most cases, pain has been smoldering for several days. There is associated nausea, vomiting, constipation, diarrhea, or urinary symptoms like dysuria, urgency, and frequency. Diverticular bleeding is uncommon in the presence of diverticulitis.

Physical exam reveals abdominal distention, and left lower quadrant tenderness with possible tender palpable mass. Right-sided diverticulitis may be confused with acute appendicitis. Patients frequently have low-grade temperature. Presence of peritoneal signs is an ominous sign.

Extra-GI associations include arthritis, pyoderma gangrenosum, leg pain/cramps, and renal disease.

Diagnosis

A CBC shows leukocytosis in majority of the cases. The rest of the routine labs including hepatic and pancreatic enzymes are normal. A urine analysis will be normal or may show sterile pyuria because of adjacent inflammation. The diagnosis is usually made on clinical grounds.

Abdominal x-rays may help exclude an intestinal obstruction or perforation. Further testing is only needed if the diagnosis is in doubt or if patients do not respond to empiric therapy. The diagnostic accuracy of a CT scan is between 95 and 100%. A CT scan can also help exclude the presence of obstruction, fistula, peritonitis, or abscesses.

Although used in the past for diagnosis, a barium enema is relatively contraindicated in acute diverticulitis. If needed, a water-soluble contrast enema may be performed in atypical cases. Similarly, colonoscopy is contraindicated especially in acute severe diverticulitis and should only be undertaken in atypical cases if colonoscopic findings may affect management. The role of compression ultrasonography is evolving.

Differential Diagnosis

It includes acute appendicitis, Crohn's disease, endometriosis, pelvic inflammatory disease, ischemic colitis, and peptic ulcer disease.

Complications

These include obstruction that is rarely complete; perforation and abscess, which occurs in 20% of the cases without diffuse peritonitis; and fistulae (colovescicular or colovaginal). Jaundice and hepatic abscess may occur.

Treatment

ANTIBIOTICS

Young healthy patients with mild symptoms may be treated as outpatients with ciprofloxacin 500.0 mg PO bid plus metronidazole 500.0 mg PO tid for 10 days. Hospitalized patients may be treated with single agents like piperacillin-tazobactam (Zosyn), ampicillin-sulbactam (Unasyn), or ticarcillin-clavulanate (Timentin). Combination therapy using metronidazole or clindamycin combined with a third generation cephalosporin or quinolone is equally effective. Patients with right-sided diverticulitis can be treated medically if the diagnosis can be made preoperatively.

GENERAL MEASURES

Patients should be closely monitored. Bowel rest and antibiotics are effective in uncomplicated cases. Most patients start improving within 2 to 3 days. Outpatients should receive clear liquids for 2 to 3 days until clinical response is evident and then diet can be advanced slowly. Hospitalized patients should be made NPO, along with intravenous fluid administration. Meperidine is superior to morphine for pain relief.

FAILURE OF THERAPY

Risk factors for failure of medical therapy include immune-suppressed patients including those with history of diabetes, renal failure, and collagen vascular disorders, as well as those undergoing chemotherapy or taking corticosteroids.

Clinical deterioration or lack of improvement suggests an abscess. Options include percutaneous drainage under CT guidance or laparotomy. Worsening of clinical situation with increasing pain and peritonitis prompts surgical intervention.

POSTHEALING MANAGEMENT

The role of dietary therapy after resolution is controversial. Most physicians recommend a high fiber diet. Avoiding particular foods like seeds, corn, and nuts is controversial.

A full evaluation of the colon about 4 to 8 weeks after resolution should be undertaken to rule out the possibility of colon cancer, which may occur in up to 5 to 10% of the cases.

ROLE OF SURGERY

Recurrence occurs in about 30 to 40% of the cases and elective surgery and should be considered after the second episode. The role and timing of surgery in young patients remains controversial. Surgery is recommended after the first attack of complicated diverticulitis and after the second attack in most cases. The role of laparoscopic surgery is evolving. Many experts recommend surgery in young patients after the first attack of uncomplicated diverticulitis.

DIVERTICULAR BLEEDING

Epidemiology

Diverticular bleeding occurs in about 5% of the patients with diverticulosis and is usually seen in elderly subjects with comorbid conditions. Diverticular bleeding is the cause of about half the patients admitted for severe lower GI bleed.

Pathogenesis

Bleeding occurs due to injury to the artery supplying the diverticulum. Because of the herniation of the sac, the artery is covered only with mucosa and a localized injury predisposes it to rupture into the lumen. A minor or occult bleed is unusual and presence of occult blood in stool should not be ascribed to diverticulosis.

Clinical Features

Bleeding is painless, massive, and usually requires blood transfusions. There may be nausea, weakness, dizziness, and palpitations. Abdominal pain is absent except for abdominal cramps related to the cathartic effect of the blood trying to expel the colonic contents.

Physical examination reflects hypovolumia, dehydration, and anemia. Abdominal exam is unremarkable.

Management

GENERAL MANAGEMENT

This includes initial resuscitation, localization of the source of bleeding, and appropriate treatment. Hematochezia may be due to an upper GI source in about 5 to 10% of the cases, and as such, nasogastric aspirate should be done to exclude an upper GI source.

LOCALIZING THE SOURCE OF BLEEDING

The most commonly-used modality to localize the source of lower GI hemorrhage is colonoscopy. Although colonoscopy in an unprepared colon may be performed, it is better to cleanse the colon via 1 gallon of polyethylene glycol (GoLytely, CoLyte) given over 2 hours through a nasogastric tube along with metoclopramide 10.0 to 20.0 mg IV or erythromycin 250.0 mg IV to expedite the gastrointestinal transit and hasten bowel cleansing. While a colonoscopy can be potentially therapeutic, it is uncommon to visualize an actually bleeding diverticulum at the time of colonoscopy. The appropriate timing of colonoscopy (ie, urgent versus emergent) is also a matter of debate among gastroenterologists.

ROLE OF ARTERIOGRAPHY AND RADIONUCLIDE SCAN

Colonoscopy may be difficult in patients with active and severe bleeding. Arteriography is recommended in such cases. It requires greater than 0.5 to 1.0 mL/minute bleeding rate and should only be performed if active and ongoing bleeding is present.

Radionuclide bleeding scan may be performed in patients in whom bleeding site can not be localized by colonoscopy and if the bleeding is suspected to be slow or intermittent. It may help to localize the general region of bleeding, as well as to document whether the bleeding is active so that arteriography may be performed, thereby decreasing the frequency of negative arteriograms.

METHODS TO CONTROL BLEEDING

Endoscopic treatment for bleeding diverticulum includes injection of epinephrine in four quadrants along with endoscopic tamponade and cautery of the active bleeding diverticulum. The nonbleeding diverticular vessel may be treated with cautery at 10 to 15 watts of power with moderate pressure. Angiographic treatment of diverticular bleeding includes intra-arterial vasopressin. If vasopressin fails, embolization of the bleeding vessel should be undertaken.

ROLE OF SURGERY

Elective surgery is recommended after two or more transfusion requiring episodes of bleeding or if the source of bleed has not been identified. Unless an actual bleeding diverticulum has been identified by colonoscopy or arteriography, it is usually a good idea to perform an upper endoscopy to definitely exclude a upper gastrointestinal source prior to undertaking the surgery. A notation of "clear NG aspirate" in the chart should not preclude a preoperative upper endoscopy.

Prognosis

A recurrence of bleeding occurs in 20 to 30% of the patients after the first episode, which rises to 50% after the second episode of bleeding.

SEGMENTAL COLITIS

Patients with left-sided diverticulosis may develop segmental colitis mimicking IBD. Whether this is a true entity related with diverticulosis, or an atypical form of IBD, remains controversial. Patients complain of abdominal pain, diarrhea, hematochezia, and even weight loss. Etiology may be ischemic. Histology may or may not mimic IBD, but patients may be empirically treated with immune-modulators. Surgery may rarely be required.

PEARLS

○ Diverticular bleeding is uncommon during an acute episode of acute diverticulitis.

○ Occult GI bleeding should not be attributed to diverticulosis.

○ Colonoscopy is relatively contraindicated in the presence of acute diverticulitis, especially acute severe diverticulitis.

BIBLIOGRAPHY

Stollman NH, Raskin JB. Diagnosis and management of diverticular disease of the colon in adults. *Am J Gastroenterol.* 1999;94 P 3110-3121.

Chapter
79   *Colorectal Polyps* ▬▬▬▬

POLYPS

Colon polyps are of various types based on histology. Only adenomatous polyps have malignant potential, whereas hyperplastic, inflammatory, and juvenile polyps or hamartomas do not increase the risk. Most adenomas are tubular (about 80%), whereas less than 5% are villous. Approximately 15 to 20% have mixed tubulovillous histology.

CANCER RISK

1. About 95% of colorectal cancer (CRC) arises in adenomas. Adenoma transforms into cancer usually in about 7 to 10 years.

2. Polyps greater than 1.0 cm in size or with villous or tubulovillous histology especially if multiple, increase the risk by about 4 to 6 fold.

3. Other features of the polyps that confer increased risk include high-grade dysplasia or multiple (three or more) polyps.

4. Initial data suggested that adenomas greater than 2.0 cm in size may have greater than 50% risk for CRC, but that does not appear to be the case.

5. Tubular adenomas less than 1.0 cm in size, especially if single, do not increase the risk.

6. Management strategies for benign tubular adenoma are detailed in Chapter 81.

7. Patients with familial adenomatous polyposis have markedly increased risk for CRC (see Chapter 81).

PREVENTION OF POLYPS

Patients with initial or recurrent colorectal adenomas should consume diet low in fat and high in fruit, vegetables, and fiber; maintain normal body weight; avoid smoking and excessive alcohol use; and take dietary supplementation of 2.0 to 3.0 g/day of calcium carbonate. Data on the beneficial role of NSAIDs, including COX-2 inhibitors, folic acid, and selenium supplementation, is evolving.

MANAGEMENT OF MALIGNANT POLYPS

1. Malignant polyps with favorable features or histology may be managed endoscopically. Polyps with high-grade dysplasia require no further therapy if endoscopic resection margins are free of cancer.

2. Polypectomy is adequate for invasive carcinoma in a pedunculated polyp if the stalk and polypectomy margins are not involved, there is no lymphatic or venous invasion and there are no features of poorly differentiated carcinoma. Surgery should be undertaken if the histology shows poor differentiation, evidence of lymphatic or venous invasion, invasion into the submucosa, invasive carcinoma or involvement of the stalk, or incomplete polypectomy.

3. Patients with malignant polyp with favorable features should undergo repeat colonoscopy in 3 months with follow-up surveillance colonoscopy at standard intervals for nonmalignant adenomas, once a negative colonoscopy has been accomplished.

MANAGEMENT OF BENIGN POLYPS

1. Management of adenomas is described in Chapter 81.

2. Hyperplastic polyps are the most common, and do not increase the risk for concurrent adenomas. They rarely undergo malignant transformation. It should be followed up as any normal colonoscopy unless they are numerous (>20) and large.

3. Mucosal polyps are usually small with no clinical significance.

4. Inflammatory pseudopolyps are usually seen in the IBD scattered throughout the colon. These are not dysplastic and do not increase the risk for cancer.

5. Submucosal polyps may occur due to lipoma, leiomyoma, pneumatosis cystoides intestinalis, hemangioma, fibroma, and carcinoid.

6. Juvenile polyps increase the risk for bleeding; however, they do not transform into cancer. Familial juvenile polyposis on the other hand does increase the risk for CRC when synchronous adenomas or mixed histology polyps are present.

7. Peutz-Jeghers syndrome is associated with increased risk for GI and extra-GI cancers. The GI cancers predominantly occur in the small intestine followed by stomach, colon, and pancreas. Extra-GI cancers occur in lungs, breast, uterus, ovary, and testes.

PEARLS

○ Over 95% of the colon cancers arise from pre-existing adenomas.

○ Decision for surgical or endoscopic management of a malignant polyp depends upon the histologic features and the presence of cancer-free margins.

BIBLIOGRAPHY

Winawer S, Fletcher SR, Rex D, et al. Clinical guidelines and rationale—update based on new evidence. *Gastroenterology.* 2003;124:544.

Grady WM. Genetic testing for high-risk colon cancer patients. *Gastroenterology.* 2000;124(6):1574-94.

Chapter
80 Colorectal Cancer

CRC is primarily a disease of Western society. Over 98% of the CRC are adenocarcinomas. Metastatic lesions in colon from other cancer sites including breast, ovaries, prostate, lungs, and stomach may occur. CRC generally refers to adenocarinomas unless otherwise specified.

EPIDEMIOLOGY

Almost 150 000 new cases of colon cancer and 79 000 cases of rectal cancer are diagnosed in the United States each year. It is the second leading cause of cancer-related mortality in the United States. The prognosis in the United States has been improving over the last two decades, perhaps because of increased screening and better treatments. The overall 5-year survival is 61% in the United States, compared to about 30% in the China.

Over 95% of the CRC occurs beyond age 40. Age-adjusted incidence, as well as mortality, is higher among men. The lifetime incidence for a patient with average risk is 5%. African Americans have the highest incidence for CRC in the United States, as well as the highest mortality.

PATHOGENESIS

Although there is a markedly increased risk because of genetic influences, most CRC is sporadic rather than familial. About 95% arise as polyps and then go on to form cancer. This follows a normal mucosa to adenoma to adenocarcinoma sequence. Adenoma transforms into cancer in about 7 to 10 years.

A mutation of the APC gene, which is also known as gate keeper gene, is seen in about 85% of CRC. Familial adenomatous polyposis (FAP) is associated with a germline mutation in the APC gene that resides on chromosome 5q21-22. Several hundred mutations of the APC gene have been identified. The DNA mismatch repair genes are called "caretaker" genes and include hMSH2, hMLH1, hPMS1, hPMS2, and hMSH6. The caretaker gene mutations are seen in about 10 to 20% of sporadic CRC and are associated with microsatellite instability and hereditary nonpolyposis colon cancer (HNPCC). K-ras gene mutation is present in over 50% of large adenomas and carcinomas. The p53 gene mutations are involved in the latter processes of carcinogenesis in about 70 to 80% of the CRC.

RISK FACTORS

1. Patients with gate-keeper gene and caretaker gene mutations have markedly increased risk for CRC.

2. A personal history of large polyps or CRC, as well as a family history, confers increased risk.

3. Involvement of first-degree relative (ie, parent, sibling, or child) increases the risk 1.7-fold. The risk is further increased if two first-degree relatives have colon cancer or the index case is diagnosed below the age of 55.

4. Polyps greater than 1.0 cm in size or with villous or tubulovillous histology, especially if multiple, increase the risk by about 4- to 6-fold. Tubular adenomas less than 1.0 cm in size do not increase risk—especially if there is only one present.

5. The coexistence of diabetes mellitus increases the risk by 1.5-fold, especially amongst women. Increased insulin due to hyperinsulinemia, as well as elevated insulin-like growth factor concentrations, perhaps stimulate colonic tumor cells.

6. Prior cholecystectomy may result in a modestly increased risk of right-sided CRC.

7. Other risk factors include cigarette smoking, ureterocolic anastomoses after bladder surgery, prior pelvic irradiation, and acromegaly. The impact of BRCA1 gene mutations remains unclear.

PREVENTATIVE FACTORS

These include a high fruit, vegetable, and fiber diet; a low fat or low cholesterol diet; folic acid supplementation; high calcium intake; and regular physical activity. Drugs like aspirin, sulindac, COX-2 inhibitors, and HMG-CoA reductase inhibitors also offer protection, but their role in management remains to be established. The role of hormone replacement therapy in pathogenesis of CRC is controversial.

CLINICAL MANIFESTATIONS OF COLORECTAL CANCER

The predominant symptoms include abdominal pain, change in bowel habit, and hematochezia or melena. Weakness, anemia, and weight loss are only seen in a minority of cases. Alteration in bowel habit reflects a left-sided lesion. Similarly hematochezia occurs due to rectal rather than colon cancer.

Patients with advanced disease may have right upper quadrant pain, abdominal distention, early satiety, and umbilical metastasis. Unusual presentations include perforation and fistula to bladder or small intestine, fever of unknown origin with intra-abdominal abscess, and Streptococcus bovis bacteremia.

METASTASIS

About 20% of the cases have distant metastasis at the time of diagnosis. The spread occurs by local, transperitoneal, lymphatic, and hematogenous routes. The most likely sites include lymph nodes, liver, and lungs. CRC accounts for about 6% of adenocarcinoma of unknown origin.

SYNCHRONOUS AND METACHRONOUS CANCER

Synchronous cancers at another site in the colon occur in about 5% of the cases. Metachronous CRC occurs in 1 to 3%.

DIAGNOSIS

Diagnosis is made upon symptomatic presentation or on screening through endoscopic evaluation and confirmation by histology. Most appear as mass-like lesions upon colonoscopy.

A small fraction of CRC arises de novo without prior adenoma. These cancers appear as small reddish slightly elevated flat or with central depression lesions.

STAGING

Staging is done on clinical grounds. Dukes' classification is being increasingly replaced by TNM pathological classification.

Duke's Classification

Dukes' Stage A lesion implies a mucosal lesion above muscularis propria without involvement of lymph nodes. Stage B-1 suggests involvement of muscularis propria but not into serosa or pericolic or perirectal tissues and without involvement of lymph nodes. Stage B-2, on the other hand, involves serosa and pericolic or perirectal tissues without any involvement of lymph nodes. Stage C-1 is the same as Stage B-1 but with lymph node involvement. While Stage C-2 is the same as B-2 with lymph node involvement, Dukes' Stage D suggests distant metastasis.

Tumor-Node-Metastasis Classification

Tumor-node-metastasis (TNM) classification is based on the primary tumor, regional lymph nodes, and the presence or absence of distant metastasis. Stage T*is* suggests carcinoma in situ or intramucosal carcinoma, while T1 implies invasion into the submucosa. Stage T2 suggests invasion of muscularis propria, whereas in T3 the tumor has invaded through the muscularis propria into the subserosa or into nonperitonealized pericolic or perirectal tissues. T4 is assigned when the tumor invades other adjacent organs and/or perforates visceral peritoneum.

For regional lymph nodes, N0 is assigned when there is no evidence of regional metastasis, N1 if one to three regional lymph nodes are involved, and N2 if metastasis involves four or more regional lymph nodes. M0 implies absence of distant metastasis and M1 is just the opposite.

The cancer can thus be grouped based on above classification. Stage 0 is T*is*, N0M0, Stage 1 is T1 or 2, N0M0, Stage 2A is T3, N0M0, Stage 2B is T4, N0M0. Similarly Stage 3A implies any T, N1M0, whereas 3B is any T with N2M0. Stage 4 implies M1 or distant metastasis.

Staging Strategy

Preoperative staging is done by physical examination, as well as a CT scan of the chest and abdomen. Liver enzymes may be normal in spite of hepatic metastasis. The use of MRI is not routinely recommended. A PET scan may be helpful in patients who are thought to be candidates for resection of isolated colorectal cancer metastasis to liver, as well as for localizing site of disease recurrence in patients with elevated carcinoembryonic antigen (CEA) levels.

Endoscopic ultrasound is helpful in staging of rectal cancer. Intraoperative evaluation may also be undertaken as part of staging process. The use of tumor marker CEA is not recommended for diagnosis but does have prognostic utility in patients with newly diagnosed CRC, as well as for postoperative follow up. Persistently elevated CEA levels that do not normalize following surgical resection suggest presence of persistent disease.

TREATMENT OF COLON CANCER

Surgery is the only known cure. Resection of the colonic tumor with adequate tumor-free margins, as well as regional lymphadenectomy, is usually undertaken. Malignant polyps can be managed endoscopically in many cases (see Chapter 79). Patients with resectable primary colonic tumor and limited distant metastasis may undergo resection of metastasis as part of resection of primary tumor. This includes isolated liver or pulmonary metastasis.

Palliative surgery is indicated in patients with unresectable primary tumors with evidence of obstruction or uncontrolled hemorrhage. The role of laparoscopic colectomy is evolving.

Surgery is sometimes needed for diagnosis of recurrence of cancer in patients with persistently rising CEA levels, but without evidence of cancer on a CT scan.

Adjuvant Therapy for Colon Cancer

Adjuvant therapy for resected colon cancer is indicated in patients where all visible disease has been resected for Stage 3 colon cancer. Treatment includes 5-FU with leucovorin. Adjuvant therapy for Stage 2 colon cancer is not routinely recommended. Addition of radiation therapy to adjuvant chemotherapy for Stage 3 colon cancer is controversial. Adjuvant infusion therapy directly into the liver is investiga-

tional. The role immunotherapeutic adjuvant therapy using mono-
clonal antibody edrecolomab as part of 5-FU chemotherapy appears
promising. Patients undergoing surgery for limited hepatic metastasis
may benefit from adjuvant chemotherapy.

Chemotherapy for Metastatic Colon Cancer

Systemic chemotherapy is helpful in metastatic rectal and colon
cancer. A combination of 5-FU plus leucovorin and irinotecan is
approved as first line therapy. Patients who are refractory to the above
treatment may undergo salvage therapy with oxaliplatin along with 5-
FU and leucovorin.

TREATMENT OF RECTAL CANCER

Low anterior resection is the treatment of choice for patients with
upper- and midrectal cancers along with postoperative adjuvant radiation and chemotherapy for patients with transmural or node positive
disease.

Local excision is undertaken for early superficial (T1 or T2) distal
rectal cancer, whereas abdominoperineal resection may be needed in
advanced cases or when the anal sphincter is involved. A down-stag-
ing preoperative radiation and chemotherapy may be undertaken
prior to planned resection, which permits a sphincter preserving low-
anterior resection rather than abdominoperineal resection.

SURVEILLANCE AFTER CANCER RESECTION

Recommendations for surveillance are a matter of debate among
different specialty organizations. In general, surgeons and oncologists
tend to recommend more frequent follow-up exams than gastroenterologists. A postresection colonoscopy at 1 to 3 years is recommended. Further surveillance is recommended at 3 to 5 year intervals.
In addition, a CEA level should be examined every 3 months for 2 to
3 years. In case of rectal cancer, flexible sigmoidoscopy should be performed every 3 to 6 months for 3 years.

PROGNOSIS

The 5-year survival rate for Stage 1 colon cancer is 95%, Stage 2 is
75%, Stage 3 is 37 to 66%, and Stage 4 is less than 5%. For rectal cancer
the 5-year survival rate are as follows: Stage 1 (72%), Stage 2 (52%),
Stage 3 (37%), and Stage 4 (4%).

PEARLS

○ Over 95% of colon cancers arise from pre-existing adenomas.

○ Colorectal cancer, if detected in early stages, is curable.

○ The surgical, oncologic, and postresection management is different for colon and rectal cancer.

BIBLIOGRAPHY

Wiggers T. Surgery for rectal cancer. *Scand J Surg.* 2003;92(1):53-6.

Rao S, Cunningham D. Adjuvant therapy for colon cancer in the new millennium. *Scand J Surg.* 2003;92(1):57-64.

Grady WM. Genetic testing for high-risk colon cancer patients. *Gastroenterology.* 2003;124(6):1574-94.

Chapter 81 *Familial Polyposis/Cancer Syndromes*

HEREDITARY NONPOLYPOSIS COLORECTAL CANCER (LYNCH SYNDROME)

Epidemiology

HNPCC is associated with about 3 to 5% of all CRCs.

Clinical Features

In contrast to sporadic colon cancer, HNPCC occurs much earlier and predominantly involves the right colon. The mean age at initial diagnosis is 40 to 50 with 70% of initial cancers occurring proximal to the splenic flexure. As many as 5 to 18% of the patients may have synchronous or metachronous cancers.

Extracolonic Malignancies

There is a high risk of extracolonic cancers especially endometrial cancer, which occurs in 40% of females. Other sites include ovary, stomach, small intestine, hepatobiliary system, and urinary system.

The HNPCC patients who also develop benign or malignant sebaceous gland tumors are called *Muir-Torre syndrome*.

Turcot's syndrome is the development of glioblastoma in association with HNPCC. Turcot's syndrome may also involve central nervous tumors in association with FAP.

Pathogenesis

HNPCCs usually arise from pre-existing colorectal adenomas that are few in number and hence the label "nonpolyposis." However, they have increased malignant potential compared to sporadic adenomas. HNPCCs tend to have better prognosis than the sporadic colon cancer.

Diagnosis

The diagnosis is based on Amsterdam I and II criteria and Bethesda guidelines. Amsterdam I criteria involves a rule of 3, 2, 1 (ie, at least three relatives with CRC, one of whom must be first degree relative of the other two, involvement of two or more generations with at least one case diagnosed before the age of 50, and FAP has been excluded). Amsterdam criteria II modification includes extracolonic cancers (stomach, small intestine, hepatobiliary tract, endometrium, ovaries, renal pelvis, ureters, and skin) that can be substituted for colorectal cancer as part of three cancers required by initial criteria.

Bethesda guidelines suggest that screening for HNPCC should be considered in patients meeting any of the following criteria:

1. Subject meeting the Amsterdam criteria.
2. Subject with two HNPCC-related cancers (stomach, small intestine, hepatobiliary tract, endometrium, ovaries, renal pelvis, ureters, and skin), including a synchronous or metachronous CRC.
3. A patient with CRC who has a first-degree relative with colorectal or HNPCC-related cancer or colorectal adenoma, with one of the cancers diagnosed before 45 years of age and the adenoma diagnosed before 40 years of age.
4. A patient with CRC or endometrial cancer diagnosed at an age below 45.
5. Patient with right-sided CRC with undifferentiated pattern before the age of 45.
6. Patients with signet-ring cell-type CRC diagnosed before the age of 45.
7. Patient with adenoma diagnosed before age 40 years.

Modified Bethesda criteria advocated by the American Gastroenterological Association (AGA) changes the age of adenocarcinoma diagnosis from less than 45 to less than 50 years.

Genetic Testing

It involves DNA sequencing of hMSH2 and hMLH1 for germline disease causing mutations, as well as microsatellite instability (MSI) testing upon the tumor tissue. Commercial testing is available and sensitivity varies from of 50 to 95%.

Interpreting the Results of Genetic Testing

Screening for HNPCC in family members reduces the death rate significantly. The presence of the gene mutation in an affected member allows precise genetic testing of family members. Analysis for MSI in tumor or adenoma tissue should be used as the screening test in patients suspected of having HNPCC. Only the patients with MSI high in the tumor should undergo specific testing for mutations of hMSH2 and hMLH1; patients with MSI-low or MSI-stable are unlikely to test positive for these mutations.

MSI testing may be skipped and germline mutation testing undertaken directly in families in which tumor tissue is not available and in families or individuals who meet any of the first three of the modified Bethesda criteria. Patients harboring disease causing mutations in one of the HNPCC genes are at 70 to 90% risk for developing colorectal cancer.

Management of Genetic Diagnosis of HNPCC

Patients with a genetic diagnosis of HNPCC should undergo colonoscopy every 1 to 2 years starting between the ages of 20 to 25 or ten years earlier than the index case. An annual colonoscopy should be performed after the age of 40.

Although the efficacy for screening for other cancers remains to be established, experts recommend that patients with HNPCC diagnosis should also undergo annual screening for extracolonic cancers, including annual screening for endometrial (pelvic examination and endometrial aspirate with or without transvaginal ultrasound) beginning at age 25 years. Some experts also perform 1) annual urinalysis and cytologic examination for renal tumors beginning at age 25; 2) annual transvaginal ultrasound and serum CA-125 for ovarian cancer; and 3) annual skin surveillance.

Periodic upper endoscopy is generally recommended only in patients with a family history of gastric cancer. Screening for gastric cancer in patients without a family history of gastric cancer is controversial.

FAMILIAL ADENOMATOUS POLYPOSIS

FAP is an autosomal dominant disorder. It is responsible for less than 1% of colon cancer in the United States.

Extracolonic Malignancies

Extracolonic malignancies sometimes seen with FAP include ampullary carcinoma, thyroid cancer, hepatoblastoma, gastric carcinoma, and cental nervous system (CNS) tumors. Adenomas may also be seen in the gallbladder and small intestine.

Turcot's syndrome is FAP-associated with brain tumors whereas Gardner's syndrome implies additional benign extraintestinal tumors like osteoma, lipoma, and desmoid tumor.

Pathogenesis

It is caused by germline mutations in the APC gene located on chromosome 5q21. Attenuated form of APC may be seen.

Polyps develop in the second or third decade of life in most cases, with an average age of 16. Nearly 100% of the patients with FAP develop colon cancer by the age of 45. Patients with FAP have hundreds of colorectal adenomas, whereas patients with attenuated FAP have variable number of adenomas (with an average of 30 polyps) and occur approximately 10 years later than FAP.

Indications for Genetic Testing

1. Patients with FAP should be tested to identify a detectable mutation. Presence of a particular mutation in the relatives makes a diagnosis. If no mutation is identified, testing of relatives at risk is inconclusive.

2. Patients with greater than 20 adenomas suspected of FAP or attenuated FAP.

3. First-degree relatives of patients with attenuated FAP.

Colonic Screening Based on Genotyping

At-risk relatives who test positive for APC mutation, should undergo a flexible sigmoidoscopy every year starting at the age of 10 to 12 until the age of 35 if the exams are negative. Sigmoidoscopy is adequate although some people prefer colonoscopy. In at-risk relatives of patients who are negative for APC gene mutation, sigmoidoscopy is undertaken starting at age 25.

In case genotyping is not available, the at-risk relatives should undergo sigmoidoscopy every year starting at age 12, then every 2 years after the age of 25, every 3 years starting at the age 35, and then continue testing as one would with average risk after the age of 50.

Upper Gastrointestinal Screening

Upper endoscopy using front and/or side-viewing scopes for gastroduodenal polyps is recommended initially for those in their late teens or early 20s, and then again every 3 years. Duodenal adenomas should be sampled and removed if possible. Biopsies should be obtained from ampulla even if it appears normal endoscopically. If no adenoma is detected, repeat exam should be undertaken in three years. On the other hand, if a periampullary adenoma is found, surveillance endoscopy and biopsy should be performed every 1 to 3 years.

Patients with high-grade dysplasia in the ampullary region should undergo surgery or more frequent surveillance. On the other hand, a low-grade dysplasia should be followed by more frequent surveillance (eg, EGDs every 6 months for 1 year and then every 12 months). Patients with ampullary carcinoma should have surgical consultation.

Fundic gland polyps do not increase risk for cancer, whereas gastric adenoma have low but definite risk.

Screening Recommendations

Regular surveillance of retained rectum every 6 months in patients with subtotal colectomy, or every 1 to 2 years in case of ileoanal pouch anastomosis, is recommended. Some experts recommend surveillance of terminal ileum, although no guidelines have been established

Additional recommendations include careful palpation of thyroid annually and abdominal palpation with serum alpha-fetoprotein every 6 months for detection of hepatoblastoma until the age of 7 years.

Treatment

Once polyposis is found in patients with FAP, a colectomy is recommended after the initial diagnosis if polyps are multiple, large, or with villous histology and/or high-grade dysplasia. Patients with few small polyps in the second decade of life may be followed endoscopically with the surgery timed according to school schedule. Patients with FAP should undergo total proctocolectomy with ileoanal anastomosis, whereas a subtotal colectomy with ongoing surveillance is adequate in patients with attenuated FAP who have little rectal involvement.

Medical Treatment

Although sulindac causes a regression of colorectal adenomas, it is incomplete and should not replace colectomy as treatment of choice. COX-2 inhibitors may also be effective.

PEUTZ-JEGHERS SYNDROME

Peutz-Jeghers syndrome (PJS) is a rare autosomal dominant disorder characterized by hyperpigmented spots on lips and buccal mucosa plus multiple gastrointestinal hamartomas. These polyps occur most commonly in the small intestine but may also occur in the colon and stomach. A locus for this disorder has been mapped to chromosome 19p.

Clinical Features

In addition to hyperpigmented spots, the manifestations include intestinal obstruction, bleeding, and recurrent bouts of small bowel intussusception.

Risk for Malignancy

There is a 15-fold increased risk for GI, as well as non-GI cancers. Potential sites of malignancy include stomach, small intestine, colon, pancreas, breast, ovaries, uterus, and the lung. The GI cancers occur due to adenomatous transformation within the hamartomas.

Surveillance of Patients

Patients should undergo EGD every 2 to 3 years with a biopsy of all polyps in a search for adenoma and a complete excision of polyps greater than 1.0 cm. In addition, colonoscopy should be undertaken every 3 years with biopsy of all polyps and complete excision of polyps greater than 1.0 cm.

Patients should also undergo small bowel series beginning at the age of 10 years. Surgery should be undertaken for symptomatic small bowel polyps or those greater than 1.5 cm in size.

Other recommendations include 1) an annual history and physician exam with routine tests; and 2) an annual gynecologic exam starting with abdominal and pelvic ultrasound, as well as biannual Papanicolaou smear starting at the age of 25. Some experts recommend gynecologic surveillance starting in adolescence.

In addition, breast surveillance in women should be undertaken beginning at age 25 years in women with mammography beginning at age 35. Some experts suggest starting baseline mammography at 25 and then yearly after the age of 40.

Patient self-examination of breast and testicles should be part of surveillance program.

Screening of Relatives

Genetic testing is now available and involves detection of mutations in a gene encoding serine threonine kinase (LKB1 or STK11).

However, mutations are seen in only 50 to 60% of families with PJS, suggesting that other genetic abnormalities are involved.

First-degree relatives should undergo an EGD and enteroscopy, or upper GI series and small bowel series at least once during the second decade of life.

FAMILIAL JUVENILE POLYPOSIS

Familial juvenile polyposis is an autosomal dominant disorder characterized by 10 or more juvenile polyps in the colon. Gene mutations on multiple chromosomes have been identified. Clinical features include rectal bleeding, anemia, abdominal pain, intestinal obstruction, and rectal prolapse. Adenomatous transformation may occur within the hamartomas leading to an increased risk for CRC.

Screening of Relatives

At-risk family members should undergo a fecal occult blood testing plus sigmoidoscopy or colonoscopy starting at the age of 12 to 15 and repeated every 1 to 5 years between the ages of 30 to 40, and thereafter the interval may be extended. Colonoscopy should be performed anytime lower gastrointestinal symptoms occur.

Patients with a finding of solitary juvenile polyp and no family history of CRC have the same risk of cancer as general population. Patients with multiple juvenile polyps, (ie, more than five) are candidates for surveillance.

Surveillance of Patients

There are no clearly defined recommendations for surveillance. Documented cases should undergo surveillance (colonoscopy every 1 to 3 years) until the age of 70 years. Prophylactic surgery should be considered for:

1. Patients with large number of polyps.
2. Those with multiple polyps with adenomatous change and high-grade dysplasia.
3. In cases polyps cannot be removed endoscopically.
4. Persistent bleeding.
5. In patients with family history of CRC.

In addition, an EGD with small bowel biopsy or an upper GI series and small bowel follow-through should be undertaken every 1 to 2 years after the age of 25.

PEARLS

○ Females with the HNPCC gene also have a high-risk for endometrial and ovarian cancer. Screening for HNPCC family members reduces death rate significantly.

○ Although sulindac causes a regression of colorectal adenomas in FAP, it is incomplete and should not replace colectomy as the treatment.

BIBLIOGRAPHY

Winawer S, Fletcher R, Rex D, et al. Clinical guidelines and rationale—update based on new evidence. *Gastroenterology*. 2003;124:544.

Grady WM. Genetic testing for high-risk colon cancer patients. *Gastroenterology*. 2003;124(6):1574-94.

Boardman LA. Heritable colorectal cancer syndromes: recognition and preventive management. *Gastroenterol Clin North Am*. 2002;31(4): 1107-31.

McGarrity TJ, Kulin HE, Zaino RJ. Peutz-Jeghers syndrome. *Am J Gastroenterol*. 2000;95(3):596-604.

Chapter

82 *Colorectal Cancer Screening* ▬

SCREENING OPTIONS

Fecal Occult Blood Test

Fecal occult blood testing reduces CRC mortality by 20 to 30%. In addition to reducing mortality, it also reduces the incidence of CRC. However, it can not detect polyps that are not bleeding and leads to many false positive results. Two samples from three consecutive stools should be examined without hydration. Dietary restrictions do not reduce the positivity rate while at the same time reduce compliance, as such may not be necessary.

Sigmoidoscopy

Sigmoidoscopy reduces incidence and mortality of colorectal cancer within the reach of a simoidoscope by about 60%. Patients with a tubular adenoma seen on flexible sigmoidoscopy, unless it is diminutive and single, should undergo full colonoscopy.

FOBT Plus Sigmoidoscopy

The combination of FOBT plus sigmoidoscopy has been studied with mixed results and appears to impart only a marginal benefit.

Barium Enema

A double contrast barium enema can detect about half of the polyps greater than 1.0 cm, which must then be followed by colonoscopic evaluation and excision. The effectiveness of this modality for prevention of CRC mortality has not been studied.

Colonoscopy

Colonoscopy results in the reduction of incidence of colorectal cancer by 70 to 90%. Colonoscopy is not perfect and can miss about 25% of diminutive polyps, 13% of adenomas polyps from 6.0 to 9.0 mm, and 6% of large adenomas or even cancers. It is offered as one of the screening options by nongastroenterological specialties, although gastroenterologists consider this as the screening test of choice.

Virtual Colonoscopy

The results of studies regarding its effectiveness vary. It probably is not cost-effective since patients with any suspicious lesions on virtual colonoscopy would then need the full colonoscopic evaluation.

Stool Tests for Genetic Mutations

The commercially available test (PreGen Plus) looks for 23 molecular markers and includes 21-point mutations in APC, K-ras, p53 genes; one microsatellite instability marker, BAT-26; as well as a DNA integrity assay. However, the exact role of this test in the screening strategies remains to be established.

SCREENING STRATEGIES

The optimal screening strategy has not been determined although most gastroenterologists prefer colonoscopy. Discussion between the physician and patient should include the evidence of effectiveness of various modalities and the effect on outcome, safety, convenience, and cost, as well as cost per saved year of life.

AVERAGE RISK PATIENTS

A cafeteria approach needs to be applied. Patients should undergo screening at or after the age of 50. Unless colonoscopy has been undertaken, a positive test on any other test should prompt evaluation of the entire colon by colonoscopy. In case of negative results on any of the strategies chosen, annual FOBT plus flexible sigmoidoscopy every 5 years, DCBE every 5 years, or a colonoscopy every 10 years is recommended.

All polyps on sigmoidoscopy should be biopsied, and if histology shows adenoma, a colonoscopy should be performed. A colonoscopy for a single tubular adenoma less than 5.0 mm in size is controversial.

The use of virtual colonoscopy is controversial and its exact role in the screening strategy needs to be determined.

Medicare reimburses for annual fecal occult blood tests, flexible sigmoidoscopy every 4 years, and colonoscopy every 10 years for average patients. Medicare also pays for colonoscopy every 2 years for high-risk patients. Barium enema may be reimbursable if an attending physician provides a written certification.

MODERATE TO HIGH RISK PATIENTS

This involves initiating the screening at an early age as well as performing more exams frequently, preferably with procedures that visualize the entire colon.

Positive Family History

1. In patients with a first-degree relative diagnosed with adenoma or CRC after the age of 60, screening should begin at age 40, and performed at the same interval as average-risk persons.
2. In case a first-degree relative was diagnosed before the age of 60 or more than one first-degree relatives have CRC, the screening should be by colonoscopy beginning at age 40 or 10 years before the index case and repeated every 3 to 5 years.
3. Patients with one second-degree relative or third-degree relative with adenoma or CRC should be screened as average-risk subjects.

Familial Polyposis/Cancer Syndromes

Please see Chapter 81 for details.

Inflammatory Bowel Disease

Chronic IBD is a risk factor; the degree of risk depends upon the extent and duration of the disease. While there is no increased risk to patients with proctitis or proctosigmoiditis, left-sided colitis increases the risk by 3-fold where as extensive or pancolitis increases the risk by 5- to 15-fold. Some studies suggest the risk of left-sided colitis and extensive/pancolitis is similar. The incidence of CRC is 0.5% in subjects with UC of 10 to 20 years duration and increasing to 1% per year thereafter. The coexistence of UC with PSC further potentiates the risk.

Patients with pancolitis have as high as a 30% risk for CRC. Those with Crohn's colitis probably have a similar risk for CRC as UC. Colonoscopy is recommended every 1 to 3 years starting at age 7 or 8 with the occurrence of left-sided colitis and pancolitis. Some experts start screening in patients with left-sided colitis at 12 to 15 years of the disease. The evidence for effectiveness of these strategies in IBD remains to be established.

SURVEILLANCE

Surveillance in patients with polyps should be undertaken based on the risks.

1. The American College of Gastroenterology (ACG) and the AGA recommend that patients with one or two adenomas less than 1.0 cm in size each should have a repeat colonoscopy in 5 years. The American College of Surgeons (ACS) recommends a follow-up colonoscopy at 3 to 6 years in patients with a single adenoma less than 1.0 cm in size.

2. According to ACG/AGA, patients with greater than a 1.0 cm polyp or multiple adenomas (3 or more) or high-grade dysplasia or villous elements should have follow-up colonoscopy in 3 years. After one negative 3-year surveillance colonoscopy, subsequent colonoscopy may be undertaken at 5-year intervals. ACS recommends that patients with more than one adenoma, high-grade dysplasia or villous elements should have two follow-up colonoscopies at 3-year intervals.

3. Patients with numerous adenomas may have follow-up colonoscopy at 1 year.

4. Patients with large sessile adenoma (>2.0 cm) should be re-endoscoped in 2 to 6 months after piecemeal removal. Persistence of residual adenomatous tissue for two to three therapeutic colonoscopies should prompt surgical consultation.

5. Hyperplastic polyps, mucosal polyps, inflammatory polyps and juvenile polyps (except juvenile polyposis syndrome, Peutz-Jeghers syndrome) do not increase the risk for cancer and should be followed as average risk patients.

6. Patients with personal history of colorectal cancer should undergo colonoscopy at the time of diagnosis. If a full colonoscopy is not possible prior to surgery, an examination

should be undertaken thereafter. Recommendations for further surveillance are a matter of ongoing debate between different professional organizations. A repeat colonoscopy should be undertaken initially at 1 to 3 years and then every 3 to 5 years. A routine CT scan for follow-up of colon cancer is not recommended. Please see Chapter 80 for details.

SECONDARY PREVENTION OF POLYPS

Patients with initial or recurrent colorectal adenomas should consume a diet low in fat and high in fruit, vegetables, and fiber; maintain normal body weight; avoid smoking and excessive alcohol use; and take dietary supplementation of 2.0 to 3.0 g of calcium carbonate. The role of NSAIDs, folic acid, selenium, and aspirin supplementation is evolving.

PEARLS

○ Over 95% of colon cancers arise from pre-existing adenomas.

○ Colonoscopy for CRC screening is effective and reduces incidence of CRC by as much as 90%. However, there is a lack of data on the effectiveness of barium enema for screening for CRC. Results of studies on effectiveness of virtual colonoscopy are conflicting.

○ Different professional organizations have published different guidelines for screening and surveillance.

BIBLIOGRAPHY

Winawer S, Fletcher R, Rex D, et al. Clinical guidelines and rationale—update based on new evidence. *Gastroenterology*. 2003;124:544.

Grady WM. Genetic testing for high-risk colon cancer patients. *Gastroenterology*. 2003;124(6):1574-94.

Chapter

83 *Anorectal Disorders*

Anorectal disorders are one of the most common causes for self-medication by patients. Because of lack of knowledge, patients tend to attribute almost all their symptoms to hemorrhoids.

COMMON COMPLAINTS

Common symptoms that occur include pain, bleeding, rectal protrusion, fecal incontinence, perianal itching, and altered bowel habit. Pain can vary from sharp, dull, or burning to constant, and may be associated with bleeding. Bleeding is usually bright red blood on the toilet paper or on the side of the stool and may be associated with pain. A proximal source, such as cancer, cannot be excluded in many patients, and as such, some sort of endoscopic evaluation of the lower colon and rectum should be carried out.

HEMORRHOIDS

Epidemiology

About 5% of the US population seeks medical attention for hemorrhoids.

Anatomical Features

Hemorrhoids are normal vascular cushions arising from hemorrhoidal veins. They are submucosal and are called external or internal depending upon whether they exist below or above the dentate line. While internal hemorrhoids arise from superior hemorrhoidal cushion, the external hemorrhoids rise from inferior hemorrhoidal plexus. Both communicate with each other and often coexist. They do not have direct communication with the portal system and are not more common in portal hypertension. Hemorrhoids aid in normal continence.

Pathogenesis

While most hemorrhoids are asymptomatic, hemorrhoidal disease or "hemorrhoids" occur more commonly in the elderly. Other risk factors include chronic diarrhea, pregnancy, pelvic tumors, chronic constipation, and weight lifting. The factors contributing to hemorrhoidal disease may be multifactorial, including loss of connective tissue anchoring hemorrhoids to the underlying sphincters, increased tone of internal anal sphincters, and swelling of hemorrhoidal cushions.

Clinical Features

Patients have painless bleeding associated with bowel movements, especially bright red blood on the side of the stool or on the toilet paper. Blood may occasionally drip into the toilet. Although blood loss is usually small, it can be alarming, and chronic blood loss can cause iron deficiency anemia. On rare occasions, the bleeding can be severe, especially in patients with coagulopathy. Bleeding associated with a painful defecation suggests the possibility of an anal fissure. Pain may be present in case of thrombosed external hemorrhoids.

Pruritus ani is usually related to other causes such as suboptimal perianal hygiene, but hemorrhoids may contribute to it by permitting leakage of rectal contents, as well as difficulty in cleaning skin tags. Aggressive cleaning especially in cases of diarrhea may also contribute to itching.

Differential Diagnosis

These include anal fissure, condylomata acuminata, rectal prolapse, and Crohn's disease.

Clinical Classification

Internal hemorrhoids may be classified from Grade I through Grade IV. Grade I hemorrhoids may bulge into the lumen but do not extend below the dentate line. Grade II hemorrhoids may prolapse on defecation or straining but reduce spontaneously. Grade III hemorrhoids are associated with prolapse and require patient manipulation to reduce them. Grade IV hemorrhoids are irreducible and prone to strangulate.

Management

Fiber supplementation is effective in reducing acute episodes and should be administered at 20.0 to 30.0 g/day with increased fluid intake. Bulking effect of fiber may prevent perianal irritation by reducing seepage.

Topical analgesic creams, steroid creams, suppositories, and warm sitz baths are effective for pruritus. Use of steroid cream for longer than 1 week at a time should be avoided. Sitz baths should be performed three times a day and help by reducing inflammation and relaxing the internal anal sphincter.

Patients nonresponsive to simple measures are candidates for minimally invasive procedures. These include rubber band ligation, infrared coagulation, bipolar diathermy (Bicap), laser photocoagulation, sclerotherapy, and cryosurgery. The choice of the procedure depends upon local expertise.

Rubber band ligation is one of the best options for Grade I, II, and III disease, but is associated with a high incidence of post-treatment pain if the bands are applied too close to the dentate line.

Surgical therapy is indicated in patients with acute thrombosed hemorrhoids, severe hemorrhage, and hemorrhoids that are refractory to medical treatment. Grade III or Grade IV hemorrhoids frequently require surgery.

Mixed hemorrhoidal disease (ie symptomatic external and internal hemorrhoids) also require surgery, since large external hemorrhoidal tags that are symptomatic can only be effectively treated by excision. Closed hemorrhoidectomy is the most common surgical procedure for internal hemorrhoids. Stapled hemorrhoidectomy is suitable for symptomatic internal hemorrhoids without a significant external hemorrhoidal component. Serious infectious complications have however been reported with this technique.

In patients with concomitant fissure, once the fissure is treated, the constipation should improve and hemorrhoidal symptoms may resolve without surgery. Some surgeons perform lateral internal sphincterotomy for patients with hemorrhoids and concomitant anal fissure.

Thrombosed Hemorrhoids

Thrombosed external hemorrhoids present with excruciating pain and surgical evacuation provides prompt relief. Medical management should be undertaken if the patient presents after 48 hours. This includes oral and topical analgesics, stool softeners, and sitz baths.

External Hemorrhoids

Patients with external hemorrhoids are not candidates for minimally invasive procedures or surgery except for patients with thrombosed external hemorrhoids. Symptomatic external hemorrhoidal tags that interfere with hygiene are treated with surgical excision. These frequently recur in women following pregnancy.

ANAL FISSURE

An anal fissure is a tear in the lining of anal mucosa usually in the posterior midline distal to the dentate line.

Pathogenesis

It occurs because of trauma due to large hard stools or in association with IBD, tuberculosis, leukemia, and other conditions. Ischemia may contribute to the chronicity of fissure.

Clinical Features

Patients present with throbbing pain (most frequently occurring during or made worse following defecation), bleeding, seepage, and difficulty with evacuation. There may be perianal itching. A digital rectal exam is painful and should be avoided.

Diagnosis

This is made by inspection of the anal region by separating the buttocks. While acute fissure looks like a fresh tear, chronic fissures have raised edges and are associated with a sentinel tag. The fissure is usually located posteriorly. Consider Crohn's disease and tuberculosis in patients with fissures at other locations.

Treatment

Medical management involves sitz baths, fiber supplements, stool softeners, analgesics, topical nitroglycerin (0.2% ointment bid), as well as botulinum toxin (eg, BOTOX) injection.

Injection of botulinum toxin 20 units on each side of the fissure into the anal sphincter improves healing. Repeated therapy with botulinum toxin may be required because of a short-term response or in those who do not respond to treatment. Botulinum toxin may be superior to topical nitroglycerin and is associated with fewer side effects. Oral calcium channel blockers diltiazem 60.0 mg bid or nifedipine 20.0 mg bid for 8 weeks may be beneficial, but may have associated systemic side effects.

Surgery is undertaken for patients who fail to respond to medical therapy. Complications of surgery include minor fecal incontinence.

ANAL WARTS

Condylomata acuminata or anal genital warts is a sexually transmitted disease caused by the human papilloma virus. Women with multiple sex partners, homosexual men, and individuals infected with HIV are at high-risk.

Clinical Features

Patients may be asymptomatic or present with pruritus, leakage, bleeding, discomfort, and visible or palpable masses in the perianal region. These may interfere with defecation and intercourse.

Diagnosis

Lesions appear as flat, smooth or verrucous, papilliform masses. The extent should be documented by endoscopic evaluation. Anal canal lesions are present in about 40% of the patients. Biopsy should be undertaken if diagnosis is uncertain.

Differential Diagnosis

Differential diagnosis includes internal hemorrhoids, condylomata lata, and squamous cell carcinoma.

Treatment

Options for local chemical treatments include podophyllin, which can only be used externally; trichloroacetic acid for both internal and external lesions, as well as during pregnancy; and intralesional injection of 5FU/epinephrine. All topical treatments are associated with a high recurrence rate. Repeated applications are frequently necessary. Cryotherapy using liquid nitrogen spray may also be performed. Laser therapy is effective but very expensive.

Immune-modulator imiquimod 5% topical cream is effective but can be used only for external lesions. Subcutaneous or intramuscular alpha-interferon injections are effective but have a high rate of side effects, as well as recurrence.

Topical application of cidofovir and BCG is investigational.

Role of Surgery

Surgery is indicated in patients when medical or ablative therapy fails or when lesions are amenable to surgical removal. If there are condylomata in the anal canal or rectum, these must be treated in the operating room since it is too painful do in an awake patient; they need to be excised, cauterized, or otherwise destroyed. Excisional therapies are done under anesthesia.

PEARLS

- Hemorrhoids are not painful except in case of thrombosed hemorrhoids. Look for a fissure in cases where pain is the predominant symptom.
- Itching, although frequently attributed to hemorrhoids, is usually related to suboptimal hygiene.

REFERENCES

Gopal DV. Diseases of the rectum and anus: a clinical approach to common disorders. *Clin Cornerstone.* 2002;4(4):34-48.

Mazier WP. Hemorrhoids, fissures, and pruritus ani. *Surg Clin North Am.* 1994;74(6):1277-92.

Chapter 84 *Miscellaneous Colorectal Disorders*

MELANOISIS COLI

It is a reversible hyperpigmentation of the colon or rectum occurring as a result of prolonged use of anthraquinone containing laxatives or some herbal teas. The use of osmotic or diphenolic laxatives does not lead to this condition. The incidence is rising. Histologically the pigment is seen in the macrophages of lamina propria. It may be a marker for potential development of cathartic colon. Its association with an increased risk for CRC is controversial. There is no treatment.

CATHARTIC COLON

It occurs as a result of chronic constipation and longstanding laxative abuse, leading to a tortuous and redundant colon. Initially, a destruction of the myenteric plexus by anthraquinones was suggested as the cause; however, this concept is controversial. Barium studies may show a loss of haustral folds.

DIVERSION COLITIS

Diversion colitis is characterized by inflammation in colon/rectum due to exclusion from fecal stream after surgery (eg, Hartmann procedure).

Pathogenesis

It occurs due to a deficiency of short-chain fatty acids (SCFA) that are normally produced from bacterial fermentation of dietary carbohydrates. SCFAs feed the colonic cells; in addition, they modulate fluid and electrolyte transport, as well as regulate colonic motility and mucosal circulation.

Clinical Features

Symptoms occur only in minority of patients and include rectal bleeding and mucus discharge, severe diarrhea, or sepsis.

Diagnosis

Histologic and/or endoscopic changes can be documented after fecal exclusion in most cases. Pathology shows an expansion of submucosa and mucosa with an increase in lymphocytes and plasma cells. Crypt abscesses may occur. Differential diagnosis includes antibiotic-induced colitis and chronic idiopathic IBD.

Treatment

Restoration of the colonic continuity with reanastomosis is a definitive cure. In cases where that cannot be accomplished, SCFA enemas should be used. These consist of 60 mL bid of sodium acetate, sodium propionate, and sodium n-butyrate, along with sodium chloride for 4 to 8 weeks. After improvement occurs, the enemas are tapered to a maintenance schedule. Patients with diversion colitis not responding to SCFAs may be tried on 5-ASA enemas or suppositories or rectal administration of sucralfate suspension.

SOLITARY RECTAL ULCER SYNDROME

Solitary rectal ulcer syndrome is a misnomer, since it may not be solitary, it may not be in the rectum, and there may not be frank ulceration.

Epidemiology

It is an uncommon disorder usually associated with constipation especially in the elderly or developmentally challenged subjects.

Pathogenesis

Pathogenesis is not well-understood; it probably relates to chronic straining and internal rectal prolapse leading to trauma associated with ischemic changes.

Clinical Features

Presentation is variable and includes rectal bleeding, rectal pain, incomplete evacuation, mucus, tenesmus, and occasional incontinence.

Diagnosis

Diagnosis is based upon history, clinical and endoscopic findings, as well as characteristic histology. Endoscopic findings may include a frank ulceration usually in the distal rectum. Instead of an ulcer, the lesion may be polypoidal or just an erythematous patch. The ulceration or erythema may be present proximally. Endoscopic ultrasound shows a thickened rectal wall. Defecography, may show internal rectal prolapse. Histology is characteristic.

Differential diagnosis includes IBD, ischemic colitis, NSAID colitis, and endometriosis.

Treatment

Management is conservative with bulk laxatives, bowel retraining, reassurance, and plenty of fluids—unless otherwise restricted. Biofeedback may be helpful in obstructive defecation. Surgery should not be performed in these patients, unless there is full-thickness overt rectal prolapse. Surgery is considered as a last resort only when conservative treatment options have failed and symptoms are disabling. Options include local incision, rectopexy, and fecal diversion.

PEARLS

- ○ Melanosis coli is associated with longstanding laxative abuse. It is reversible and has no pathologic significance.
- ○ Solitary rectal ulcer syndrome may not be solitary, a frank ulcer may not be present, and it may be located at sites in colon proximal to rectum.

BIBLIOGRAPHY

Felt-Bersma RJ, Cuesta MA. Rectal prolapse, rectal intussusception, rectocele, and solitary rectal ulcer syndrome. *Gastroenterol Clin North Am.* 2001;30(1):199-222.

Giardiello FM, Lazenby AJ. The atypical colitides. *Gastroenterol Clin North Am.* 1999;28(2):479-90.

DIAGNOSTIC AND THERAPEUTIC MODALITIES

Chapter

85 *Antibiotic Prophylaxis*

Most antibiotic prophylaxis for endoscopies is done against bacterial endocarditis. Exceptions include prophylaxis in patients with recent synthetic vascular graft, ascites, and for procedures like percutaneous endoscopic gastrostomy and ERCP. Patients with prosthetic joints do not require prophylaxis.

CARDIOVASCULAR PROPHYLAXIS

This is based upon the type of procedure and the underlying cardiovascular condition.

Conditions Requiring Prophylaxis

Moderate to high-risk conditions include prosthetic heart valves, past medical history of endocarditis, congenital cyanotic heart disease, surgically constructed systemic or pulmonary shunts, acquired valvular defects, hypertrophic cardiomyopathy, mitral valve prolapse with regurgitation or valvular thickening, and intracardiac defects that have been surgically repaired within the preceding 6 months. Patients with synthetic vascular graft placed within the preceding 1 year should also receive prophylaxis.

Conditions Not Requiring Prophylaxis

Prophylaxis is probably not indicated for functional murmurs, atrial septal defect, mitral valve prolapse without significant regurgitation or leaflet thickening, mild tricuspid regurgitation, coronary artery disease including coronary artery bypass surgery, intracardiac lesions repaired more than 6 months prior, previous rheumatic fever without valvular defects, and cardiac pacemakers or implanted defibrillators.

Procedural Indications

Among patients at risk for infection as outlined above, prophylaxis is recommended for esophageal variceal sclerotherapy, esophageal dilation, and possibly polypectomy. Prophylaxis is not indicated for diagnostic endoscopy with or without biopsy.

Specific Recommendations

Patients undergoing upper endoscopic evaluation may be given amoxicillin 2.0 g orally 1 hour before the procedure. No postprocedure doses are required.

For patients undergoing colonoscopy or ERCP, administer ampicillin 2.0 g IV plus gentamicin 1.5 mg/kg up to 120 mg IV 30 minutes before the procedure. In penicillin-allergic patients, vancomycin 1.0 g IV should be administered. A postprocedural dose of ampicillin 1.0 g IV or amoxicillin 1.0 g PO 6 hours after the colonoscopy should be given.

NONCARDIOVASCULAR PROPHYLAXIS

SBP Prophylaxis

Patients with liver cirrhosis undergoing EGD for upper gastrointestinal (GI) bleeding should receive antibiotic prophylaxis. Cultures should be drawn. Start treatment with a third generation cephalosporin. If cultures are negative for 48 hours, switch to PO antibiotic (norfloxacin 400.0 mg PO bid). Many experts give prophylaxis to all patients with ascites prior to EGD.

Suspected Biliary Obstruction

All patients undergoing ERCP with suspected bile duct obstruction or pancreatic pseudocyst receive antibiotic prophylaxis. Options include ampicillin-sulbactam (Unasyn) 3.0 g IV, cefoxitin 1.0 g IV, cefotaxime 1.0 g IV, ciprofloxacin 400.0 mg IV, or a combination of ampicillin plus gentamicin. A follow-up dose of antibiotic after ERCP may not be needed if adequate drainage has been accomplished.

Percutaneous Endoscopic Gastrostomy

Patients undergoing percutaneous endoscopic gastrostomy should receive prophylaxis. Options include cefazolin 1.0 g IV or levofloxacin 500.0 mg IV before the procedure.

PEARLS

- ❍ Antibiotic prophylaxis is not indicated for every immune-compromised patient or for every cardiovascular condition prior to endoscopy.
- ❍ Antibiotic prophylaxis is indicated for percutaneous endoscopic gastrostomy, EGD for patients with liver cirrhosis and GI hemorrhage, and ERCP with suspected obstruction or pseudocyst.

BIBLIOGRAPHY

Dajani AS, Taubert KA, Wilson W, et al. Prevention of bacterial endocarditis. Recommendations by the American Heart Association. *JAMA*. 1997;277(22):1794-801.

Soares-Weiser K, Brezis M, Tur-Kaspa R, Leibovici L. Antibiotic prophylaxis for cirrhotic patients with gastrointestinal bleeding. *Cochrane Database Syst Rev*. 2002;(2):CD002907.

Chapter

86 *Esophagogastroduodenoscopy* ▮

Esophagogastroduodenoscopy (EGD) visualizes the esophagus, stomach, and proximal duodenum distal to the ampulla of Vater. It is a diagnostic as well as therapeutic procedure.

PREPARATION

Except in times of emergency, it is usually done after 5 to 6 hours of fasting. Most patients receive a local anesthetic spray and conscious sedation. Nonsedated EGD is being increasingly performed across the world. Patients do not need to stop aspirin or NSAIDs prior to procedure.

INDICATIONS

These include unexplained dyspepsia associated with alarm symptoms of weight loss or bleeding, dyspepsia refractory to treatment, upper GI bleeding, dysphagia or odynophagia, caustic ingestion, foreign body in esophagus or stomach (including meat impaction in esophagus), esophageal variceal sclerotherapy, or banding. Esophageal stents can be performed for palliation of esophageal cancer. Nasoenteric as well as gastrostomy feeding tubes can be placed. Endoscopic methods for treatment of gastroesophageal reflux disease (GERD) (eg, Endocinch, Stretta and Enteryx) have been approved by the United States Food and Drug Administration (FDA).

CONTRAINDICATIONS

These include hemodynamic instability, suspected perforation of esophagus, and combative patient. Issue of instability is a relative one since a heavily bleeding patient may be somewhat compromised hemodynamically, but may need endoscopy to stop the bleeding in order to improve the hemodynamic status. Diagnostic EGD with biopsies can be done in presence of coagulopathy within therapeutic range.

SPECIAL SITUATIONS

While controlled studies are lacking, recent myocardial infarction is considered a relative contraindication. Patients without arrhythmia or hemodynamic instability at the time of procedure tolerate the procedure well. Similarly, risk and benefits should be carefully weighed in cases of pregnant patients.

COMPLICATIONS

Complications relating to conscious sedation and intubation may account for as many as half of the complications related to endoscopy. These include bradycardia, hypotension, vasovagal reaction, respiratory depression, shock, and myocardial infarction. Oxygen desaturation occurs in as many as two-thirds of the patients undergoing endoscopy; severe desaturation is uncommon.

Although transient bacteremia is common, the risk for infectious complications in average risk patients is low; the risk of endocarditis is estimated to be 1 in 10 million. Difficult intubation may lead to retropharyngeal and retroesophageal abscess. Loss of teeth may occur if there is a presence of periodontal disease or loose teeth.

Risk for perforation is low for diagnostic endoscopy (0.03%); however, mortality due to perforation may be as high as 25%. Bleeding is rare and may occur in patients with significant thrombocytopenia and/or coagulopathy. A diagnostic EGD can be performed with a platelet count as low as 20 000/mm^3. In patients with leukemia or other conditions with dysfunctional platelets, a threshold of 30- to 50 000/mm^3 should be used. However, if biopsies or dilation needs to be performed, platelet transfusions should be administered. Mallory-Weiss tears occur in 1 in 1000 cases, but are usually not clinically significant.

The risk for perforation due to mercury filled dilators (Maloney) is 0.4%. The risk may be decreased by using wire-guided or through-the-scope (TTS) balloon dilators. Dilatation can cause pain, bleeding, and bacteremia. Caustic strictures and complex tortuous strictures are at high risk for perforation. Pneumatic dilation of achalasia has a perforation rate of about 5%. Perforation rate due to dilation of malignant strictures may be as high as 10%.

PEARLS

- ○ Coagulopathy in therapeutic range is not a contraindication to diagnostic EGD.
- ○ Risk for infectious complications is low.

BIBLIOGRAPHY

Mahmood Z, McMahon B, O'Morain C, Weir DG. Innovations in gastrointestinal endoscopy: endoscopic antireflux therapies for gastroesophageal reflux disease. *Dig Dis*. 2002;20(2):182-90.

Chapter 87 *Colonoscopy*

This endoscopic procedure visualizes the entire colon and in some cases the ileocecal valve is also intubated to examine the terminal ileum.

INDICATIONS

Colonoscopy is indicated for screening for colorectal cancer (CRC), surveillance for colon polyps and CRC, infectious gastroenteritis, chronic infections of the GI tract (tuberculosis), functional diarrhea, inflammatory bowel disease (IBD), angiodysplasia of intestine, blood in stool, iron deficiency anemia, acute colonic ischemia, radiation enteritis, toxic gastroenteritis, intestinal obstruction, megacolon, and foreign body in colon or rectum.

CONTRAINDICATIONS

Contraindications include perforated viscus, severe colitis, severe diverticulitis, and unstable patient.

PREPARATION

A number of cleansing regimens are used depending upon the physician preference and the population characteristics.

Polyethylene Glycol

Polyethylene Glycol (PEG) is perhaps the most common single laxative used for purgation. Flavored preparations are available. The drug is available as a powder in a jug, and is prepared as a 1-gallon solution. The solution passes through the gut without being absorbed, without damaging the colonic mucosa, and with minimal fluid shifts in the gut lumen.

The disadvantage is that a patient must take PEG in a large volume, which makes most people nauseous. Metoclopramide or prochlorperazine (Compazine) 10.0 mg PO or IM may overcome this problem. Chilling the solution before drinking and sucking on lemon slices, as well as slowing the rate of consumption, can help. Use of a nasogastric tube for administration helps in some hospitalized patients.

Polyethylene glycol is contraindicated in patients with ileus, severe gastroparesis, mechanical bowel obstruction, and dysphagia.

Sodium Phosphate

Oral fleet phospho-soda (sodium phosphate) is another common laxative preparation. The aqueous solution is available as flavored as well as unflavored form. It is given in two split doses of 1.5 oz (with three 8 oz glasses of water over 30 minutes with each dose) the day before the colonoscopy, separated by several hours prior to the exam. Another option is an evening dose the day before and then on morning of the colonoscopy.

Sodium phosphate tablets are also available. Three tablets are taken seven times every 15 minutes with 8 oz of clear liquids the night before the procedure. Twenty tablets are administered the next day in a similar fashion beginning 3 to 5 hours before the procedure.

Phosphate tablets/solution are better tolerated than PEG solution but may produce colonic damage mimicking Crohn's disease. They can also cause massive fluid and electrolyte shifts and have potential for increased phosphate and sodium absorption. Sodium phosphate laxatives should be used in caution with patients with cardiac failure, renal insufficiency, as well as ascites.

Combination Laxatives

While all of the above preparations work in the majority of the cases, the response rate is variable depending upon the patient population. As such, physicians may add additional laxatives to one of the above regimens. The most commonly used combination is perhaps PEG solution combined with magnesium citrate 1 to 2 bottles (10 oz each) given 24 to 48 hours prior to the colonoscopy. Patients in whom magnesium citrate cannot be undertaken because of renal insufficiency, may benefit from addition of one or two doses of bisacodyl 20.0 mg each (Dulcolax 5.0 mg tablets) given about 12 to 48 hours prior to colonoscopy.

Commercial Kits

Fleet bowel preparation kits are available. These include a combination of various cathartics like sodium phosphate, castor oil, laxative tablets like bisacodyl, along with a suppository and/or enema.

Adjunctive Measures

In addition to cleansing, and depending upon bowel habit of the patient, a clear liquid diet of 16 to 72 hours prior to the colonoscopy may be undertaken. Clear liquid nutritional supplements (BoostBreeze and Resource Fruit Beverage) are now available which can be taken during the period of "clear liquid diet" and can improve compliance.

Iron or iron containing preparations should be withheld for a week prior to procedure. Coumadin should be withheld for 4 to 5 days prior to endoscopy. In case patients must remain anticoagulated, intravenous heparin or subcutaneous enoxaparin (Lovenox) may be administered in the meantime.

There is no need to stop aspirin or other NSAIDs. Patients arrive in the endoscopy suite after fasting for about 6 hours. However, essential oral medications may be taken with a sip of water during this fasting period.

PEARLS

- ○ There is no need to stop aspirin or NSAIDs prior to colonoscopy.
- ○ Colonoscopy is contraindicated in the presence of acute severe diverticulitis.
- ○ Colonic evacuation regimen needs to be individualized to the patient's clinical characteristics.

BIBLIOGRAPHY

Waye JD. Colonoscopy "my way": preparation, anticoagulants, antibiotics, and sedation. *Can J Gastroenterol.* 1999;13(6):473-6.

Chapter
88 Complications of Colonoscopy ■

Overall complication rate varies from 3 to 4 per 1000 colono-scopies. However, it is higher in patients undergoing polypectomy, which may be as high as 2 to 3%. Complications include bleeding, perforation, myocardial infarction, and cerebrovascular accidents.

FOLLOW-UP BARIUM ENEMA

A same-day barium enema after failed colonoscopy is safe unless the patient has undergone deep biopsies or polypectomy in which case barium enema should be delayed for at least 5 days.

POSTPOLYPECTOMY SYNDROME

Postpolypectomy coagulation syndrome occurs as the result of transmural injury from electrocautery in 0.5 to 1.5% of patients undergoing polypectomy. It manifests as abdominal pain, fever, peritoneal signs, and elevated WBC. Plain x-rays show absence of free air. Treatment includes bowel rest, and a broad spectrum of antibiotics. Surgery is not necessary.

PERFORATION

A CT scan is superior to abdominal x-rays for detection of perforation. Although colonic perforations usually require surgical intervention, surgery may not be needed in selected cases of iatrogenic perforation, silent perforation, or those with localized peritonitis without signs of sepsis that improve with conservative management. However, surgical consultation must always be undertaken in all cases.

Patients with microperforation presenting within a few hours after procedure manifest with localized pain, tenderness but without diffuse peritoneal signs. Such patients may be treated medically with bowel rest and antibiotics.

HEMORRHAGE

Postpolypectomy hemorrhage can usually be controlled with endoscopic measures. Measures to reduce the risk for complications including proper polypectomy technique, use of saline or epinephrine injections at the base of polyps, use of metallic clips and detachable snares to prevent postexcision hemorrhage, and the correction of coagulopathy are founded on expert opinion and not based on results of scientific studies.

UNCOMMON COMPLICATIONS

Complications related to the use of oral cleansing preparations include Mallory-Weiss tear, esophageal perforation, and pulmonary aspiration. Histologic changes on the colonic mucosa including erythema and erosions may occur. Rare complications include splenic rupture, acute appendicitis, intra-abdominal hemorrhage due to tearing of mesenteric blood vessels, bacteremia, retroperitoneal abscess, subcutaneous emphysema, and even death. There is an extremely rare risk for explosion if electrocautery is performed.

PEARLS

○ Colonoscopy is a relatively safe procedure, but serious complications can occur.

○ Most currently used measures to reduce the risk for complications have not been subjected to controlled trials.

BIBLIOGRAPHY

Nelson DB. Procedural success and complications of large-scale screening colonoscopy. *Gastrointest Endosc*. 2002;55(3):307-14

Chapter 89 *Endoscopic Retrograde Cholangiopancreatography* ▬

Endoscopic retrograde cholangiopancreatography (ERCP) is a complex procedure that allows for visualization of the biliary and pancreatic ductal systems. In contrast to routine colonoscopy or upper endoscopy, a side viewing scope is used. With the advent of MRCP as an equivalent diagnostic modality, ERCP is becoming more of a therapeutic procedure.

INDICATIONS

ERCP is indicated in patients with suspected choledocholithiasis, pancreatic or biliary cancer, recurrent pancreatitis, and pancreatic pseudocysts. Its role in cases of suspected sphincter of Oddi dysfunction is controversial.

Preoperative ERCP is not routinely required in patients undergoing cholecystectomy if there is a low probability of stones in the bile duct since intraoperative exploration during laparoscopic cholecystectomy, as well as postoperative ERCP, are safe and effective. Early ERCP and sphincterotomy reduces morbidity and mortality in patients with severe biliary pancreatitis with evidence of obstruction.

PREOPERATIVE PREPARATION

Patients should be NPO after midnight and should undergo a CBC and coagulation studies.

All patients suspected of biliary obstruction should receive preoperative parenteral antibiotics. A commonly-used regimen is ampicillin 2.0 g IV plus gentamicin 1.5 mg/kg IV (up to 120.0 mg) given 30 minutes before the procedure. Vancomycin 1.0 g IV is given instead of ampicillin for patients who are allergic to Penicillin. Other options include ampicillin/sulbactam (Unasyn 3.0 g IV), cefoxitin 1.0 g IV, cefotaxime 1.0 g IV, or ciprofloxacin 500.0 mg IV.

A postprocedural dose of antibiotics is not necessary if adequate drainage has been accomplished.

COMPLICATIONS

Reactions to Contrast Media

Adverse reaction to the contrast media used during the ERCP is rare. In patients with a history of iodine dye allergy, a nonionic/low osmolality contrast medium should be used. In addition, corticosteroids with or without antihistamines are given preoperatively in such cases starting the day before the ERCP; administration of IV steroids starting just before the ERCP is another option.

Complications Related to Routine Endoscopy

Risk for complications is high as compared to routine endoscopy. These include drug reactions, hemodynamic instability, oxygen desaturation, perforation, and hemorrhage.

Complications Unique to ERCP

These include pancreatitis, sepsis, and retroperitoneal duodenal perforation. Retroperitoneal duodenal perforation is best diagnosed by a CT scan and not by plain x-ray. Some experts recommend a routine measurement of pancreatic enzymes prior to procedure and then follow-up after the ERCP although that is controversial. We recommend assessment of pancreatic enzymes only in presence of clinical manifestations suggestive of pancreatitis.

Bleeding may occur due to sphincterotomy. Inadequate use of cautery results in bleeding, whereas excessive use may lead to perforation. Complications are more with a therapeutic ERCP rather than the diagnostic alone. While the risk for pancreatitis is about 5 to 10%, bleeding occurs in about 2 to 3%, and perforation in 0.5%. The overall complication rate is 8 to 15% with a mortality rate of 0.5%.

Risk Factors for Complications of ERCP

The risk for complications increases in cases of problematic cannulation, precut sphincterotomy, combined percutaneous and endoscopic procedure, sphincter of Oddi dysfunction, liver cirrhosis, low case volume at the GI lab, inexperience of the endoscopist, advanced age of the patient, emergency procedures, and Billroth II gastrectomy.

PEARLS

O A CT scan is the test of choice for diagnosis of retroperitoneal duodenal perforation.

O The risk of pancreatitis due to ERCP is about 5 to 10% whereas the overall mortality rate is about 0.5%.

BIBLIOGRAPHY

Shah SK, Mutignani M, Costamagna G. Therapeutic biliary endoscopy. *Endoscopy*. 2002;34(1):43-53.

Cohen S, Bacon BR, Berlin JA, et al. NIH state-of-the-science conference statement: ERCP for diagnosis and therapy, January 14-16, 2002. *Gastrointest Endosc*. 2002;56(6):803-9.

Chapter 90
Endoscopic Ultrasound ▬▬

Endoscopic ultrasound (EUS) combines the endoscopic visualization with the radiological modality of ultrasound to visualize structures adjacent to the GI wall from within the gut lumen. It is usually performed for characterization of lesions already identified by previous endoscopy or imaging studies.

INDICATIONS

It is primarily used for staging of the tumor by assessing the tumor depth, as well as involvement of adjacent lymph nodes and vascular structures for cancer of esophagus, stomach, pancreas, bile duct, and rectum.

Pancreas

Because of its location adjacent to the stomach and duodenum, the pancreas can be visualized in detail and EUS can be used for localizing and characterizing even small lesions including cysts, as well as tumors that may have been missed by other imaging studies. EUS is more accurate for assessing the vascular invasion due to the pancreatic cancer. Endosonographic features suggesting differentiation between benign and malignant lymph nodes have been described; however, only an aspiration/biopsy can make a definitive diagnosis.

EUS is highly sensitive for detection of neuroendocrine tumors compared to CT. EUS-guided aspiration and biopsy can be performed with high sensitivity and specificity without seeding of the transcutaneous tract.

In addition, early changes of chronic pancreatitis can be visualized by EUS as compared to other imaging studies.

Biliary System

EUS is highly accurate for the detection of choledocholithiasis and cholelithiasis. It also assists in staging of cancers of the gallbladder and the bile duct.

Esophagus and Stomach

EUS is useful for staging the cancer of esophagus and is superior to a CT scan for tumor invasion and detection of malignant lymphadenopathy. The involvement of celiac lymph nodes makes the esophageal cancer unresectable.

EUS can differentiate between a cystic or solid structure from a vascular structure like varices. In patients with dysphagia, it is useful in differentiating a narrow lumen due to an intrinsic lesion versus an extrinsic compression like the heart or aorta. Submucosal lesions (ie, leiomyoma or GI stromal tumor can be seen arising from the muscularis propria layer). The gastric wall thickening can be identified especially in lymphoma or MALToma.

Miscellaneous

These include biopsy of mediastinal lymph nodes due to metastasis from either esophageal or nonsmall cell lung cancer, biopsy of paragastric and retroperitoneal lymph nodes, staging for lymphomas, characterization of large gastric folds, evaluation of pelvic and perianal disease (in patient with fecal incontinence to determine whether external and/or internal sphincter muscle are intact), and evaluation of lymphadenopathy of uncertain origin (FNA).

Therapeutic EUS

On the therapeutic front, EUS is useful for directing celiac plexus neurolysis in patients with unresectable pancreatic cancer.

CONTRAINDICATIONS

These include unstable or combative patient, known or suspected perforation, acute diverticulitis, or an obstructed lumen. It should be avoided by inexperienced endoscopist as well as in cases of high grade strictures. Complication rate of EUS is higher than routine upper endoscopy.

PEARLS

○ EUS is superior to CT scan for assessing tumor depth and involvement of lymph nodes and adjacent vascular structures.

○ EUS-guided aspiration and biopsy of suspicious lesions can be performed.

BIBLIOGRAPHY

Fusaroli P, Caletti G. Endoscopic ultrasonography. *Endoscopy*. 2003;35(2): 127-35.

Chapter 91
Percutaneous Endoscopic Gastrostomy and Jejunostomy

About 100 000 gastrostomies are performed each year in the United States. This technique is used to provide GI access for nutrition in patients with dysphagia. Gastrostomies can also be placed surgically as well as by interventional radiology.

METHODS OF ENTERAL ACCESS

Short-term enteral access can be obtained by nasogastric feeding tubes. PEG is used if long-term access is required. In a fashion similar to PEG, the feeding tube can directly be placed into the jejunum. A pre-existing PEG can also be converted (PEGJ), so that the feeding port is in the jejunum.

INDICATIONS

While the use of PEG/percutaneous endoscopic jejunostomy (PEJ) is clearly indicated in patients with dysphagia, its role is controversial in anorexia-cachexia syndrome (eg, AIDS, cancer) or in patients with neurological vegetative state. PEG is undertaken in patients with demonstrated rehabilitation potential or to maintain quality of life in specific cases (eg, obstructive esophageal cancer in case patient is doing well otherwise). It may be reasonable in patients with anorexia and weight loss due to cancer with the understanding that the goal is not necessarily an improvement in the nutritional status. PEG does not improve outcome in patients with dysphagia related to dementia; thus, PEG may only be undertaken with the understanding that it will not improve functional status or survival.

PROCEDURE

Patients require PT/INR and a platelet count before procedure. Patient must be NPO after midnight. Routine preparation is the same as in cases of EGD except that preoperative antibiotic (example cefazolin 1.0 g IV) is administered. After transillumination and finger indentation of the appropriate gastric or jejunostomy site as appropriate, the feeding tube is placed. The feeding can be initiated as early as 6 hours after the procedure.

The role of prophylactic local antibiotics at the time of PEG placement is controversial. Some experts apply topical antibiotics, whereas others simply clean the tube with hydrogen peroxide and dry dressing.

SPECIAL SITUATIONS

Pregnancy

PEG tubes have been in placed safely in pregnant patients as late as 26 weeks of pregnancy.

Ascites

Large tense ascites is a relative contraindication. However, if a patient with ascites needs a PEG, a large volume paracentesis should be carried out before placement and then for the first week after the PEG placement. Antibiotics should be continued for 1 week. The risk vs benefits ratio should be weighed carefully.

OUTCOME AFTER PERCUTANEOUS ENDOSCOPIC GASTROSTOMY

Bear in mind, the mortality at 30 days is about 20 to 30%. This is usually related to the underlying disorder and not due to the procedure itself. The effect on quality of life has not been adequately studied.

COMPLICATIONS OF PERCUTANEOUS ENDOSCOPIC GASTROSTOMY

Depending upon the definition of complication, the incidence of complications varies from 15% to 70%, most of which are minor. Patients at risk for complications include elderly patients with severe comorbid illness or sepsis.

Wound Infection

Patients with wound infection (usually *Staphylococcus*) should be treated with first generation cephalosporin or a fluoroquinolone.

Visceral Perforation

Perforation of the bowel, gallbladder, and a tear of solid organ like liver may occur.

Bowel Obstruction

Dislodged catheter can lead to intestinal obstruction.

Pneumoperitoneum

Pneumoperitoneum without peritoneal signs is of no clinical significance. However, if abdominal pain, tenderness, peritoneal signs, and leukocytosis develop, a perforation should be suspected and surgical consult obtained.

Gastric Ulcers

Gastric ulcers can develop at the site of PEG tube. Loosening of the external bolster such that the internal bolster is removed from the gastric wall is of benefit.

Necrotizing Fasciitis

Necrotizing fasciitis can be prevented by making a skin incision of about 1.0 cm so that the PEG tube is not tight and maintains the external bolster about 1.0 cm from abdominal wall after PEG placement. The treatment includes surgical debridement and antibiotics.

Cologastrocutaneous Fistula

Cologastrocutaneous fistula occurs due to the interposition of the colon between the anterior abdominal wall and the gastric wall. Risk factors include elderly patients or those who have had multiple surgeries. Patients may remain asymptomatic, have transient symptoms, or may develop symptoms months later especially when the PEG tube is removed and another one is replaced at bedside.

Aspiration Pneumonia

Aspiration pneumonia is common as a result of endoscopy. However, there is no advantage of PEG vs PEJ tube for reducing the incidence of aspiration pneumonia. PEJ should be performed in patients with gastroparesis, high gastric residuals, and in those who are refluxing feeding contents into the lungs. The jejunostomy tube can be placed endoscopically or surgically just like gastrostomy tube. PEG can also be converted into PEGJ.

Peristomal Leakage

Risk factors include severe comorbid illnesses, as well as uncontrolled diabetes. Replacing the tube with another tube or a large tube is not helpful. A new PEG tube usually needs to be placed, although a trial of removal of the pre-existing tube for 12 to 24 hours, and then replacing with another tube under radiographic guidance may be undertaken.

Tube Dysfunction

Clogging can be reduced by dissolving as much medications as possible in water. Administration of bulking agents and cholestyramine through the tube should be avoided. Flushing should always be undertaken after medication use. Irrigation with 60 cc warm water is superior to carbonated beverages. The gastrostomy tube can also be cleared with a brush.

Since most clogging is due to proteinaceous precipitates, meat tenderizers have been recommended; however, there is potential for ulceration.

Tube dysfunction due to deterioration of the tube occurs frequently over the long-term. A daily administration of 3 to 5 cc of alcohol through the tube may help reduce the deterioration.

TUBE REPLACEMENT

The endoscopically placed gastrostomy tube can be removed or replaced at the bedside. However, the replacement should be done within 1 to 2 hours of removal. If replacement is delayed, radiographic confirmation should be obtained prior to feeding.

Bedside replacement of the tube should be avoided if it occurs within 2 weeks of the initial PEG tube placement. If it is undertaken, a radiographic confirmation should be obtained before feeding.

Do not replace PEJ without fluoroscopy.

PEARLS

○ There is a 30-day mortality of 20 to 30% after PEG placement and is related to the underlying disorder. Consider this prior to placing PEG as to whether it is justified on the basis of improving quality of life or outcome.

○ If PEG tube is inadvertently removed, it may be replaced at the bedside if done within 1 to 2 hours. Otherwise, it should be done under radiological guidance.

BIBLIOGRAPHY

Nicholson FB, Korman MG, Richardson MA. Percutaneous endoscopic gastrostomy: a review of indications, complications and outcome. *J Gastroenterol Hepatol.* 2000;15(1):21-5.

Minocha A, Rupp TH, Jaggers TL, Rahal PS. Silent Colo-gastrocutaneous fistula as a complication of percutaneous endoscopic gastrostomy. *Am J Gastroenterol.* 1994;89(12):2243-2244.

Chapter
92 *Gastrointestinal Radiology*

PLAIN X-RAY ABDOMEN

Ideally, a posterior/anterior chest x-ray, in combination with supine and upright abdomen views, should be ordered. In patients with limited mobility, an anterior/posterior view of chest, supine abdomen, and left lateral decubitus x-ray series should be undertaken. An upright chest x-ray is essential for excluding pneumoperitoneum. Fluid levels and bowel dilation is seen obstruction. If the air is seen all the way to the rectum, pseudo-obstruction should be suspected. Mechanical obstruction is suggested by dilatation of the bowel only to the point of a transition.

Intestinal gas with or without air fluid levels may be normal. Normal abdominal x-rays do not exclude the possibility of bowel obstruction. Pneumatosis cystoides intestinalis or simply pneumatosis intestinalis may be seen in intestinal ischemia.

Air seen in the hepatic region may represent portal venous gas or pneumobilia. The portal venous gas is seen towards the periphery of the liver whereas pneumobilia is seen towards the hilum and is potentially a less serious condition.

CONTRAST AGENTS IN GASTROENTEROLOGY

Barium is the contrast agent of choice in most studies of the luminal gut. A water-soluble contrast should be used if perforation is suspected but is less sensitive. While aspiration of barium is not a problem in most people, aspiration of water-soluble contrast can result in chemical pneumonitis, pulmonary edema, and even death.

BARIUM SWALLOW

Depending on the institution and local nomenclature, a barium swallow may mean evaluation of oropharyngeal and proximal esophageal region for the swallowing problems or may be used strictly for esophagus. Terms like oropharyngeal esophogram, videoesophogram, dysphagiagram, or modified barium swallow are frequently used for assessment of oropharyngeal or transfer dysphagia.

On the other hand, the usual barium swallow is performed for looking at anatomic defects in the esophagus, as well as part of preoperative evaluation for reflux disease.

Benign stricture may be seen in GERD. Stricture may be malignant. Schatzki's ring is an incidental radiological finding without any clinical significance in most cases, although it does cause dysphagia in a minority of patients.

A bird beak appearance is seen in achalasia. There is marked esophageal dilatation with air-fluid levels and diminished peristalsis throughout the esophagus along with absence of any hiatal hernia. In contrast to achalasia, esophageal dilatation is mild to moderate in scleroderma with diminished peristalsis in lower two-thirds of the esophagus.

Sliding hiatal hernia may be seen in patients with scleroderma because of the gastroesophageal reflux.

SMALL BOWEL SERIES

Small bowel enteroclysis is considered to be superior to "usual" small bowel series, which is, at best, a screening procedure; a "dedicated small bowel study" may be equally effective. Enteroclysis is more cumbersome and expensive with increased patient discomfort and radiological exposure. It is useful for suspected mechanical obstruction, evaluation of obscure GI bleeding, as well as malabsorption.

In a patient with suspected obstruction showing a dilated small bowel but not in the right lower quadrant, a small bowel series may be performed. However, in patients with dilated small bowel (including right lower quadrant involvement), a barium enema using single contrast should be undertaken. In patients without small bowel dilatation, small bowel follow-through may be the test of choice. CT is superior for evaluation of intestinal obstruction, especially when a hernia, strangulation, close loop obstruction, and abnormalities outside the gut are suspected.

BARIUM ENEMA

A double contrast study is useful for evaluation of colon polyps and cancer. A single-contrast enema should be used to evaluate fistula, sinuses tracts, and colonic obstruction. While it was used routinely before the advent of CT, a barium enema should be avoided in patients with acute diverticulitis, acute colitis, or toxic megacolon.

DEFECOGRAPHY

It is used for assessment of anorectal function in patients with functional constipation or fecal incontinence. Barium paste is introduced into the rectum and pictures are taken during attempted and simulated defecation. Lesions identified include rectocele, intussusception, rectal prolapse, enterocele, and excessive pelvic floor descent. The role of defecography in evaluation of anorectal dysfunction is controversial because many of the abnormalities may also be seen in the normal population.

FISTULOGRAPHY

It is performed for a suspected fistula between the skin and the gut. It is superior to a barium study of upper or lower GI tract for assessment of a fistula.

PERCUTANEOUS TRANSHEPATIC CHOLANGIOGRAM

A percutaneous transhepatic cholangiogram (PTC) is usually performed after a failed ERCP procedure for visualization of biliary system, as well as for any biliary drainage as appropriate. Indications include biliary obstruction at or above the level of portahepatis, biliary obstruction following biliary-enteric anastomosis, and bile duct injuries.

MESENTERIC ANGIOGRAPHY

It is performed to localize the source of bleeding, as well as to control it if needed. The patient must be bleeding at the time of the procedure and the bleeding rate should be at least 0.5 to 1 mL/minute. Embolization of the bleeding vessel using coils or gelfoam can be performed.

Pharmacological options to control bleeding include intra-arterial infusion of vasopressin. It is particularly effective for controlling bleeding from superior mesenteric, gastroduodenal, and left gastric arteries. The infusion can be continued for 12 to 24 hours while monitoring the patient for hemodynamic parameters, as well as for any cardiac complications.

TRANSJUGULAR INTRAHEPATIC PORTOSYSTEMIC SHUNT

Transjugular intrahepatic portosystemic shunt (TIPS) is useful as a treatment for variceal bleeding, refractory ascites, hydrothorax, and Budd-Chiari syndrome. It causes a reduction of the portosystemic pressure gradient to 8.0 to 12.0 mmHg by creating a shunt between the portal and the hepatic venous system in the liver. Technical success is achieved in 90% of the cases.

Lowering of pressure gradient causes the gastric and esophageal varices to decompress. If the varices continue to persistently fill at portal angiography despite the shunt, embolization may be performed.

TIPS is contraindicated in patients with right heart failure, polycystic liver disease, systemic infection, portal vein thrombosis and severe hepatic encephalopathy.

In case of recurrence of variceal bleed, shunt can be examined by angiography for possible balloon dilatation or additional stent placement. Shunt patency can be assessed by a color Doppler ultrasound or angiography. Patency of shunt is usually checked 24 hours after placement and then at intervals of every 1 to 6 months depending upon the institution. Routine checks are usually done by Doppler ultrasound and venography may be performed if there is significant interval change. Symptomatic patients directly go on to venography.

There is 5 to 15% mortality rate at 30 days, usually related to the underlying severity of liver disease. The procedure-related mortality is less than 5%. Seventy percent of the shunts remain patent at 1 year and 40% at 2 years. The shunt patency rate after revision, if occluded, is 90% at 2 years.

The most common long-term complication is hepatic encephalopathy, which occurs in about 20 to 30% of the cases. Encephalopathy may be severe enough in some cases to require complete or partial occlusion of the shunt.

ABDOMINAL CT SCAN

It is useful for imaging the solid structures. A single-contrast enhanced CT scan has a sensitivity of about 70%, whereas the sensitivity of triple-phase imaging is 80%. A CT scan with pancreatic protocol should be obtained when the pancreas is the main target of interest. It involves thin section imaging through the pancreas during the arterial, portal, and venous phases of imaging.

CT arterial portography (CTAP) is done by placing a catheter in the superior mesenteric artery for direct contrast injection during CT scanning. This increases the sensitivity for detection of liver lesions to 90%. It is infrequently used these days because of the high sensitivity of newer CT scan machines in detecting subtle liver lesions.

The CT is more sensitive than MRI for the detection of liver metastasis. It is also superior to ultrasound for the assessment of lesions of pancreas including acute and chronic pancreatitis. Normal CT scan does not exclude mild pancreatitis. CT scan detects pancreatic necrosis with the sensitivity of 80%.

A CT scan has a sensitivity of greater than 95% for imaging of a liver abscess which appears as a low density lesion. The lesion may be multilocular.

Finding of increased iron deposition findings can be seen on CT, as well as MRI scan, and a radiographic diagnosis of iron overload can be made. Toxic levels of amiodarone can mimic iron overload on CT scan.

A CT scan is useful in diverticulitis, IBD, ischemic colitis, as well as for staging colonic tumors and the assessment of lymphoma. Thickened appendiceal wall with luminal distension equal to or greater than 6.0 mm suggests acute appendicitis.

ULTRASOUND

Ultrasound is usually ordered for lesions of the liver, as well as biliary and pancreatic systems.

Liver

The sensitivity of ultrasound in detecting metastasis is 60%.

Ultrasound of the liver is normal in hemochromatosis unless there is superimposed liver cirrhosis.

"Hemangioma" is a frequent incidental finding. If hemangioma is detected on ultrasound and it is less than 3.0 cm in an otherwise asymptomatic patient with normal liver chemistries, a repeat ultrasound at 3 months should be performed. However, if the findings are atypical or the patient has abnormal chemistries and the lesion is greater than 2.0 cm in size, a tagged RBC scan should be undertaken. If the findings on the RBC tagged scan are equivocal, an MRI may be undertaken with a CT scan as the last option. If, however, the initial lesion is found on a CT with its classical features, further work-up is optional and may be undertaken with a tagged RBC scan or ultrasound. In case the findings on the CT scan are atypical for hemangioma, a tagged RBC scan or MRI should be undertaken.

Bile Ducts

Normal intrahepatic ducts are 1.0 to 2.0 mm in diameter and are not seen on ultrasound. The common bile duct is 5.0 mm or less usually. Diameter greater than 6.0 to 7.0 mm warrants investigation or explanation. Common bile duct diameter may increase with age, after cholecystectomy, as well as in patients with previously resolved biliary obstruction. In equivocal cases, obstruction may be excluded by intravenous cholecystokinin injection or by radionuclide liver scan (HIDA scan). A dilated bile duct that doesn't decrease in size upon CCK injection indicates a biliary obstruction.

Gallbladder

Thickening of the gallbladder wall greater than 3.0 mm in diameter in a distended gallbladder is abnormal and can occur due to acute cholecystitis, congestive heart failure, hypoalbuminemia, portal hypertension, veno-occlusive disease, hepatitis, AIDS cholangiopathy, PSC, leukemic infiltration, and gallbladder cancer.

Pancreas

Ultrasound is less sensitive than a CT scan for detection of chronic pancreatitis. Dilation of the pancreatic duct is a classical finding of a chronic pancreatitis seen on ultrasound. Pancreas may not be visualized because of the overlying bowel gas.

Appendix

Appendicitis may be diagnosed by a distended, noncompressible appendix with an adjacent fluid collection, and/or a phlegmon or an abscess on ultrasound. A CT scan is superior to ultrasound for diagnosis of acute appendicitis.

TRANSABDOMINAL SONOGRAPHY

In contrast to the usual ultrasound exam, transabdominal sonography (TABS) examines the bowel while disregarding the solid structures. It can assess the thickness of bowel wall, sites and extent of bowel inflammation, location and length of strictures, intra-abdominal abscess, and any postoperative recurrence.

MRI SCAN

This is useful for lesions of solid structures as well as biliary and pancreatic systems. A Gadolinium MRI scan can help assess bowel inflammation and differentiate between active inflammation and fibrotic strictures. The role of MRI in assessing the defecation dynamics is evolving.

MRCP is an alternative way to examine the biliary tract as well as pancreatic duct. It is comparable to ERCP in its diagnostic accuracy, but does not offer therapeutic option. It is superior to ERCP for detection of pseudocysts. Besides being noninvasive, it avoids a radiation exposure.

CHOLESCINTIGRAPHY

It is indicated for the diagnosis of acute cholecystitis, biliary dyskinesia, bile duct obstruction, and biliary leak. The test is commonly called a HIDA scan, and can be undertaken with bilirubin levels as high as 20.0 mg/dl. Failure to opacify gallbladder at one hour suggests acute cholecystitis. Morphine infusion may be undertaken in case of failure of opacification in order to increase the sensitivity. HIDA scan has sensitivity and specificity of 95% for acute cholecystitis. Patients with prolonged fasting as in TPN may have false positive test. In such cases, patient may be given intravenous cholecystokinin 30 minutes before the study.

Findings of common bile duct obstruction on HIDA scan include lack of visualization of small intestine. HIDA scan can also identify bile duct leaks, although the exact location can not be determined.

A significant reduction in gallbladder ejection fraction upon injection of cholecystokinin (CCK) suggests gallbladder dyskinesia. Normal ejection fraction exceeds 35 to 40%. However, most gastroenterology experts believe that the ejection fraction between 20 and 40% represents a gray zone. Patients with ejection fraction less than 20% and typical biliary symptoms and after exclusion of other potential etiologies may be candidates for cholecystectomy.

GASTRIC EMPTYING

It can be performed for both solid and liquid food; however, solid emptying alone is sufficient for practical purposes. A standard radiolabeled solid meal is administered—a liquid meal is used in cases of infants. A 4-hour test is the method of choice. Normal is less than 6% retention at 4 hours, whereas values between 6 to 10% represent a gray zone.

"Rapid" gastric emptying may also cause problems. Preliminary data suggests that less than 37% of the standardized meal remaining at 1 hour may be abnormal.

LIVER-SPLEEN SCAN

It is an anatomic, as well as a functional test. It can detect focal inflammatory, infectious, and neoplastic lesions. However, its use has largely been replaced by ultrasound and CT because of their superiority.

SCHILLING'S TEST

It is indicated for work-up of vitamin B_{12} malabsorption, although modifications can be used to exclude other disorders also. Vitamin B_{12} therapy should not be withheld prior to doing this test. Patient is administered as a pill containing radioactive cyanocobalamine. Two hours later, nonradio-labeled vitamin B_{12} is administered intramuscularly which binds to vitamin B_{12} receptors. Urine is collected over 24 hours. Radioactive cobalamine excretion less than 10% of the oral radioactive dose over 24 hours suggests vitamin B_{12} malabsorption.

Stage II of the test is undertaken in case of an abnormal test; a patient is administered oral Intrinsic Factor (IF) along with a pill containing radioactive vitamin B_{12}. Normalization of radioactive B_{12} excretion at 24 hours on Stage II suggests the diagnosis of pernicious anemia.

If pernicious anemia is not the cause, further stages may be undertaken after administration of a course of antibiotics to correct possible small bowel bacterial overgrowth (SBBO) or with coadministration of pancreatic enzymes to normalize the exocrine pancreatic deficiency.

RADIONUCLIDE BLEEDING SCAN

Tagged RBC scan is usually used. The radionuclide labeled RBCs are injected and scans are obtained at various intervals during the next 24 hours. Tagged RBC scan can detect slow intermittent bleeds as compared to angiography, which requires active brisk bleeding at the time of examination.

RBC scan requires bleeding at the rate of at least of 0.1 mL/minute for a positive result. Results of delayed scans obtained at 12 to 24 hours after injection should be interpreted with caution since there may be pooling of blood from different sites in the GI tract.

OCTREOTIDE SCAN

This allows for accumulation of radionuclide material by binding to the somatostatin receptors in neuroendocrine tumors. It is useful for diagnosis and localization of gastrinoma, glucagonoma, carcinoid, pheochromocytoma, and VIPoma.

RADIONUCLIDE-LABELED WBC SCAN

It is useful for assessing the extent of active inflammation in the colon. It may be undertaken in patients with IBD in cases where colonoscopy has not been complete or not performed. It cannot distinguish IBD from other causes of colitis like *C. difficile* colitis or ischemic colitis.

PEARLS

○ The choice of radiological test depends upon the indication and the question being asked. A discussion with the radiologist about the case helps get the most out of the test.

○ MRCP is similar in accuracy to a diagnostic ERCP but does not offer the therapeutic option.

○ Positive results on delayed images on RBC bleeding scan should be interpreted with caution.

BIBLIOGRAPHY

Fayad LM, Kowalski T, Mitchell DG. MR cholangiopancreatography: evaluation of common pancreatic diseases. *Radiol Clin North Am.* 2003; 41(1):97-114.

MISCELLANEOUS TOPICS

Chapter
93 *AIDS Patients*

EPIDEMIOLOGY

The incidence of opportunistic infections amongst AIDS patients has been declining recently because of the advent of highly effective antiretroviral therapy.

Diagnostic Clues:
1. Opportunistic infections are uncommon if CD4 count is greater than 200/mcL.
2. Multiple infections may occur simultaneously.
3. Side effects of the antiretroviral therapy should be taken into account in the differential diagnosis since many of those medications will cause gastrointestinal (GI) upset, nausea, vomiting, diarrhea, abdominal pain, oral ulcers, pancreatitis, and lactic acidosis.

ORAL MANIFESTATIONS

Oral lesions are present in up to 80% of the patients with HIV. Painful aphthous ulcers may occur and no organism can frequently be identified. Treatment includes local anesthetics, as well as topical dexamethasone. Systemic corticosteroids and thalidomide may be needed. Oral thrush (candidiasis) may be treated with oral nystatin (500 000 units swish and swallow) five times a day.

ESOPHAGEAL MANIFESTATIONS

Esophageal manifestations include dysphagia, odynophagia, and chest pain. Differential diagnosis includes infections (*Candida*,

Cytomegalovirus [CMV], Herpes), gastroesophageal reflux disease (GERD), idiopathic esophageal ulcer, and pill esophagitis. The most common infection is *Candida*, whereas the most common viral infection is *CMV*. Esophageal candidiasis can be asymptomatic.

Candida Esophagitis

About 25% of these patients may have superimposed viral infection. Empiric therapy with fluconazole is recommended for patients with mild symptoms and presence of oral thrush. Standard regimen is 200.0 mg/day for 2 weeks. Many physicians use a loading dose of 200.0 mg followed by 100.0 mg/day for 2 to 4 weeks. The treatment yields a symptomatic response within 3 to 5 days and the medication is then continued in such cases. In case of severe symptoms and/or those not responding to treatment, endoscopy should be performed. Brush cytology for candida is superior to biopsy although endoscopic findings are highly specific.

While mild cases may respond to topical nystatin (500 000 units, swish and swallow five times per day), many experts caution against the use of topical therapy even in mild cases. Ketoconazole is not recommended because of erratic absorption depending upon gastric acidity. Rarely will intravenous amphotericin-B be needed. Primary antifungal prophylaxis is not recommended. Secondary prophylaxis may be undertaken in rare cases of frequent severe recurrences using fluconazole 100.0 to 200.0 mg/day.

Cytomegalovirus Esophagitis

It causes odynophagia. EGD shows ulcers of various sizes and depth and are usually located in the middle to distal third of the esophagus. As many as 15% of the patients may have concomitant *CMV* retinitis. Diagnosis is made upon endoscopy and the biopsies should be taken from the base of the ulcer. Serology and culture studies for *CMV* are not helpful. Ganciclovir or vanganciclovir is the treatment of choice. Foscarnet is used for resistant cases; however, it is expensive. Although primary prophylaxis with ganciclovir has been advocated in patients with CD4 count of less than 50/mcL, it is not routinely recommended because of high cost, toxicity, and lack of effect on survival. Secondary prophylaxis is usually recommended for the rest of life.

Herpes Esophagitis

Herpes simplex esophagitis presents with multiple, small superficial ulcers in the esophagus. The biopsies from the edge of the ulcer provide the best yield for diagnosis. Histopathology of the ulcer shows multinucleated cells, ground glass nuclei and intra-nuclear inclusion bodies. Treatment involves acyclovir. Primary prophylaxis is not recommended. Secondary prophylaxis may be given to patients with frequent and severe recurrences.

Idiopathic Esophageal Ulcer

These may be single or multiple. Diagnostic studies for infectious etiologies are negative. Treatment includes prednisone starting at 40.0 mg/day and tapered over 6 to 8 weeks after resolution of symptoms. Thalidomide is another option.

GASTRIC MANIFESTATIONS

Gastric involvement in AIDS is uncommon. Dyspeptic symptoms are more likely to be related to GERD, peptic ulcer disease, or gastroparesis. Gastric lymphoma presents with anorexia, nausea, vomiting, weight loss, or bleeding. Kaposi sarcoma is usually asymptomatic.

Existence of AIDS gastropathy as a distinct clinical entity consisting of hypochlorhydria with gastric atrophy and antiparietal cell antibodies is controversial. Infection due to *Cryptosporidium, Histoplasma, Herpes zoster*, and *MAI* is rarely seen. Occasionally idiopathic aphthous ulcers are identified.

AIDS DIARRHEA

Etiology

Antiretroviral therapy, especially protease inhibitors, is a frequent cause of diarrhea. Opportunistic infections are seen if CD4 count is less than 100 to 200/mcL. Other infections can also be seen as in any non-AIDS patient.

Small Bowel vs Large Bowel Diarrhea

Diarrhea is common among patients with HIV. Patients with small bowel diarrhea present with large volume, watery stools associated with nausea, vomiting, bloating, abdominal cramps, and weight loss. On the other hand, colonic diarrhea is characterized by small volume stools associated with abdominal pain, urgency, and incontinence. Fecal leukocytes are usually positive.

Investigations

Work-up includes freshly collected stools for fecal leukocytes, ova and parasites; *C. difficile toxin* test; special studies for *Giardia, Cryptosporidia,* and *Microsporidia*; and routine bacterial cultures for *Salmonella, Shigella, Campylobacter*, and *Yersinia*. Blood cultures for enteric pathogens, as well as *MAI*, should be undertaken as needed.

Endoscopic evaluation is indicated if the preliminary work-up is negative, or if the patient is sick and immune-compromised. This includes sigmoidoscopy or colonoscopy (with or without EGD) and a small bowel biopsy, including duodenal aspirate for parasites.

Management Strategy

Patients with mild to moderate symptoms and CD4 count greater than 200/mcL are unlikely to have an opportunistic infection. They can be treated with antidiarrheal medications if a small bowel diarrhea is suspected. Colonoscopy with or without ileoscopy and biopsy should be performed if a colonic source is suspected.

1. Diagnosis of *Cryptosporidium* is made by examining the stool for oocysts or upon small bowel biopsy. Anti-HIV therapy offers best chance for resolution of symptoms.

2. Clinical presentation and diagnosis of *Microsporidia* is similar to *Cryptosporidia*. Some species may be amenable to treatment with albendazole.

3. *Isosopora* is diagnosed by identification of multiple large intracellular forms, mild villous atrophy, and eosinophilia on small bowel biopsy. Stool examination shows large oocysts and Charcot-Leyden crystals. Trimethoprim-sulfamethoxazole is effective although recurrences are common and may require secondary prophylaxis.

4. *Cyclospora* is diagnosed and treated similar to Isosopora and may need secondary prophylaxis.

5. While *Giardia* infection is not more common in HIV-infected patients than in the general population, it is more common among those who practice oral-anal sex. Diagnosis is made via examination of duodenal aspirate and stools for cysts and trophozoites, in addition to stool test for *Giardia* antigen. Treatment with metronidazole is effective. Secondary prophylaxis may be needed.

6. Small bowel infection with *CMV* is uncommon.

7. Diarrhea due to colonic involvement with *Salmonella, Shigella,* or *Campylobacter* occurs frequently in HIV-infected patients. Secondary prophylaxis (ciprofloxacin 500.0 mg bid, or TMP/SMZ DS 1 tablet BID for several months) may be undertaken in a patient with advanced AIDS and a very low CD4 count who has just been treated for primary salmonellosis. Secondary prophylaxis is not used in cases of *Shigella* or *Campylobacter*.

8. Other infections in patients with AIDS include *Yersinia*, *Aeromonas*, *E. coli*, *Vibrio vulnificus*, and *Listeria*. Precautions to avoid exposure to sources of these organisms are important (ie, reptiles, young or sick pets, raw or undercooked eggs, meat, shell fish, unpasteurized diary products and apple cider, poorly washed produce, ready-to-eat cold cuts or hot dogs, etc). Also avoid exposure to human or animal feces, contaminated water, travel to parts of the world with poor sanitary conditions, refrigerated meats spreads, deli foods, and food from street venders. Frequently, empiric treatment using ciprofloxacin or trimethoprim-sulfamethoxazole is prescribed before a particular agent can be identified.

9. *CMV* infection of the colon may be asymptomatic or the patient may present with abdominal pain, nausea, vomiting, diarrhea, bleeding, weight loss, ulceration, and perforation. Diagnosis is made by biopsy. About 20% of the patients may have only right colonic involvement and will be missed upon flexible sigmoidoscopy.

10. Other colonic problems in AIDS patients include *C. difficile*, *MAI*, *Mycobacterium tuberculosis*, *Bartonella*, *Cryptosporidium*, *Entameba histolytica*, *Cryptococcus*, *Pneumocystis*, and *Candida*. The role of nonhistolytica *Entamoeba*, *Blastocystis hominis*, *Adenovirus*, and *Rota* virus in pathogenesis of AIDS-diarrhea is controversial.

11. Uncommon colonic problems may include lymphoma, Kaposi sarcoma, toxic megacolon, pneumatosis cystoides intestinalis, idiopathic ulcers, and intussusception.

12. *Herpes simplex* may lead to anorectal disease. Similarly *CMV*, gonorrhea, syphilis, and anal warts may be seen.

PANCREATIC MANIFESTATIONS

Pancreatitis may occur due to antiretroviral therapy especially didanosine, infections as well as the HIV virus. Hyperamylasemia may be asymptomatic. Lymphoma may also involve pancreatitis.

PEARLS

○ Opportunistic infections are uncommon at a CD count greater than 100 to 200/mcL.

○ Empiric treatment is frequently undertaken in patients with mild symptoms.

BIBLIOGRAPHY

Oldfield EC III. Evaluation of chronic diarrhea in patients with human immunodeficiency virus infection. *Rev Gastroenterol Disord*. 2002; 2(4):176-88.

Chapter 94 *Food Allergies*

Food allergy and food intolerance are two different entities. Food allergy or hypersensitivity implies an IgE-mediated immunologic response to proteins in foods, whereas food intolerance suggests an nonimmunologic, adverse reaction to certain food. Food intolerance may occur as a result of toxins as seen in food poisoning or lactose intolerance.

EPIDEMIOLOGY

Food allergies are more common in children than adults, but can develop in adulthood. Food allergies are most common in children less than 3 years of age and often occur in the presence of other atopic diseases, especially atopic dermatitis and asthma. The prevalence in children is believed to be 4 to 8%. A family history of atopic diseases is common.

About 20% of adults perceive they have food allergies, but the true prevalence is unknown.

Although any food has the potential to cause allergic reactions, a short list of foods accounts for 90% of the significant hypersensitivity reactions. Most hypersensitivity reactions in infants are caused by cow's milk, but allergy to soy proteins also occurs. In case of early introduction of solids into the diet, reactions to eggs and wheat are not uncommon, especially in patients with atopic dermatitis. In children, cow's milk, eggs, peanuts, soy, wheat, tree-nuts (walnuts, hazelnut), fish, and shellfish account for most of the problems. Peanuts, tree-nuts, fish, and shellfish account for most of the food allergy in adults. Fatal allergic reactions to food in children occur predominantly in those with persistent asthma who are known to be peanut allergic and who ingest peanut protein in prepared foods.

CLINICAL FEATURES AND PATHOGENESIS

Food hypersensitivity is not one particular disease but involves numerous immunopathophysiologic mechanisms leading to poorly defined gastrointestinal symptom complexes. True food allergic reactions involve specific-IgE production against various food antigens and manifest with allergic symptoms as seen with other forms of IgE mediated immediate hypersensitivity (anaphylactic) reactions. These include pruritus, urticaria, angioedema, laryngospasm, bronchospasm (asthma), hypotension, acute diarrhea, or shock. These symptoms occur as a result of IgE-mediated release of mediators from mast cells in the skin, GI and respiratory tract, and from basophils in the blood.

On the other hand, non-IgE mediated hypersensitivity reactions are involved in proctitis/proctocolitis, enteropathy, and food-protein-induced enterocolitis, and are likely to be delayed or chronic reactions. Primary cell mediated reactions are instrumental in such reactions.

The *oral allergy syndrome* is characterized by oral itching and edema usually seen in patients with allergy to pollens that share similar protein allergens to the culprit foods. For instance, some ragweed allergic individuals have oral allergy syndrome to cantaloupe, honeydew melon, watermelon, and banana.

Individuals with *food-associated exercise-induced anaphylaxis* only develop symptoms of anaphylaxis after eating certain foods (eg, celery and others in the ragweed family) and then vigorously exercising.

Food allergy can be an etiologic factor in gastroesophageal reflux. It is a cause of eosinophilic esophagitis in infants and eosinophilic gastroenteritis in adults and children.

Other forms of food hypersensitivity are rare, do not appear to be IgE mediated, and are not associated with pruritus or urticaria. These syndromes may result in anemia, chronic diarrhea, or pulmonary hemorrhage.

Accurate identification and strict elimination of the offending allergenic proteins results in resolution of symptoms in all forms of food hypersensitivity.

DIFFERENTIAL DIAGNOSIS

Food hypersensitivity should be part of the differential diagnosis of a variety of disorders when food proteins cause clinical symptoms. These include syndromes of nausea/vomiting and acute or chronic diarrhea. Individuals with eosinophilic gastroenteritis have abnormalities of gastrointestinal motility, eosinophil products (Charcot

Leyden crystals) in their stools, and food specific IgE. Celiac disease and mastocytosis can masquerade as food allergy. The role of food allergy in constipation is not established.

DIAGNOSIS

The diagnosis of food hypersensitivity is suggested by the history of reproducible allergic reactions coincident with, or within hours of ingestion of a particular food/foods. Avoidance of that food and foods of the same family should prevent similar reactions in the future. The standard for the diagnosis of food allergy is a double-blind food challenge. See Figure 94-1.

If avoiding certain food prevents further symptoms, no further evaluation is necessary. If the culprit food is uncertain, diagnostic testing may be useful. CBC, total eosinophil counts, and stool studies may be performed as indicated. When eosinophilic gastroenteropathy is suspected, GI biopsies are necessary to confirm the diagnosis of eosinophilic esophagitis or gastroenteritis.

Studies for malabsorption are rarely undertaken in the evaluation of food allergy. Commercial food allergens (vaccines) used for *in vitro* and *in vivo* testing are not standardized and do not always provide reliable results.

RAST or skin tests with commercial food allergens are particularly useful in the evaluation of patients who experience food related allergic reactions and the causative food is unclear. The presence of food specific IgE also provides support for the diagnosis of allergy to a specific food. However, the presence of food specific IgE does not make the diagnosis of food allergy; many highly allergic individuals have specific IgE, but do not react when the food is ingested. Patients with chronic symptoms not associated with food allergy usually test negative for food specific IgE.

Tests of unproven utility include intradermal skin tests with food, food specific IgG4 antibodies, provocation and neutralization tests, cytotoxicity tests, and applied kinesiology.

Elimination diets are rarely required in the management of food allergy as identification of the culprit food from the history is usually straight forward. However, in some highly atopic individuals with food allergy and IgE to a variety of food proteins, the removal of foods thought to be responsible for symptoms from the diet and observation of the patient for improvement may be a surrogate to the more specific, but more risky, double-blind food challenge.

Carefully performed double-blind food challenges are the standard for the diagnosis of food allergy. Standardized protocols for double-blind food challenges exist. History and skin-testing determine the

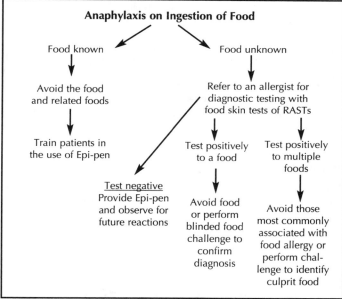

Anaphylaxis on Ingestion of Food

Food known → Avoid the food and related foods → Train patients in the use of Epi-pen

Food unknown → Refer to an allergist for diagnostic testing with food skin tests of RASTs

<u>Test negative</u>
Provide Epi-pen and observe for future reactions

Test positively to a food → Avoid food or perform blinded food challenge to confirm diagnosis

Test positively to multiple foods → Avoid those most commonly associated with food allergy or perform challenge to identify culprit food

Figure 94-1. An algorithm for evaluation of food allergy.

timing and doses of the food challenges. Resources for treatment of anaphylaxis including epinephrine, antihistamines, corticosteroids, and fluids must be available for food challenge. Elemental diets and amino acid-based hypoallergenic formulations that provide total nutrition may be useful for short-term treatment of infants with multiple food allergies.

In eosinophilic gastroenteritis, resolution of symptoms upon elimination of the offending dietary protein from the diet may occur over weeks or even months. Repeat endoscopy and biopsy may be useful in some cases to document resolution of pathology.

PEARLS

- O Mothers of children from atopic families should be encouraged to breast feed so as to prevent or delay food allergy in infants.
- O A working diagnosis of allergy to a specific food may be made in any patient who develops symptoms of anaphylaxis after food ingestion. That food should be avoided and the patient

given an epinephrine delivery device (Epi-pen, Epi-pen Jr) to keep with them at all times in case of an inadvertent ingestion of the culprit food.

○ In individuals with signs and symptoms of eosinophilic enteropathy, biopsy of the gastrointestinal tract is warranted. Determination of food-specific IgE responses in a given patient may be useful in identifying those foods that may trigger this syndrome and should be avoided.

○ Referral to a certified allergist may be useful in the evaluation of individuals with food allergy where the culprit food is unclear.

BIBLIOGRAPHY

Sampson HA, Sicherer SH, Birnbaum AH. AGA technical review on the evaluation of food allergy in gastrointestinal disorders. *Gastroenterology*. 2001;120(4):1026-40.

Sampson H. Food allergy. *J Allergy Clin Immunol*. 2003;111(2 Suppl):S540-7. Review.

Chapter 95 *Gastrointestinal Cancer Screening and Surveillance* ▬

1. *Achalasia*: Most cancers are squamous cell carcinoma. Start EGD at 15 years after the initial onset of symptoms, or 10 to 15 years after treatment. Repeat every 1 to 3 years.

2. *Barrett's esophagus* (BE): Risk of cancer is 10 to 40% depending upon dysplasia. Patients with longstanding reflux disease (especially those older than 50) and White males should be screened for BE. Risk of cancer in BE is increased only if specialized intestinal type epithelium is seen. Biopsies should be done every 1.0 to 2.0 cm starting at or 1.0 cm below gastroesophageal junction and extending 1.0 cm above the extent of columnar mucosa. Role of chromoendoscopy is controversial (see Chapter 22).

3. *Caustic injury to esophagus*: There is 1000 times increased risk for esophageal cancer in patients with caustic stricture. Cancer occurs about 15 to 50 years after ingestion, mostly in mid-esophagus at the site of stricture. EGD should be done 15 years

after the ingestion and then repeated every 1 to 3 years (see Chapter 28).

4. *Tylosis*: It is a genetic disorder with features of hyperkeratosis of the palms and soles. Ninety percent of the patients develop esophageal cancer by 65 years of age. EGD should be started at 30 years of age and repeated every 1 to 3 years.

5. *Gastric polyps*: No cancer screening is recommended for hyperplastic or sporadic fundic gland polyps. The risk for malignant transformation is less than 3% for hyperplastic and zero for fundic gland polyps. Gastric adenomas recur in about 15% of the cases. EGD should be repeated for gastric adenoma at 1 year and then repeated every 3 to 5 years. *H. pylori* (Hp) should be eradicated if present (see Chapter 34).

6. *Familial adenomatous polyposis*: Annual sigmoidoscopy should be started at 10 to 12 years of age. Full colonoscopy should be done when polyps are seen. Once multiple adenomas are identified, colectomy is recommended. Surveillance EGD should be done preferably with end and/or side-viewing endoscopes. Screening for family members is recommended based on their genetic profile (see Chapter 81).

7. *Postgastrectomy patients*: Gastric stump cancer risk is increased 2- to 4-fold in patients with gastroduodenal surgery. It is more with Billroth II, compared to Billroth I, and usually occurs at the site of gastroenteric anastomosis. EGD should be done fifteen years after gastric surgery. Further surveillance may be undertaken at intervals of 2 to 5 years. No evidence-based guidelines have been established. Presence of dysplasia necessitates a more frequent surveillance.

8. *Pernicious anemia*: Gastric cancer occurs in about 2 to 10% of patients with pernicious anemia. Patients should be screened with EGD at the time of initial diagnosis to look for any gastric polyps. Further surveillance is only recommended if an adenoma is found on initial exam.

9. *Colon cancer screening*: Various options are available. While gastroenterologists consider colonoscopy as the screening method of choice, other expert groups offer colonoscopy as one of the screening options. The beneficial effects of screening using barium enema have not been established (see Chapter 82).

10. *Hereditary nonpolyposis colorectal cancer* (HNPCC): Genetic testing should be done in all family members. Colonoscopy should be undertaken between the the ages of 20 to 25 (or 10 years before the age of onset in index case) and repeated every 2 years until the age of 40, and then annually (see Chapter 81).

11. *Ulcerative colitis* (UC): Surveillance colonoscopy should be started after 7 to 9 years in pancolitis and in left-sided colitis. Some recommend exams beginning at 12 to 15 years in cases of left-sided colitis. Colonoscopy is then repeated every 1 to 2 years. No surveillance is needed for proctitis or proctosigmoiditis because of the low-risk for malignancy (see Chapter 75).

12. *Crohn's disease*: The risk for colon cancer is only increased in cases of Crohn's colitis. Patients should undergo a colonoscopy screening program as for UC (see Chapter 75).

13. *Liver cirrhosis*: There is an increased risk of hepatocellular carcinoma. Recommendations for screening are not evidence based but are founded on expert opinion. Serum alpha-fetoprotein level every 6 months and a liver ultrasound every 6 months has been recommended. Some experts do ultrasound annually; others use a CT scan.(see Chapter 49).

PEARLS

○ Most cancer screening guidelines are based on expert opinion and not randomized controlled trials.

○ Different professional organizations have made different recommendations for screening and surveillance of various cancers including colorectal cancer.

BIBLIOGRAPHY

Thomson CA, LeWinn K, Newton TR, Alberts DS, Martinez ME. Nutrition and diet in the development of gastrointestinal cancer. *Curr Oncol Rep.* 2003;5(3):192-202.

Chapter 96 Gastrointestinal Problems in Systemic Disorders

SOURCES OF COMMON GASTROINTESTINAL COMPLAINTS

Dysphagia

This may occur in patients with sarcoidosis, esophageal graft-vs-host disease (GVHD), scleroderma, diabetes, etc. Oropharyngeal dysphagia is common in cerebrovascular disease, cerebral palsy, multiple sclerosis, Parkinson's disease, and dementia.

Nausea and Vomiting

Besides the common etiologies, nausea and vomiting may occur due to medications (narcotics, digoxin, chemotherapy, nonsteroidal anti-inflammatory drugs [NSAIDs]), alcohol, hyperemesis gravidarum, upper respiratory infections, vestibular disorders, metabolic disorders (Reye's syndrome, uremia, diabetic ketoacidosis), hyperthyroidism, sepsis, Addison's disease, cardiac disorders (myocardial infarction), congenital hepatic fibrosis, and radiation therapy.

Diarrhea

Diarrhea may occur due to numerous drugs, toxins, alcohol, radiation therapy, hypoparathyroidism, hyperthyroidism, Addison's disease, collagen vascular diseases, malignancies (especially neuroendocrine tumors), amyloidosis, and diabetes mellitus.

Constipation

It may be caused by numerous drugs, toxins, endocrine disorders (hypothyroidism, hyperparathyroidism), electrolyte abnormalities, hypopituitarism, diabetes mellitus, collagen vascular disease, amyloidosis, pregnancy, and neurological disorders.

Abdominal Pain

Extra-gi causes of abdominal pain include myocardial infarction, pulmonary embolism, pneumonia, pericarditis, diabetic ketoacidosis, Addison's disease, uremia, *Herpes zoster*, abdominal epilepsy and abdominal migraine, porphyria, angioedema, sickle cell crisis, acute leukemia, drug withdrawal, and heat stroke.

Abnormal Liver Chemistries

Abnormal liver chemistries including hyperbilirubinemia may occur due to congenital hepatic fibrosis, Hodgkin's disease, sepsis, drugs, and TPN, etc.

SYSTEMIC DISORDERS WITH GASTROINTESTINAL MANIFESTATIONS

Dermatological Disorders

1. Blue rubber bleb nevus syndrome may cause intestinal hemangiomas leading to GI bleeding and occasionally intussusception.

2. Bullous disorders like epidermolysis bullosa, pemphigus vulgaris, and bullous pemphigoid may cause vesicles and bullae in the oral cavity, esophagus, and anorectal region leading to webs, strictures, dysphagia, GI bleeding, and constipation. Dilation of strictures causes worsening of stricture in epidermolysis bullosa because of the trauma; as such, soft diets are recommended and corticosteroids may be helpful.

3. Lichen planus may involve oropharynx and esophagus. It manifests as dysphagia and esophageal stricture. Lichen planus is also associated with hepatitis C (HCV). Tylosis is associated with markedly increased risk for squamous cell carcinoma of esophagus requiring screening and surveillance.

Immunologic Disorders

1. There is increased prevalence of *Campylobacter*, *Giardia*, *Rotavirus* infections, and perirectal abscesses in X-linked hypogammaglobulinemia.

2. IgA deficiency is associated with increased prevalence of giardiasis, celiac sprue, pernicious anemia, and nodular lymphoid hyperplasia.

3. Common variable hypogammaglobulinemia is associated with an increased risk for gastrointestinal infections including parasitic, bacterial and viral infections, small bowel bacterial overgrowth (SBBO), malabsorption syndrome, pancreatic insufficiency, pernicious anemia, gallstone disease, autoimmune hepatitis (AIH), sclerosing cholangitis, as well as cancer of the stomach and small or large bowel.

4. Chronic mucocutaneous candidiasis leads to oropharyngeal and/or esophageal candidiasis and pernicious anemia.

5. Hereditary angioedema may manifest with acute abdominal pain, vomiting, diarrhea, as well as intestinal obstruction due to intussusception and transient ascites. Angioedema of the intestine may also be caused by ACE-inhibitor drugs.

Cardiovascular Disorders

1. Congestive heart failure frequently leads to enlarged liver, right upper quadrant pain, mild elevations of alanine aminotransferase (ALT)/aspartate aminotransferase (AST), ascites with increased serum-ascites albumin gradient (SAAG), anorexia, nausea, diarrhea, protein-losing enteropathy, and ischemic bowel disease.

2. Aortic stenosis is *not* associated with an increase risk for arteriovenous malformations in the GI tract.

3. There is an increased risk for intestinal perforation, pancreatitis, and cholelithiasis in patients with cardiac transplantation.

Pulmonary Diseases

1. Alpha$_1$ antitrypsin (AAT) deficiency leads to abnormal liver tests, cirrhosis, and an increased risk for liver cancer.

2. Chronic obstructive pulmonary disease causes an increased risk for peptic ulcer disease.

3. Patients with chronic respiratory problems, especially those on bronchodilators have an, increased risk for GERD.

4. Sarcoidosis frequently involves liver but may also involve luminal gut causing dysphagia due to dysmotility, stricture, or extra esophageal compression; peptic ulcer disease; pyloric stenosis; gastroparesis; malabsorption syndrome; and even protein-losing enteropathy.

5. Vagus nerve injury in patients with lung transplantation may cause esophageal and gastric dysmotility, GERD, and gastroparesis.

Renal Disorders

1. Patients with chronic renal failure may present with a wide spectrum of gastrointestinal involvement, including altered sensation of taste, anorexia, nausea, vomiting, GERD, GI bleeding (especially due to increased incidence of angiodysplasia), peptic ulcer disease, abdominal pain, constipation, ulceration and intussusception of the small or large bowel, diarrhea, and bacterial overgrowth.

2. Patients on hemodialysis may develop refractory ascites.

3. Patients with renal transplantation have increased risk for infections, peptic ulcer disease, and perforation of colonic diverticula.

4. Polycystic kidney disease is associated with hepatic cysts and Caroli's disease.

Endocrine Disorders

1. Diabetes mellitus affects digestive system in most patients. Patients may present with esophageal infections, GERD, gastric bezoar, SBBO, celiac disease, constipation, diarrhea, incontinence, cholelithiasis, nonalcoholic fatty liver disease

(NAFLD), or mesenteric ischemia. Abdominal pain may be a manifestation of diabetic neuropathy or diabetic ketoacidosis.

2. Acromegaly carries an increased risk of colonic adenomas.

3. Addison's disease causes anorexia, nausea, vomiting, weight loss, abdominal pain, and diarrhea.

4. Cushing's disease is associated with peptic ulcer disease.

5. Patients with hyperthyroidism may complain of increased appetite, weight loss, diarrhea, abdominal pain, and dysphagia. There may be atrophic gastritis, malabsorption syndrome, liver enzymes abnormalities, as well as AIH and primary biliary cirrhosis.

6. Although patients with hypothyroidism may complain of anorexia, it is usually associated with weight gain, constipation, dysphagia, heartburn, intestinal pseudo-obstruction, and ascites. Other GI diseases associated with hypothyroidism include pernicious anemia, inflammatory bowel disease (IBD), primary biliary cirrhosis, autoimmune hepatitis (AIH), and celiac disease.

7. Hyperparathyroidism is associated with abdominal pain, nausea, vomiting, peptic ulcer disease, and pancreatitis.

8. Manifestations of hypoparathyroidism include abdominal pain, diarrhea, malabsorption syndrome, and intestinal pseudo-obstruction.

Hematological Disorders

1. Sickle cell crisis presents with acute abdominal pain with fever and abnormal liver chemistries. Black pigment gallstones are common in sickle cell disease.

2. Hypercoagulable states including malignancies may cause Budd-Chiari syndrome and portal vein thrombosis, as well as ischemic bowel disease.

3. Bleeding and coagulation disorders like hemophilia and platelet dysfunction may precipitate or exacerbate GI bleeding.

4. Porphyria may present with acute abdominal pain, nausea, vomiting, or constipation. Acute intermittent porphyria is the most common and is not associated with the dermatological findings.

5. Porphyria cutanea tarda is associated with iron overload and HCV infection.

6. Mastocytosis may manifest with chest or abdominal pain, nausea, vomiting, diarrhea, malabsorption syndrome, peptic ulcer disease, GERD, and hepatosplenomegaly.

7. Involvement of GI tract and liver by leukemia and lymphoma is common.

8. Graft versus host disease occurs in patients after bone marrow transplantation (BMT). Acute GVHD occurs within first 100 days after BMT and presents with abdominal pain, diarrhea, nausea, vomiting, bleeding, malabsorption syndrome, and cholestatic liver disease. Dysphagia due to strictures or webs and cholestatic liver disease are seen in chronic GVHD.

11. Conditioning therapy with radiation and chemotherapy may lead to veno-occlusive disease of the liver usually within 8 to 23 days after BMT.

Neurological Disorders

1. Acute head injury predisposes to stress ulceration and GI bleeding.

2. Migraine and temporal lobe epilepsy may cause abdominal pain, nausea, and vomiting.

3. Neurological disorders like multiple sclerosis may cause GERD, gastroparesis, constipation, and fecal incontinence.

Rheumatological Disorders

1. Scleroderma causes GERD, gastroparesis, chronic intestinal pseudo-obstruction, SBBO, constipation, diarrhea, malabsorption syndrome, and BE. Arteriovenous malformations are also common in scleroderma and other rheumatological disorders and may cause GI bleeding. Other manifestations include oropharyngeal dysphagia, pancreatitis, and increased risk for digestive malignancies.

2. NSAIDs carry an increased risk for pill-induced esophagitis, as well ulceration and strictures throughout GI tract. Anal strictures may occur.

3. Nodular regenerative hyperplasia is seen in scleroderma, polymyalgia rheumatica, vasculitis, Felty's syndrome, and myeloproliferative disorders.

4. AIH and primary biliary cirrhosis may be seen with Sjogren's syndrome and rheumatoid arthritis.

Amyloidosis

Amyloidosis may present with an enlarged tongue, gastrointestinal dysmotility, GERD, gastroparesis, peptic ulceration, bleeding, constipation, diarrhea, SBBO, intestinal ischemia, hepatomegaly, and pancreatic insufficiency. Diagnosis can be made by rectal or gastric biopsies. Liver transplantation has been used in some cases of liver failure due to amyloidosis.

Obesity

Obesity can lead to an increased risk for cancer of esophagus and colon, cholelithiasis, NAFLD, and pancreatitis. Rapid weight loss or "yo-yo" dieting also increases the risk for cholelithiasis, nausea, vomiting, diarrhea, or constipation.

Eating Disorders

Patients with anorexia nervosa or bulimia may present with nausea, vomiting, abdominal pain, hematemesis due to Mallory-Weiss tear, constipation, pancreatitis, and abnormal liver chemistries.

PEARLS

- ○ Digestive system is affected in most cases of longstanding diabetes and rheumatological disorders.
- ○ Medications used to treat systemic disorders should be considered in the differential diagnosis as cause for patients' gastrointestinal complaints.

BIBLIOGRAPHY

Minocha A, Mandanas R, Kida M, Jazzar A. Bullous esophagitis due to chronic graft versus host disease. *Am J Gastroenterol.* 1997;92: 529-530.

Mesiya SA, Minocha A. Gastrointestinal disease in diabetes mellitus (monograph). *Southern Med J.* 1998/1999;Winter:33-38.

97 *Systemic Manifestations of Gastrointestinal Diseases* ▬▬

RHEUMATOLOGICAL MANIFESTATIONS

Inflammatory Arthritis

It is seen in patients with IBD, microscopic colitis, infectious gastroenteritis, celiac sprue, and Whipple's disease. Peripheral arthritis in IBD occurs in patients with extensive colonic involvement and correlates with a flare-up in two-thirds of the patients. IBD patients with HLA-B27 have an increased risk for inflammatory sacroilietis or spondylitis, but it does not correlate with disease activity.

Sero-negative oligoarthritis or polyarthritis is seen in Whipple's disease and may precede the onset of intestinal symptoms. Patients with celiac disease may have arthritis and osteomalacia.

Reactive Arthritis

Reactive arthritis may be seen in patients with GI infections due to *Yersinia, Salmonella, Shigella,* or *Campylobacter* in about 1 to 3% infected patients; the prevalence may be as high as 20% in case of Yersinia infection. Postenteric reactive arthritis occurs more often in males in their third or fourth decade and the onset is acute. Presence of HLA-B27 increases the risk for reactive arthritis. Reiter's syndrome may also develop in these patients.

Intestinal Arthritis-Dermatitis Syndrome

Intestinal arthritis-dermatitis syndrome occurs in 20 to 80% of patients undergoing jejunoileal or jejunocolic bypass for morbid obesity. These surgeries are rarely done these days. The cause is most likely bacterial overgrowth in the blind loop.

Miscellaneous

Other rheumatological problems including planter fasciitis, hypertrophic osteoarthropathy, osteoporosis, vasculitis, and amyloidosis may be seen in IBD.

PANNICULITIS

Pancreatic panniculitis syndrome occurs in patients with pancreatitis or pancreatic malignancies. It manifests with tender red nodules, arthritis, weight loss, fever, eosinophilia, osteolytic bone lesions, and serositis. Serum pancreatic enzyme concentrations are elevated. Biopsy of the skin shows fat necrosis.

MALNUTRITION

Vitamin D malabsorption in pancreatic insufficiency of chronic pancreatitis may cause osteomalacia. Malnutrition is also seen in chronic liver disease, IBD, and malabsorption syndrome.

HEMATOLOGICAL MANIFESTATIONS

Gastroduodenal Surgery

Gastroduodenal surgery leads to iron deficiency anemia due to hypochlorhydria and impaired iron absorption. Vitamin B_{12} deficiency is seen in patients with a subtotal or total gastrectomy because of a loss of intrinsic factor and hydrochloric acid. Intravenous administration of iron or intramuscular administration of vitamin B_{12} corrects the iron deficiency anemia and B_{12} deficiency anemia respectively in such postsurgical syndromes.

Malabsorption Syndrome

Malabsorption syndrome due to celiac disease, tropical sprue, Whipple's disease, and Crohn's disease may lead to anemia due to deficiency of iron, folic acid, and vitamin B_{12}.

Acute and Chronic Liver Disease

Acute viral hepatitis may cause pancytopenia and aplastic anemia. Spur cell anemia occurs in patients with liver cirrhosis, and transfusions do not help since the transfused cells acquire the same abnormality. However, splenectomy can slow down the process. Other causes of anemia in patients with chronic liver disease include hemolysis, GI bleeding, and folic acid deficiency.

Chronic Alcoholism

Macrocytic anemia in alcoholics occurs due to folate deficiency, reticulocytosis, chronic liver disease, and chronic alcoholism. Both acute and chronic alcoholism results in thrombocytopenia. Thrombocytopenia due to acute alcoholism reverses quickly after withdrawal.

Sickle Cell Disease

Hepatic crisis of sickle cell disease presents with right upper quadrant abdominal pain, fever, leukocytosis, and abnormal liver chemistries, but resolves within 1 to 2 weeks.

Management of asymptomatic cholelithiasis in patients with sickle cell disease is controversial and prophylactic cholecystectomy may be undertaken in patients with recurrent abdominal crisis.

Gastrointestinal Malignancies

Microangiopathic hemolytic anemia is seen as a paraneoplastic syndrome in patients with mucin producing adenocarcinoma like gastric cancer. These malignancies also predispose to migratory superficial thrombophlebitis, also known as *Trousseau's syndrome*.

Enteric Infections

GI infections caused by *E. coli O157:H7*, *Shigella*, *Salmonella*, *Yersinia*, and *Campylobacter* may be lead to hemolytic-uremic syndrome, which may be further complicated by gastrointestinal ulceration, perforation, toxic megacolon, acalculous cholecystitis, and pancreatitis. The risk is increased in patients who receive antibiotics.

DERMATOLOGICAL MANIFESTATIONS

Chronic Liver Disease

Patients may have dilated abdominal veins, palmar erythema, purpura, spider angiomata, hyperpigmentation, and jaundice. The number of spider angiomata on a patient correlates with the severity of alcohol-related liver disease.

Differential diagnosis of jaundice includes carotenoderma, due to excessive ingestion of carotene (yellow or orange vegetables like carrots and squash); lycopenoderma, due to excessive intake of lycopenes (red vegetables like tomatoes); and quinacrine administration.

Moderate to severe pruritus occurs in about 40% of the patients with chronic liver disease. Pyoderma gangrenosum may occur in patients with infectious hepatitis.

Inflammatory Bowel Disease

UC and Crohn's disease are associated with pyoderma gangrenosum, erythema nodosum, and aphthous ulcers.

Acute Pancreatitis

Turner's sign (hemorrhagic discoloration in the flank) or Cullen's sign (ecchymosis of periumbilical region) due to intra-abdominal hemorrhage are seen in less than 1% of the cases. Pancreatic fat necrosis may be seen in acute pancreatitis. Fat necrosis may also be associated with arthritis.

Celiac Disease

Celiac disease is associated with dermatitis herpetiformis (DH). Although almost all patients with a DH show some degree of histological findings of celiac disease, only about one-third of the patients may be have clinical manifestations related to sprue. Patients with DH are treated with dapsone in addition to gluten-free diet.

ENDOCRINE MANIFESTATIONS

Hypoglycemia may occur because of fasting as well as insulinoma. Reactive hypoglycemia occurring a few hours after meal may be functional or may represent early diabetes. Alcoholism may cause hypoglycemia. Hypo- or hyperglycemia may be seen in patients with chronic liver disease.

PEARLS

❍ Peripheral arthritis in inflammatory bowel disease correlates with disease activity whereas axial arthritis does not.

❍ Abnormalities of CBC are seen in patients with gastroduodenal surgery, malabsorption syndrome, acute and chronic liver disease, sickle cell disease, enteric infections, and gastrointestinal malignancies.

BIBLIOGRAPHY

Ochoa TJ, Cleary TG. Epidemiology and spectrum of disease of Escherichia coli O157. *Curr Opin Infect Dis.* 2003;16(3):259-63.

Storch I, Sachar D, Katz S. Pulmonary manifestations of inflammatory bowel disease. *Inflamm Bowel Dis.* 2003;9(2):104-15.

Chapter

98 *Gastrointestinal Infections*

ACUTE GASTROENTERITIS

Viruses are the most common cause of gastroenteritis in the United States. The illness is usually brief and self-limited.

CLINICAL FEATURES

Clinical features of gastroenteritis depend upon the region of the digestive tract involved. Typically there is nausea, vomiting, diarrhea without fever, abdominal pain, and occasional bloody diarrhea.

PATHOGENESIS

The small intestine is involved in *Salmonella, Vibrio cholera, E. coli, Yersinia, Rotavirus, Norwalk virus, Adenovirus, Giardia,* and *Cryptosporidia. Salmonella, Yersinia,* and *E. coli* can involve both small and large bowel. Large bowel pathogens include *Campylobacter, Shigella, C. difficile,* amebiasis, and *CMV*.

Rotavirus accounts for most cases of diarrhea amongst children worldwide. Illness in adults is usually asymptomatic unless patient is immune-compromised or chronically ill. Norwalk viruses are the second most common cause of nonbacterial diarrhea in the United States.

Although *Adenovirus* usually causes respiratory infection, it can also cause diarrhea especially amongst children. Infection may involve both the respiratory and GI systems with respiratory symptoms followed by GI symptoms.

DIAGNOSIS

Diagnosis of gastroenteritis is usually clinical. Stool tests may occasionally be needed to identify the pathogen. Some labs routinely culture the stool specimen only for *Salmonella, Shigella,* and *Campylobacter*; other pathogens are cultured only upon request.

TREATMENT

The treatment is usually symptomatic including antiemetics, antidiarrheals, and fluids. Oral hydration is sufficient in most cases and antibiotics are usually not needed.

Antibiotics are effective and usually indicated in patients with *Salmonella* enterocolitis, typhoid fever, *Shigella, C. difficile* colitis, *Yersinia* sepsis, moderate to severe traveler's diarrhea, *Campylobacter* dysentery or sepsis, cholera, symptomatic giardiasis, amebiasis, *Vibrio parahemolyticus,* enteroinvasive, as well as enteropathogenic, *E. coli*.

Antibiotics are unlikely to be effective in ETEC, including *E. coli O157:H7, Salmonella,* or *Yersinia* without sepsis and mild to moderate traveler's diarrhea.

Specific Infections

Salmonella

Manifestations are varied and include gastroenteritis which may be mild diarrhea; bacteremia with or without gastroenteritis; and enteric fever. Typhoid fever refers to *S. typhi*, whereas enteric fever refers to both *S. typhi* and *S. paratyphi*.

Salmonella Gastroenteritis

Salmonella gastroenteritis is the most common manifestation. It occurs via ingestion of contaminated eggs, chicken, meat, and dairy products. Patients with hemolytic anemia (sickle cell disease), malignancy, immune-suppression (AIDS, corticosteroid therapy), and achlorhydric states (gastric surgery, proton pump inhibitor [PPI] therapy), and IBD are more prone to *Salmonella* infection.

Symptoms occur within 48 hours of exposure. Features include nausea, vomiting, diarrhea which may be bloody, fever, abdominal pain, and abdominal tenderness. Most cases resolve within 5 days except colitis, which may last several weeks. About 1% of patients with gastroenteritis become chronic carriers. Treatment is focused on rehydration.

Antibiotics are only used in patients with colitis or those at risk for bacteremia including young children, elderly, immune-compromised patients, and those with endovascular prosthesis, hemoglobinopathy, or orthopedic implants. Options for antibiotics include ampicillin, TMP-SMX, quinolone and should be guided by sensitivity. Due to increasing resistance, empiric therapy with ciprofloxacin (500.0 mg bid) is recommended. Ciprofloxacin could be switched to trimethoprim/sulfamethoxazole (TMP/SMZ DS 1 tablet bid), if the organism turns out to be susceptible.

Typhoid Fever

Third generation cephalosporins and quinolones are effective for typhoid fever. Options include fluoroquinolone ciprofloxacin (500.0 mg bid) or ofloxacin (400.0 mg bid), either orally or parenterally for 7 to 10 days. Ceftriaxone (2.0 to 3.0 g qd) parenterally for 7 to 14 days is another option.

About 3% patients with typhoid fever become chronic carriers. Carriers may be treated with norfloxacin 400.0 mg bid for 4 weeks. Cholecystectomy may be needed to eradicate the infection.

Shigella

Shigella usually occurs via person-to-person spread, whereas outbreaks occur due to contaminated food and water. Patients typically have abdominal pain, low- to high-grade fever, and diarrhea that can eventually become bloody. The watery diarrhea is due to Shiga toxin, whereas dysentery suggests mucosal invasion. Hydration is the cornerstone of therapy and antibiotics are not needed in most cases.

Depending on severity and underlying illness, antibiotics may be used. Options include quinolones, TMP-SMX, or ampicillin for 1 to 5 days especially amongst elderly, daycare workers, health care workers, food handlers, and immune-compromised patients. Unless guided by sensitivity, quinolones are the drugs of choice.

E. Coli

Enterohemorrhagic E. Coli O157:H7

It causes bloody diarrhea and colitis within 3 to 5 days of ingestion of undercooked hamburger, salami, or unpasteurized milk or juice. Diarrhea is initially watery and progresses to bloody diarrhea within a few hours to a few days. Infection is often associated with nausea, vomiting, and abdominal pain. Fever is uncommon. Differential diagnosis includes ischemic colitis and other forms of infectious colitis.

Hemolytic-uremic syndrome (HUS) and thrombotic thrombocytopenic purpura (TTP) occur in 5% of the cases. Most labs do not routinely test for *Enterohemorrhagic E. coli* (EHEC) and should be specifically requested.

Antibiotics do not have any role in treatment and may increase the risk for HUS and TTP. Antidiarrheals and narcotics should be avoided.

Children should not return to school unless three stool cultures have been negative.

Enterotoxigenic E. Coli

Enterotoxigenic E. coli (ETEC) is a common cause of traveler's diarrhea. There is mild to moderate diarrhea with abdominal pain and may be associated with mild nausea and vomiting. Rehydration is the mainstay of therapy. Patients are usually treated empirically with quinolones, trimethoprim-sulfamethoxazole (TMP-SMX), or tetracycline.

Enteropathogenic E. Coli

Enteropathogenic E. coli (EPEC) is usually seen in infants, and is most common in the underdeveloped countries. Treatment includes intravenous hydration and TMP-SMX.

Enteroinvasive E. Coli

Enteroinvasive E. coli (EIEC) rarely causes diarrhea and the clinical features resemble *Shigella*. Treatment includes intravenous hydration and quinolones.

Campylobacter

Campylobacter is the most common bacterial cause of gastroenteritis in the United States. It occurs due to ingestion of contaminated poultry or milk. Symptoms occur within 1 to 4 days and include fever, malaise, abdominal pain, headache, and diarrhea. The diarrhea may become bloody.

Symptoms usually resolve within 1 to 2 weeks. However, in a few cases, they can continue for several months. The recurrence rate is high. *Campylobacter* can be complicated by HUS and *Guillain-Barre syndrome.*

Antibiotics are needed if symptoms persist beyond one week or in cases of special populations (pregnant women or immune-compromised patients), worsening symptoms, high fever, and bacteremia. Erythromycin may be used if started within first 3 days of illness. Quinolones can be started later.

Vibrio

Vibrio infection is a common cause of gastroenteritis in the coastal areas.

Vibrio parahaemolyticus can cause bloody diarrhea. Infection is self-limited and lasts 2 to 5 days. The role of antibiotics is controversial.

Vibrio cholerae results in watery diarrhea only. Oral hydration is the cornerstone of therapy for *Vibrio cholerae* infection and antibiotic treatment may include tetracycline, doxycycline, or quinolones.

Vibrio vulnificus can cause diarrhea, wound infection and septicemia. Infection occurs via ingestion or wound contamination. Immune-compromised patients (eg, liver cirrhosis) should avoid raw seafood and should not go into water if they have an open wound.

Yersinia

Y. enterocolitica infection occurs due to ingestion of contaminated food, milk, or water and can affect the small and/or large intestine. Symptoms vary from mild to severe. They include nausea, vomiting, diarrhea, abdominal pain, bleeding, and skin rash, and usually resolve within 1 to 3 weeks.

Yersinia ileocolitis may be complicated by aphthous ulcers, arthralgias, or erythema nodosum, and as such, may mimic Crohn's disease.

Antibiotics are used in immune-compromised patients, as well as in those with liver cirrhosis, iron overload, prolonged symptoms, and bacteremia. Options include tetracycline, quinolones, or TMP-SMX with or without aminoglycosides.

Giardia

G. duodenalis or *G. intestinalis* is the commonest of parasitic infections in the United States. It occurs via ingestion of contaminated food or direct person to person contact especially in daycare centers and nursing homes. Homosexual men and patients with immunoglobulin deficiency are particularly at risk.

Symptoms may be acute or subacute, intermittent, or chronic. These include nausea, vomiting, abdominal pain, increased flatulence, bloating, and diarrhea. They usually occur 1 to 2 weeks after infection. Malabsorption syndrome may occur. Stool test for cysts and trophozoites are useful in acute diarrhea. Duodenal aspirate and biopsy or stool test for *Giardia* antigen is preferred in chronic cases.

Treatment is indicated only in symptomatic cases and includes metronidazole 250.0 mg tid for 7 days. Asymptomatic subjects who work in daycare or health care system coming in contact with other patients should also be treated.

Cryptosporidium

Cryptosporidium parvum infection occurs both in immune-competent and immune-compromised hosts due to contaminated water or person to person spread. The disease is usually self-limited in immune-competent patients. Symptoms include nausea, vomiting, diarrhea, flatulence (that may last as long as 6 weeks), along with headache, fever, and myalgias. Abdominal pain, jaundice, hepatitis, and pancreatitis may occur in cases of biliary involvement.

The parasite can be detected in biopsies of the involved region, stool specimens, as well as duodenal aspirates. The diagnostic yield of the stool specimen can be enhanced by 1) examining three stool specimens; and 2) using ELISA test for antibodies against *Cryptosporidium* in stool.

Biliary involvement is confirmed by examining the bile, since stools may be negative in such cases. Liver enzymes may be elevated. Ultrasound may show thickened gall bladder, dilated bile ducts, and pancreatitis.

Antibiotics are usually recommended in children only. Antidiarrheal agents plus supportive care including intravenous hydration, as well as enteral or parenteral nutrition are important. Antibiotics are not required in immune-competent adults. In immune-deficient patients, the best treatment is to enhance the immune status (eg, use of effective anti-retroviral therapy in HIV-positive patients). Other treatments that have been tried include paromomycin, clarithromycin, azithromycin, metronidazole, and octreotide. ERCP and sphincterotomy may be needed in cases of biliary involvement.

Prognosis in HIV-positive patients without an ability to enhance immune status is poor. Prophylaxis for *Cryptosporidium* is not recommended.

Amebiasis

Entamoeba histolytica is a common cause of parasitic diarrhea in developing countries and occurs through ingestion of contaminated food or water. The spectrum of clinical manifestations varies from asymptomatic state to mild to severe nausea, vomiting, diarrhea, abdominal pain, fever, and even dysentery.

Bowel perforation can occur and the risk is increased by corticosteroid therapy. Parasites may reach the liver through portal circulation and cause liver abscess although many of these patients do not give history of colitis. Pulmonary and central nervous system (CNS) involvement may occur.

Diagnosis is made by stool examination on at least three separate occasions for cysts and trophozoites. Stool antigen for amoebae and PCR testing are superior. Metronidazole 750.0 mg tid for 7 to 14 days is effective for both intestinal and hepatic infection. Amebic hepatic abscess usually resolves on medical treatment and does not require drainage.

Blastocystis

Blastocystis hominis is occasionally identified on routine stool studies; however, its role in pathogenesis of sickness is unclear. A trial of metronidazole may be appropriate in select cases.

UNCOMMON INFECTIONS

Toxoplasmosis

Twenty to 40% of the US population has been exposed to this parasite. Infection occurs due to undercooked meat or through soil contaminated with feline feces. Most immune-competent patients remain asymptomatic.

Some patients develop cervical lymphadenopathy with mononucleosis-like symptoms. Course is self-limited and may last a few weeks to several months. Brain, lungs, eyes, and occasionally liver, bladder, heart, and testes may be involved in HIV-infected patients.

Diagnosis is made by serology in immune-competent hosts. In case of HIV-positive patients, the demonstration of tachyzoites in tissue or fluid is needed. Multiple ring enhancing lesions may be seen on a CT scan of brain. Brain biopsy may be required to diagnose cerebral involvement.

Antibiotics are required in severe cases as well as in case of pregnant or immune-compromised patients. Pyrimethamine plus sulfadiazine for 4 to 6 weeks along with leucovorin are usually administered. Alternate option is pyrimethamine plus clindamycin.

Ascariasis

Ascaris lumbricoides infects approximately 25% of the population worldwide. Infection occurs usually in children via ingestion of contaminated water or food. GI, hepatobiliary, or pulmonary involvement may be seen. Stool examination may show the eggs. Peripheral eosinophilia is seen. Treatment options include mebendazole 500.0 mg, albendazole 400.0 mg, or pyrantel pamoate 11.0 mg/kg (up to 1.0 g) as a single dose.

Toxocariasis

T. canis or *cati* occurs worldwide. Infection occurs due to exposure to dogs and cats, especially among young children with history of pica through ingestion of contaminated soil or food. Symptoms occur only in a minority of patients.

Visceral larva migrans presents with fever, hepatomegaly, urticaria, and eosinophilia. Asthma, pneumonia, seizures, and encephalopathy may be seen. Eye involvement can cause strabismus and blindness.

Diagnosis is made by identification of larvae in the involved tissues. A positive serology against larva antigens is supportive.

Most patients don't require treatment. Treatment is usually supportive. Mebendazole 200.0 mg bid or albendazole 400.0 mg bid for 5 days may be used in severe cases and is effective for killing the larvae and preventing larval migration. Diethylcarbamazine 3.0 mg/kg/day tid for 21 days is another option. Steroids are recommended in cases of pulmonary or CNS involvement.

Strongyloides

It is asymptomatic in most individuals although some patients may suffer from chronic intermittent gastrointestinal symptoms (anorexia, nausea, vomiting, diarrhea), skin itching with rash and pulmonary problems for years. Liver involvement leads to jaundice and cholestasis. Hyperinfection syndrome occurs especially in immune-compromised patients due to dissemination of larvae into multiple organs.

Diagnosis is made by detection of larvae in stool, duodenal aspirate or intestinal biopsy. Positive serology tests (ELISA) are supportive. Treatment options include ivermectin 200.0 mcg/kg/day for 1 to 2 days, albendazole 400.0 mg/day for 3 days, or thiabendazole (25.0

mg/kg bid up to 3 g/day for 2 days). Prognosis is good except in hyperinfection syndrome.

Schistosomiasis

Different parts of the body including liver, lungs, bladder, and CNS may be involved depending upon species. Clinical presentation depends upon the site of involvement. Praziquantel is the treatment of choice.

Echinococcus (Hydatid Cyst Disease)

Humans are accidental hosts in this infection caused by various species of the tapeworm, *Echinococcus*. Infection occurs by ingestion of dog feces or by permitting dogs to lick in a person's mouth. Patients may have fever, hepatomegaly, and eosinophilia. Enlarging hepatic cyst may cause abdominal pain, jaundice, portal hypertension or portal vein obstruction. Cysts may rupture, get infected or may communicate with biliary system. Rupture into lungs may lead to dyspnea and hemoptysis.

Rupture into biliary system causes cholangitis while rupture of cyst into peritoneal cavity may cause anaphylactic shock.

Diagnosis is made by ELISA and indirect hemagglutination assay along with imaging of abdominal lesions by ultrasound or CT. Heavily calcified and asymptomatic cysts may not require intervention and may be watched clinically.

Treatment is usually open surgical drainage of the cyst and removal of cyst *in toto* combined with albendazole. Exceptions include very sick patients, extremes of age, multiple cysts, and pregnancy. Adjunctive chemotherapy is given before and after surgery to reduce the risk of recurrence. Albendazole for 8 weeks combined with a percutaneous drainage and hypertonic saline irrigation of the cyst has been used with success.

PEARLS

- ○ Hydration is the mainstay of treatment of acute diarrhea.
- ○ Most cases of acute gastroenteritis resolve without specific treatment.
- ○ Uncommon infections should be part of differential diagnosis especially in immigrant populations and immune-compromised hosts.

Bibliography

Black RE, Morris SS, Bryce J. Where and why are 10 million children dying every year? *Lancet*. 2003;361(9376):2226-34.

Curtis V, Cairncross S. Effect of washing hands with soap on diarrhea risk in the community: a systematic review. *Lancet Infect Dis*. 2003;3(5): 275-81.

Chapter 99 Acute Intestinal Ischemia

Mesenteric ischemia is caused by reduction of intestinal blood flow. This may occur as a result of vascular occlusion, vasospasm, or hypoperfusion of the mesenteric vasculature. Early diagnosis and treatment are important since sepsis, bowel infarction, and death may occur.

Anatomic Considerations

Celiac axis supplies the stomach and proximal duodenum, whereas the superior mesenteric artery nourishes the distal duodenum, entire small intestine, and proximal half of colon. The inferior mesenteric artery supplies blood to distal colon and rectum. The rectum also receives blood from internal iliac arteries. The venous drainage is accomplished through superior and inferior mesenteric veins.

Less than 75% reduction of mesenteric blood flow and diminished oxygen consumption for less than 12 hours does not result in any gross or histologic damage to the gut.

Factors Regulating Intestinal Circulation

These include cardiovascular factors (blood pressure and volume), autonomic nervous system (ANS) (sympathetic, parasympathetic, and nonadrenergic noncholinergic nerves), circulating hormones (norepinephrine, angiotensin II, and vasopressin), and local tissues (mast cells and leukocytes), as well as their mediators.

While blood flow is impacted by numerous factors, the sympathetic nervous system is the most important in maintaining resting splanchnic arterial tone.

SITES OF INVOLVEMENT

Ischemic damage is rarely seen in the stomach, duodenum, or rectum because of an abundance of collateral circulation. In contrast, ischemic injury is more commonly seen at the splenic or hepatic flexure of the colon because of few anastomoses.

ISCHEMIC STATES

Intestinal ischemia may be acute or chronic, arterial or venous, and occlusive or nonocclusive. Two kinds of ischemic syndromes are recognized: acute and chronic. Acute mesenteric ischemia occurs as a result of the sudden onset of intestinal hypoperfusion, which may be the result of occlusive or nonocclusive obstruction of arterial or venous blood flow. Chronic mesenteric ischemia or intestinal angina implies an episodic or constant intestinal hypoperfusion and occurs usually in patients with established atherosclerotic arterial disease.

Generally, mesenteric ischemia is classified as 1) acute mesenteric ischemia; 2) chronic mesenteric ischemia; and 3) colonic ischemia. Some experts assert that ischemia due to vasculitis of the splanchnic circulation should be separate category. Chronic mesenteric ischemia and colonic ischemia are discussed separately in Chapter 100 and Chapter 101 respectively.

RISK FACTORS

These include advancing age, atherosclerosis, congestive heart failure, cardiac arrhythmias, severe valvular heart disease, recent massive myocardial infarction, and intra-abdominal malignancy. Other conditions predisposing to primary mesenteric ischemia include sarcoidosis, myocardial dyskinesia and intracardiac thrombosis, cardiac catheterization, aortic dissection, systemic hypotension, drugs (vasopressors and birth control pills), and abdominal trauma. Mesenteric ischemia may also be caused by adhesions, herniation, intussusception, mesenteric fibrosis, retroperitoneal fibrosis, amyloidosis, intra-abdominal malignancy, and neurofibromatosis.

There is no role of inherited coagulation defects in the pathogenesis of acute mesenteric artery thrombosis.

Mesenteric venous thrombosis (MVT) is more likely to occur in hypercoagulable states (inherited or acquired), portal hypertension, abdominal infection or trauma and pancreatitis. Up to 75% of the patients with a hypercoagulable state have an inherited thrombotic disorder, mostly likely Factor V Leiden. Acquired hypercoagulable states may occur due to paroxysmal nocturnal hemoglobinurea and myeloproliferative diseases.

PATHOPHYSIOLOGY

Acute Arterial Occlusive Ischemia

A major vessel occlusion stimulates an immediate opening up of the collateral vessels. If the occlusion persist for several hours, vaso-constriction results in reduction of the collateral flow. A sustained obstruction for a more prolonged period results in an irreversible vasoconstriction.

Mesenteric Venous Occlusive Ischemia

Mesenteric venous occlusion is a rare cause of mesenteric ischemia. MVT results in increased resistance in the mesenteric venous blood flow causing bowel wall edema and fluid efflux into the lumen, result-ing in systemic hypotension and increased blood viscosity. There is a concomitant reduction in arterial blood flow causing submucosal hemorrhages and bowel infarction.

Nonocclusive Mesenteric Ischemia

Nonocclusive Mesenteric Ischemia (NOMI) occurs as a result of splanchnic hypoperfusion (especially in patients with significant ath-erosclerosis), CHF, sepsis, cardiac dysrhythmia, and cocaine use. Medications including diuretics, digoxin and alpha-agonists have also been implicated. The prevalence of NOMI has been declining perhaps due to advancements in management of critically ill patients.

Focal Segmental Ischemia

Focal segmental ischemia (FSI) may be caused by an embolic dis-ease, strangulated hernia, vasculitis, abdominal trauma, segmental venous thrombosis, radiation therapy, or oral contraceptives. Presence of adequate collateral circulation in such patients prevents transmural infarction. However, there may be partial bowel necrosis allowing translocation of intestinal bacteria.

ACUTE MESENTERIC ISCHEMIA

Prevalence

As many as 70% of the cases of mesenteric ischemia fall into this category. It carries a mortality that may exceed 60%.

The incidence is rising because of the increased recognition of this disorder, an aging population, and improved medical care that suc-ceeds in prolonging the life of patients with severe cardiovascular dis-ease (who often go on to develop acute mesenteric ischemia). About

50% of the cases of intestinal ischemia are caused by embolism of the superior mesenteric artery. Twenty-five percent occur as a result of nonocclusive mesenteric ischemia, 10 to 20% due to superior mesenteric artery (SMA) thrombosis, 5 to 10% due to mesenteric venous thrombosis, and 5% to focal segmental ischemia.

Symptoms of Gut Ischemia

Presentation varies depending upon the underlying etiology. SMA occlusion presents with a rapid onset of severe periumbilical pain out of proportion to the physical exam with associated nausea and vomiting. Pain may be insidious or chronic. Previous history of abdominal pain due to mesenteric angina may be elicited. Patients may also have weight loss.

Patients with mesenteric venous thrombosis present with pain that may be acute or chronic, lasting from days to months, along with anorexia, nausea, vomiting, diarrhea, constipation, abdominal distention, or bleeding.

FSI presents as a small bowel obstruction (SBO) with intermittent abdominal pain, distention, vomiting, and protein-losing enteropathy (in rare cases).

Physical Signs

Abdomen may be normal or distended with reduced or absent bowel sounds. Involuntary evacuation of bowel contents may occur due to intense contractions of the gut. Abnormal examination findings and heme positive stools may be the only clues in a critically ill patient unable to complain of pain.

Peritoneal signs develop as the ischemia progresses and transmural bowel infarction develops. Patients may develop a fecal odor to their breath. High index of suspicion is required (especially in patients with known risk factors) for rapid diagnosis since early signs are nonspecific and a delay in diagnosis carries catastrophic consequences.

Physical findings in FSI may suggest an acute abdomen and the presence of an inflammatory mass. Limited necrosis may present as acute enteritis, chronic enteritis, and stricture. Acute cases of FSI simulate acute appendicitis. In chronic cases, Crohn's disease may be suspected because of cramping, abdominal pain, diarrhea, fever, and weight loss.

Diagnosis of Acute Gut Ischemia

Acute ischemia should be suspected in patients with severe abdominal pain out of proportion to physical findings.

LABORATORY STUDIES

A CBC may be normal or show only leukocytosis with significant left shift. Hemoconcentration results in increased hematocrit. Serum amylase, LDH, and CPK may be elevated along with evidence of metabolic acidosis. Any patient with presentation of an acute abdomen with associated metabolic acidosis (even if a diabetic) should be presumed to have intestinal ischemia unless proven otherwise.

NONINVASIVE IMAGING STUDIES

Plain x-rays of the abdomen are initially normal, but may show a thickened bowel wall with thumb printing. Pneumatosis intestinalis may be present. Barium studies are contraindicated.

Doppler flow ultrasound can show stenosis or occlusion in celiac and superior mesenteric artery. Its utility is limited because the view is frequently obstructed due to overlying air-filled loops of distended bowel. It may be useful for diagnosis of multi-vessel stenosis in mesenteric angina but is not recommended in acutely ill patients.

Although a CT scan is frequently obtained in abdominal pain syndromes, the early signs of acute intestinal ischemia are nonspecific, whereas in late stages they show a necrotic bowel. The findings may include bowel thickening, bowel dilation and intramural gas; mesenteric and portal venous gas may be seen occasionally.

A CT of the abdomen with intravenous contrast is diagnostic for mesenteric venous thrombosis; angiography is less reliable for MVT.

ANGIOGRAPHY

Angiography is the standard for the diagnosis of acute arterial ischemia. Venous phase may demonstrate a venous occlusive disease; however angiography is less sensitive for SMV thrombosis. In nonocclusive mesenteric ischemia, angiography reveals narrow, irregular, or beaded major branches with decreased or absent blood flow in small vessels.

ROLE OF ENDOSCOPY

Enteroscopy to examine small bowel for suspected acute ischemia may be dangerous and should be avoided. Sigmoidoscopy or colonoscopy may however be useful in acute colonic ischemia (see Chapter 101).

ROLE OF LAPAROSCOPY

Findings of normal appearing serosa are seen in early reversible cases and as such can be misleading.

Treatment of Acute Arterial Ischemia

GENERAL MEASURES

The goal is to restore intestinal blood flow as quickly as possible. It involves aggressive hemodynamic monitoring and support, fluid replacement, correction of metabolic acidosis, broad spectrum antibiotics, and nasogastric suction for GI decompression. Medications that may worsen the disease including vasoconstricting agents and digoxin should be avoided.

MEDICAL MANAGEMENT

Patients without peritoneal signs who have good collateral flow on angiography may benefit from thrombolytic therapy, anticoagulation, and/or intra-arterial papaverine. Role of antiplatelet agents such as aspirin in the perioperative period remains to be established in patients with thrombotic occlusion.

THERAPEUTIC ANGIOGRAPHY

Angiography can be of therapeutic value. Vasodilators (papaverine, tolazoline, nitroglycerine) and thrombolytics can be administered. In addition, angioplasty, stent placement, and embolectomy can be undertaken.

SURGERY

If mesenteric arteriography is not available for diagnosis, a laparotomy is indicated. For SMA embolus, surgery is usually required, which may include embolectomy. Some experts administer intra-arterial papaverine before and for 24 hours after the operation. Intraoperative duplex ultrasound can help identify the persistently ischemic segments. Necrotic segments are resected. A second look operation at 24 to 48 hours is indicated if there is any doubt about viability of the bowel left intact.

LONG-TERM MANAGEMENT

Patients with mesenteric artery thrombosis should receive aspirin. Clopidogrel (Plavix) may be another option.

Treatment of Mesenteric Venous Thrombosis

ASYMPTOMATIC MVT PATIENTS

Patients with an incidental diagnosis of MVT in an otherwise asymptomatic patient, should undergo either observation or anticoagulation for 3 to 6 months.

ACUTE MVT

Management includes heparinization and resection of the necrotic portion of the bowel. Administration of heparin in the presence of GI bleeding is controversial. Some acute onset cases may benefit from initial thrombolytic therapy followed by heparin. Until more data develops, the use of thrombolytic therapy is not recommended for routine use at this time. Papaverine infusion should be administered during angiography to counter the concomitant arterial spasm. Second look laparotomy may be undertaken to confirm the viability of small bowel.

LONG-TERM MANAGEMENT

All patients with an episode of acute mesenteric venous thrombosis, except those considered to be high risk (eg, elderly or those with portal hypertension), should be anticoagulated with warfarin for 3 to 6 months, or for life—if there is a hypercoagulable state or atrial fibrillation.

Treatment of Acute Nonocclusive Mesenteric Ischemia

This involves reversing the underlying condition that caused the splanchnic vasoconstriction, optimization of hemodynamic parameters, avoiding offending medications, and prolonged selective intra-arterial infusion of vasodilators like papaverine. Patients with peritoneal signs should undergo surgery along with postoperative papaverine infusion. In patients without peritoneal signs, angiography should be repeated in 24 hours to confirm resolution of vasoconstriction. Concomitant use of heparin to prevent thrombosis in an involved vessel has been recommended. Long-term treatment involves the use of aspirin.

Treatment of Focal Segmental Ischemia

Surgery with resection of the involved bowel segment is needed.

PEARLS

- ○ Ischemic damage is rarely seen in the stomach, duodenum, or rectum because of abundance of collateral circulation.
- ○ A high index of suspicion for intestinal ischemia, especially in high-risk individuals, is important since a delay in treatment may lead to catastrophic consequences.
- ○ A plain x-ray and CT scan of abdomen are not helpful for early diagnosis of acute arterial occlusive ischemia.

BIBLIOGRAPHY

Nehme OS, Rogers AI. Small bowel ischemia. *Curr Treat Options Gastroenterol*. 2001;4(1):51-56.

Brandt LJ, Boley SJ. AGA technical review on intestinal ischemia. *Gastroenterol.* 2000;118:954-968.

Chapter 100 *Chronic Mesenteric Ischemia*

PATHOGENESIS

Chronic mesenteric ischemia, also known as intestinal angina, occurs due to an insufficient splanchnic blood flow during periods of heightened intestinal demand that occur after eating. The hypoperfusion and ischemia are further exacerbated by the shunting of blood from the intestine to the stomach.

RISK FACTORS

Frequently there is history of smoking, underlying atherosclerosis, hypertension, diabetes, or renal insufficiency.

CLINICAL FEATURES

Patients usually present with postparandial mid-abdominal pain starting within 1 hour of eating. Pain lasts for 1 to 3 hours and may radiate to the back. Symptoms gradually get worse as time progresses. In over 75% of cases, patients develop a fear of eating resulting in weight loss. There may be concomitant nausea, vomiting, diarrhea, constipation, and bloating.

Abdominal bruit may be heard in about half of the patients but is not diagnostic. Over time, symptoms may culminate into an acute mesenteric ischemia due to acute thrombus formation and occlusion.

INVESTIGATIONS

Plain x-rays may reveal calcification of mesenteric vessels. Screening tests include doppler ultrasound, MRI, and a spiral CT of abdomen. The negative predictive value of duplex ultrasound approaches 99% and higher; if it is positive, prompt angiography should be undertaken. In patients with high index of suspicion, angiography should be undertaken.

Angiography is the procedure of choice and usually shows two or more major blood vessel involvement. SMA is always involved in mesenteric angina. Of note, a significant stenosis of two of the three major vessels (celiac axis [CA], SMA, inferior mesenteric artery [IMA]) may be seen in an otherwise healthy patient. It is therefore important to exclude other causes of abdominal pain and weight loss (eg, pancreatic cancer, gastric cancer, gastroparesis, intermittent SBO, and biliary disease, etc).

Newer diagnostic modalities include MRI angiography and tonometry, etc.

TREATMENT

Surgical reconstruction, and in some cases angioplasty with or without stent placement, may be helpful. Surgery is usually helpful in patients with at least two major blood vessels involved, including the SMA.

Angioplasty in intestinal angina results in relief of abdominal pain in 75 to 100% of patients. Half of these patients also gain weight. Arterial stenosis and recurrence of symptoms occur in 30 to 50% of patients within 1 year.

PROGNOSIS

Cumulative 5-year survival rate of the patients who survive surgical revascularization exceeds 80%.

PEARLS

- ○ Surgery is usually helpful in patients with at least two major blood vessels involved, including the SMA.
- ○ It is important to exclude other causes of abdominal pain and weight loss before embarking on surgery, since significant stenosis of two of the three major vessels (CA, SMA, IMA) may be seen in otherwise healthy subjects.

BIBLIOGRAPHY

Nehme OS, Rogers AI. Small bowel ischemia. *Curr Treat Options Gastroenterol.* 2001;4(1):51-56.

Brandt LJ, Boley SJ. AGA technical review on intestinal ischemia. *Gastroenterol.* 2000;118:954-968.

Chapter 101 *Ischemic Colitis*

Ischemic colitis represents about half of all the cases of mesenteric ischemia. It is usually seen in elderly patients.

RISK FACTORS

These include embolization, vasculitis, hypercoagulable states, aortic surgery and colonic obstruction due to cancer, and diverticulitis. An episode may be precipitated by vasospasm due to the release of vasoactive substances when blood is shunted away from the gut to the brain. This occurs during periods of systemic hypotension, or any period of transient hypotension due to dehydration, heart failure, sepsis, drugs, or hemorrhage.

Ischemic colitis may also be seen following aortic surgery, in long distance runners, intra-abdominal infections, IBD, and patients using drugs (birth control pills, danazol, digoxin, diuretics, alosetron, barbiturates, vasopressin, psychotropic drugs, ergot, amphetamines, cocaine, and sumatriptan). Inadvertent ligation of IMA may occur during aortic surgery.

Other risk factors include coronary artery bypass surgery, hemodialysis, mesenteric venous thrombosis, sickle cell disease, and acquired-inherited thrombotic conditions—especially in young patients.

PATHOGENESIS

The episode is usually precipitated by an operative or nonpostoperative, nonocclusive low-arterial flow situations in IMA and, occasionally, SMA circulation. Colonic ischemia can infrequently be a component of IMA, SMA, SMV, and IMV-occlusive disease. Right-sided ischemic colitis usually occurs due to nonocclusive disease.

There is transient reduction in blood flow which is insufficient to meet the metabolic demands of certain regions of the colon. The ischemic injury of the superficial colonic mucosa can be detected within one hour. Prolonged ischemia results in necrosis leading to transmural infarction within 8 to 16 hours.

DIAGNOSIS

Diagnosis is based upon the clinical presentation, physical exam, and endoscopic studies.

Clinical Features

These depend upon the extent and duration of ischemia, as well as the cause. There is a sudden onset of abdominal pain and tenderness, usually on the left side, with mild to moderate rectal bleeding and loose stools within 24 hours. In contrast to diverticular bleeding, the blood loss is usually not massive and patients usually do not require transfusions.

Over 80% of the patients resolve with conservative measures. In a minority of patients, the pain becomes more continuous and diffuse. There is abdominal distension, tenderness, and a reduction or absence of bowel sounds.

In severe cases, massive fluid, protein, and electrolyte leakage through the gangrenous mucosa occurs. This results in dehydration, shock, and acidosis requiring urgent surgical consultation.

Laboratory Studies

Laboratory studies are nonspecific but elevation of lactate, LDH, and CPK suggest advanced tissue damage. Gangrene is suggested by a WBC greater than $20,000/mm^3$ and metabolic acidosis. Assessment for hypercoagulability should be undertaken in young patients and in those with recurrent ischemic colitis.

Imaging Studies

Plain x-ray findings are nonspecific and may show distended loops of bowel. A CT of the abdomen may show thickened bowel wall, pneumatosis intestinalis, and gas in the mesenteric veins in advanced cases. Barium enema should be avoided. Experience with MR-arteriography is limited. Duplex ultrasound is an involving noninvasive technique.

Invasive Studies

Angiography is not helpful since colonic blood flow has already returned to normal by the time the tests are undertaken. In addition, ischemic colitis involves usually the arterioles, whereas the large vessels are patent. Angiography and laparoscopy may be useful when the presentation is atypical, diagnosis is unclear, and to follow patients after surgery for the development of any further ischemia. Angiography may also be helpful when concomitant acute superior mesenteric artery ischemia is suspected.

Endoscopic Evaluation

Colonoscopy should be considered when diagnosis is unclear and there is no clinical or radiological evidence of perforation or peritonitis. Usually the lesions are segmental in distribution and there is a abrupt transition between injured and noninjured mucosa. Splenic flexure, descending colon, and sigmoid colon involvement is seen in majority of cases. The rectum is involved in only 5% of the cases.

Endoscopic findings include pale mucosa with petechial hemorrhages and bluish hemorrhagic nodules, which suggest submucosal bleeding. Mucosa may appear cyanotic with ulceration and hemorrhages. Pseudomembranous colitis may be seen, although it is not associated with *C. difficile* infection.

PATHOLOGY

Mucosal biopsies show nonspecific changes such as hemorrhages, crypt destruction, capillary thrombosis, granulation tissue with crypt abscesses, and pseudopolyps. Biopsies of the ischemic stricture may show extensive transmural fibrosis and mucosal atrophy.

DIFFERENTIAL DIAGNOSIS

It includes infectious colitis especially *CMV* colitis and *E. coli 0157:H7*, *C. difficile* infection, IBD, diverticulitis, radiation enteritis, mesenteric inflammatory veno-occlusive disorder, and colon cancer.

TREATMENT

Treatment depends on the severity of the disease and is mostly conservative. Optimizing cardiovascular function is of paramount importance. Bowel rest and intravenous fluid administration should be undertaken to ensure adequate colonic perfusion. Nasogastric suction should be performed if ileus is present. Avoid any medications that may exacerbate ischemia. Empiric broad spectrum antibiotics like cefoxitin are usually recommended. Use of vasodilators like papaverine is not beneficial. Corticosteroids should not be used since they may increase the risk for perforation.

Monitoring the Patient

Patients should be carefully followed for persistent fever, diarrhea, bleeding, and the development of peritoneal signs and leukocytosis.

Role of Surgery

In patients who clinically do not improve or deteriorate (peritoneal signs, massive bleeding, and fulminant colitis), laparotomy and segmental resection are indicated. Colonic infarction requires a surgical intervention and second look operation may be undertaken in about 24 hours to assess the viability of the remaining bowel.

Other indications for surgery include failure of acute segmental colitis to heal within 2 to 3 weeks, recurrent bouts of sepsis despite apparent healing, and symptomatic colonic stricture.

Embolectomy, bypass surgery, and/or bypass graft surgery are rarely required since a large arterial obstruction is rarely involved.

Anticoagulants and Antiplatelet Agents

Role of antiplatelet agents remains to be established. Anticoagulant therapy may be administered to patients who develop ischemia due to mesenteric venous thrombosis or cardiac embolization.

COMPLICATIONS

Of all the patients, chronic colitis develops in 20 to 25%, stricture in 10 to 15%, gangrene in 15 to 20%, and fulminant universal colitis in less than 5%.

Stricture

Asymptomatic strictures without evidence of inflammation should be observed. Symptomatic strictures required segmental resection. Endoscopic dilatation or stents may be helpful in select cases.

Chronic Ischemic Colitis

Presentation of chronic ischemic colitis is variable and may include recurrent bacteremia, persistent sepsis, bloody diarrhea, weight loss or abdominal pain. Patients with recurrent episodes of bacteremia or sepsis with unhealed segmental colitis should undergo a segmental colonic resection. Patients who are misdiagnosed as IBD will respond poorly to the treatment for IBD and have increased risk for perforation when treated with corticosteroids.

PROGNOSIS

Prognosis of ischemic colitis is usually excellent with most patients improving within 1 to 2 days, and complete clinical resolution within a couple of weeks. However, right colon ischemic colitis is associated with poor prognosis.

A follow-up colonoscopy should be performed after 4 to 8 weeks of resolution of symptoms to exclude a colonic malignancy. Recurrence is unusual if predisposing conditions are adequately addressed.

The mortality for colonic infarction approaches as high as 50 to 75% despite surgical intervention.

PEARLS

○ Angiography is of limited value and is rarely needed for investigation of colonic ischemia.

○ Most patients resolve with conservative measures without long-term sequelae and recurrence is uncommon.

BIBLIOGRAPHY

Nehme OS, Rogers AI. New developments in colonic ischemia. *Curr Gastroenterol Rep.* 2001 Oct;3(5):416-9.

Lavu K, Minocha A. Mesenteric inflammatory veno-occlusive disorder: a rare entity mimicking inflammatory bowel disorder. *Gastroenterol.* 2003;125:236-239.

Linder JD, Monkemuller KE, Raijman I, et al. Cocaine-associated ischemic colitis. *South Med J.* 2000;93(9):909-13.

Chapter
102 *Obesity*

EPIDEMIOLOGY

The prevalence of obesity is rising dramatically worldwide. Reversing the previous trends, the number of obese people worldwide is greater than the number of those suffering from malnutrition.

In the United States, the number of obese people has risen exponentially during the latter half of the 20th century. Obesity is more prevalent amongst African Americans and Hispanic Americans, as compared to Whites. Since 1990 alone, the number of obese people has risen by about 60%. About two-thirds of obese adults have a body mass index (BMI) more than 25, 30% have a BMI greater than 30, whereas as many as 5% have BMI exceeding 40.

The prevalence of obesity amongst American children has more than doubled over the last 20 years. Obesity is the second leading cause of premature death in the United States. Approximately 7% of all health care costs in the United States are accounted for by obesity.

DEFINITION

It is defined as excess body fat as measured by BMI, which is the ratio of weight (kg) and height (meters-squared). It can be also be calculated as the ratio of body weight (pounds) and the height (inches) squared multiplied by 703. While normal BMI is 18 to 25, subjects with BMI between 25 and 30 are characterized as overweight, while those greater than 30 are defined as obese. Patients with BMI between 30 and 35 are classified as Class I obesity and those between as 35 and 40 Class II. Similarly, Class III refers to a BMI between 40 and 50, Class IV between 50 and 60, and Class V greater than 60. The average BMI of American adult is 28.

COMPLICATIONS OF OBESITY

Obesity is associated with increased morbidity and decreased life expectancy. It leads to a multitude of complications including metabolic, anatomic, degenerative, neoplastic, and social problems. These include hypercholestrolemia, coronary artery disease, diabetes, cholelithiasis, fatty liver, hypertension, and sleep apnea.

The physical structure of the body contributes to acid reflux, obstructive sleep apnea, stress incontinence, and venostasis. Degenerative complications include osteoarthritis and vertebral disc problems.

Obesity increases the risk for endometrial, ovarian, breast, prostate, colon, gallbladder, pancreatic, and esophageal cancer. Obesity also contributes to depression, anxiety, as well as eating disorders—some of which can exacerbate the weight problem, thereby setting up a vicious cycle. Socioeconomic consequences of obesity include lower educational achievement, and increased unemployment or underemployment.

PATHOGENESIS

Body weight is maintained by a tight regulation of caloric intake and body energy expenditure within 0.15%; any disturbance of this process leads to obesity. A combination of genetic, socioeconomic, ethnic, lifestyle, environmental, and developmental factors play a role.

Central weight control is maintained through hypothalamus. Sympathetic nervous system is also involved.

Hormonal factors include leptin, neuropeptide Y, and insulin. Role of leptin in the pathogenesis is controversial. Leptin inhibits appetite, reduces food intake, and stimulates energy expenditure. Obese patients have excess of circulating leptin suggesting functional resistance. However, human trials using leptin have shown only modest benefit. Recent studies using peptide YY have been encouraging.

Genetic influences also play a role. In a genetically predisposed individual, environmental and life style factors initiate the process of imbalance leading to obesity.

Lifestyle and environmental factors include a decrease in physical activity and exercise, increased availability of high-calorie foods, irregular meal patterns, and high stress patterns of life.

Perhaps the single most important factor in the rise of obesity in the recent years may be the exponential rise in sugar intake.

MANAGEMENT

Management options include dietary modification, exercise, behavioral therapy, medications, and surgery.

Dietary Modification

The role of dietary modification in producing a consistent and long-term weight loss is controversial. Various diet plans include the United States Department of Agriculture (USDA) food guide pyramid, a low fat diet, and a very low-fat diet as promoted by Ornish. A very low carbohydrate diet promoted by Atkins has recently been very popular. The mechanism of weight loss through dieting may be the reduced caloric intake along with inducing a regularity in otherwise irregular eating patterns. This is supported by the fact that persons in prisons or living in impoverished societies are rarely obese.

The goal should be a weight loss of no more than 1 to 2 pounds per week. Very low calorie diets of less than 800 K_{cal}/day should be avoided and if medically necessary should only be undertaken under medical supervision.

Exercise

Exercise is important for weight loss maintenance, but its effectiveness in initiating weight loss in severely obese is a matter of debate. An obese person may not be able to burn enough calories for it to be an effective method of weight loss. The above notwithstanding, exercise results in health benefits including reduced mortality.

Behavioral Approaches

Success of behavioral approach depends upon the intensity and frequency rather than any particular therapy approach. Internet-based counseling systems are in their infancy.

Medical Therapy

In case dietary and lifestyle measures fail to induce weight loss, drugs may be used if BMI is greater than 30; a threshold of greater than 27 is applied in patients suffering from weight-related medical complications. The options include phentermine, sibutramine (Meridia), and orlistat (Xenical).

Medications produce modest weight loss of less than 5% of initial body weight. Dietary and lifestyle modifications along with counseling result in the same degree of weight loss (3.0 to 5.0 kg weight loss for 1 to 2 years) with or without addition of medications. As such, many experts caution against routine long-term use of these medications. While the pharmacotherapy appears to be safe for short-term use, the long-term safety remains to be clearly established.

Phentermine suppresses appetite and its side effects include hypertension and palpitations. Sibutramine is a serotonin-norepinephrine re-uptake inhibitor that can cause suppression of appetite. It is contraindicated in patients with uncontrolled hypertension. Orlistat is a selective pancreatic lipase inhibitor that leads to reduced intestinal fat digestion. Significant weight gain is seen after 1 to 2 years of continued use. Side effects include steatorrhea with oil leakage and potential deficiency of fat-soluble vitamins.

Psychotropic agents for weight loss include bupropion (Wellbutrin, Zyban). In contrast, some psychotropic agents like citalopram (Celexa) and paroxetine (Paxil) promote weight gain.

Surgery

Surgery is an effective method for weight control. As many as 90% of patients lose greater than 20% of their body weight, and the majority of them maintain the weight loss over a period of 5 years. Indications for surgery include a BMI greater than 40; the threshold is lower (greater than 35) in cases of obesity-related medical problems.

The three most common surgeries used currently are Biliary-pancreatic diversion (duodenal Switch), Roux-en-Y gastric bypass surgery (RYGB), and laparoscopic adjustable band (Lap-Band); these can be performed laparoscopically. Bariatric surgery works by either be being restrictive (limits caloric intake) or malabsorptive (prevents calorie absorption). The duodenal switch is a malabsorptive procedure, while the Lap-Band is a restrictive procedure. The RYGB is a "hybrid" with both restrictive and malabsorptive aspects.

Vertical banded gastroplasty (VBG), creates a small proximal gastric pouch by placing a band limiting the storage capacity of the stomach. However, it is losing popularity because of long-term complications and reduction in weight loss with time.

RYGB in addition to creating a small proximal gastric pouch also involves gastrojejunostomy through this pouch; thus, the major part of the stomach is excluded from the food intake. RYGB produces a weight loss of about 65% of excess body weight. It does not lead to protein-calorie malnutrition. However, a deficiency of iron and vitamin B_{12} can be seen and transient dumping syndrome may occur.

The adjustable Lap-Band has been approved by the United States Food and Drug Administration (FDA) as a restrictive procedure. Jejuno-ileal bypass, popular in 1960s and 1970s is no longer used.

Adjunctive preoperative and postoperative measures including lifestyle adjustments plus dietary and psychological therapy help sustain results over the long-term. Bariatric surgery has a mortality of approximately 0.5%.

PEARLS

○ Drug therapy for weight loss may be no more effective than lifestyle changes over the long run.
○ Surgery is an effective method of a weight-loss in carefully selected patients.

BIBLIOGRAPHY

Klein S, Wadden T, Sugerman HJ. AGA technical review on obesity. *Gastroenterology*. 2002;123:882.

INDEX